AF726391

Stem Cells: Clinical Research

Stem Cells: Clinical Research

Edited by Ashton Silk

hayle medical

New York

Hayle Medical,
750 Third Avenue, 9th Floor,
New York, NY 10017, USA

Visit us on the World Wide Web at:
www.haylemedical.com

© Hayle Medical, 2020

This book contains information obtained from authentic and highly regarded sources. Copyright for all individual chapters remain with the respective authors as indicated. All chapters are published with permission under the Creative Commons Attribution License or equivalent. A wide variety of references are listed. Permission and sources are indicated; for detailed attributions, please refer to the permissions page and list of contributors. Reasonable efforts have been made to publish reliable data and information, but the authors, editors and publisher cannot assume any responsibility for the validity of all materials or the consequences of their use.

ISBN: 978-1-63241-866-1

Trademark Notice: Registered trademark of products or corporate names are used only for explanation and identification without intent to infringe.

Cataloging-in-Publication Data

Stem cells : clinical research / edited by Ashton Silk.
p. cm.
Includes bibliographical references and index.
ISBN 978-1-63241-866-1
1. Stem cells. 2. Stem cells--Research. 3. Cells. 4. Clinical medicine--Research. I. Silk, Ashton.
QH588.S83 S84 2020
616.027 74-dc23

Table of Contents

Preface

The main aim of this book is to educate learners and enhance their research focus by presenting diverse topics covering this vast field. This is an advanced book which compiles significant studies by distinguished experts in the area of analysis. This book addresses successive solutions to the challenges arising in the area of application, along with it; the book provides scope for future developments.

Stem cells are the cells which differentiate into other cells and thereby replenish tissues of the body. This gives them the potential for therapeutic use in tissue repair and regeneration. Stem cells can be categorized into distinct cell types- embryonic stem cells and adult stem cells. Embryonic stem cells can divide into more stem cells or any type of cell in the body. This allows embryonic stem cells to repair or regenerate diseased tissues and organs. Adult stem cells were believed to create only similar kinds of cells but emerging evidence suggests that these may also have the ability to create other types of cells. This holds immense potential in medicine. Adult stem cells are being tested in people with heart disease or neurological conditions. Adult cells have been successfully transformed into stem cells using genetic reprogramming. This can enable the use of reprogrammed cells and prevent the immune system rejection of new stem cells. This book discusses the fundamentals as well as modern approaches of stem cell therapy. It consists of contributions made by international experts. For all readers who are interested in the study of stem cells, the case studies included in this book will serve as an excellent guide to develop a comprehensive understanding.

It was a great honour to edit this book, though there were challenges, as it involved a lot of communication and networking between me and the editorial team. However, the end result was this all-inclusive book covering diverse themes in the field.

Finally, it is important to acknowledge the efforts of the contributors for their excellent chapters, through which a wide variety of issues have been addressed. I would also like to thank my colleagues for their valuable feedback during the making of this book.

Editor

1

Therapeutic Potential of Stem Cells in Follicle Regeneration

Agnieszka Owczarczyk-Saczonek,[1] **Magdalena Krajewska-Włodarczyk**,[2] **Anna Kruszewska**,[1] **Łukasz Banasiak**,[3] **Waldemar Placek**,[1] **Wojciech Maksymowicz**,[4] **and Joanna Wojtkiewicz**[5,6,7]

[1]*Department of Dermatology, Sexually Transmitted Diseases and Clinical Immunology, University of Warmia and Mazury in Olsztyn, Olsztyn, Poland*
[2]*Department of Rheumatology, University of Warmia and Mazury in Olsztyn, Olsztyn, Poland*
[3]*Department of Plastic, Reconstructive and Aesthetic Surgery, L. Rydygier Collegium Medicum in Bydgoszcz, Nicolaus Copernicus University in Torun, Toruń, Poland*
[4]*Department of Neurology and Neurosurgery, Faculty of Medical Sciences, University of Warmia and Mazury in Olsztyn, Olsztyn, Poland*
[5]*Foundation for Nerve Cell Regeneration, University of Warmia and Mazury in Olsztyn, Olsztyn, Poland*
[6]*Department of Pathophysiology, Faculty of Medical Sciences, University of Warmia and Mazury in Olsztyn, Olsztyn, Poland*
[7]*Laboratory for Regenerative Medicine, Faculty of Medical Sciences, University of Warmia and Mazury, Olsztyn, Poland*

Correspondence should be addressed to Agnieszka Owczarczyk-Saczonek; aganek@wp.pl

Academic Editor: Shibashish Giri

Alopecia is caused by a variety of factors which affect the hair cycle and decrease stem cell activity and hair follicle regeneration capability. This process causes lower self-acceptance, which may result in depression and anxiety. However, an early onset of androgenic alopecia is associated with an increased incidence of the metabolic syndrome and an increased risk of the cardiac ischaemic disease. The ubiquity of alopecia provides an encouragement to seek new, more effective therapies aimed at hair follicle regeneration and neoregeneration. We know that stem cells can be used to regenerate hair in several therapeutic strategies: reversing the pathological mechanisms which contribute to hair loss, regeneration of complete hair follicles from their parts, and neogenesis of hair follicles from a stem cell culture with isolated cells or tissue engineering. Hair transplant has become a conventional treatment technique in androgenic alopecia (micrografts). Although an autologous transplant is regarded as the gold standard, its usability is limited, because of both a limited amount of material and a reduced viability of cells obtained in this way. The new therapeutic options are adipose-derived stem cells and stem cells from Wharton's jelly. They seem an ideal cell population for use in regenerative medicine because of the absence of immunogenic properties and their ease of obtainment, multipotential character, ease of differentiating into various cell lines, and considerable potential for angiogenesis. In this article, we presented advantages and limitations of using these types of cells in alopecia treatment.

1. Introduction

Hair loss is caused by a variety of factors: hereditary (trichodystrophy, androgenic alopecia), concomitant medical conditions, hormonal disorders (thyroid gland disorders, insulin resistance), autoimmune (patchy alopecia, systemic lupus erythematosus), nutritional disorders, environmental factors (medicines, UV radiation), psychological factors (stress, trichotillomania), and ageing. The damaging factors affect the hair cycle and decrease stem cell activity and hair follicle regeneration capability.

Alopecia is commonly regarded as a defect with apparently no significant health consequences. However, hair loss affects self-acceptance, which may result in depression and anxiety [1, 2]. It is not only an aesthetic issue. An early onset of androgenic alopecia is associated with an increased incidence of the metabolic syndrome and an increased risk of the cardiac ischaemic disease [3]. The ubiquity of alopecia provides an encouragement to seek new, more effective therapies aimed at hair follicle regeneration and neoregeneration.

1.1. Stem Cells in the Hair Follicle. Hair follicles have a niche for mature stem cells—hair follicular stem cells (HFSCs)—a so-called "bulge" in the attachment region of arrector pili muscles, which contain epithelial and melanocyte stem cells. Moreover, HFSCs are also situated within the outer root sheath (ORS), within the region of the proximal end of the isthmus—this area is also known as the "bulge" [4]. HFSCs take part in the regeneration of epidermal cells and the structure of hair follicles and sebaceous glands [5] (Figure 1).

Stem cells of the "bulge" can remain in their niche where they self-regenerate, but they can also move down to the hair matrix region, where they become progenitor cells which then form an internal hair follicle and the hair stem [6]. The "bulge" region is not uniform, with two compartments distinguishable in it: the lower part, close to the hair matrix, which generates the internal hair follicle cell line, and the upper part, which self-regenerates, but which does not directly participate in the regeneration of the hair follicle [7, 8]. Since the heterogeneity of the "bulge" also depends on its relationship with the basal membrane, two populations of CD34+ cells are distinguished. One of them, the so-called suprabasal SCs, contains lower levels of a6-intergin and has a lower proliferative potential [6, 9]. The "isthmus" region is, apart from the "bulge," another one which also contains stem cells participating in the formation of interfollicular epidermis and sebaceous glands [7, 10].

Another type of stem cells within the hair follicle is dermal papilla cells (DPCs), probably originating from dermal condensation, which is the initial stage of the hair follicle development [11, 12]. DPCs play an important role in induction and regulation of hair growth and the formation of new hair follicles [11, 13, 14]. Signals from DPCs activate stem cells in the "bulge" and germinal matrix cells in the late telogen/early anagen phase [11, 15] by activating the Wnt/β-catenin pathway [11, 16]. Moreover, DPCs have potential for differentiation into lines of adipocytes and osteocytes [11, 17], and they can be transformed into pluripotential cells [11, 18].

Alopecia involves changes in two types of hair stem cells, both human hair follicle stem cells (HFSCs) and dermal papilla cells (DPCs) [19, 20]. They ensure conditions for proper hair regeneration [20]. In scarring alopecia (lupus erythematosus, lichen planus), inflammatory cell infiltration around the bulge results in an irreversible loss of HFSCs. Although the progenitor cells are damaged, HFSCs are preserved in patchy and androgenic alopecia. This is why this type of alopecia can be reversible [20].

Stem cells of the "bulge" are increasingly well characterised, especially in murine hair follicle, which facilitates their identification, although no universal marker has been found for them. One of them is cytokeratin 15 (CK15), which is why CK15+/integrin α6+ or CD34+/integrin α6+ cells have been identified as "bulge" cells [21]. Studies on murine hair follicles have also revealed expression of, inter alia,

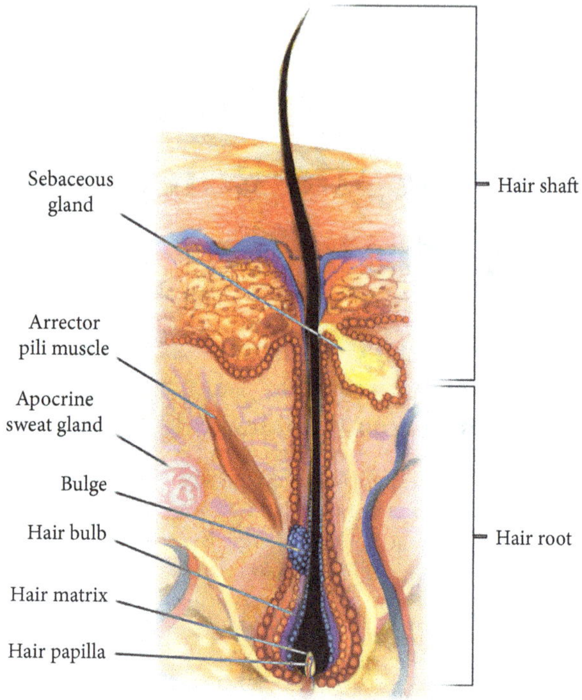

FIGURE 1: Hair follicle anatomy.

CK19 [8, 22] and numerous transcription factors, that is, Sox9, Lgr5, Gli1, Hopx, LHX2, Nfatc1, and Tcf3 [8, 25]. However, expression of certain markers depends on the hair cycle phase and on the precise location of the cells within the bulge [7, 8]. Lgr5, a receptor involved in the Wnt signaling pathway, has been identified as an actual marker of the hair follicle stem cells [25]. Stem cells of the upper and lower parts of the bulge in the telogen hair follicle affect the expression of CD34 and only of the lower part of Lgr5. Cells participating in the formation of a new anagen hair express Lgr5, but not CD34 [26]. Cells of the upper part of the "bulge" present a higher expression Nfatc1, which is associated with a state of rest [6]. Expression of Lgr6 [7, 10] and Lrig1 [7, 27] has been observed within the "isthmus." Meanwhile, progenitor cells of the germinal matrix are derived from stem cells of the bulge but, unlike them, exhibit a high level of P-cadherin [8, 28].

Human hair follicle stem cells are less known than murine HFSCs. It seems that certain markers are common to both human and mouse HFSCs, that is, CD34 [4, 23], K15 [4, 19], K19 [4, 29], and CD200 [4, 19, 23]. The presence of other markers, i.e., Sox9 and LHX2, requires further studies [30]. Markers found only in human stem cell follicles belong to PHLDA1 [4, 24] and EpCAM/Ber-EP4, which is a useful marker of the telogen secondary hair germ [4, 28].

Dermal papilla cells present different markers, including those from hair follicle cells and dermal fibroblasts [11]. Alkaline phosphatase (ALP) is the most important for both human and murine HFs and is the most specific of the markers [11, 29, 30]; its high activity is a marker of DP cell differentiation [11, 31]. Moreover, expression of α-SMA

[11, 17], laminin, and fibronectin [11] as well as CD133 [11, 32] has been observed in DPCs.

Marker expression changes in pathological states. Immunoreactivity of CK15 is decreased in people with patchy alopecia, and it is present in androgenic alopecia [21]. Hair follicles in the frontal parts of the scalp exhibit a deficit of CD34 in androgenic alopecia, and its expression is preserved in hair follicles of the occipital region [21]. Another marker CD200 of matrix cells is poorly expressed in patchy alopecia, which may be a sign of the disappearance of the immune privilege and can contribute to pathogenesis (reaction of autoreactive lymphocytes) [21, 33].

Stem cells in the bulge remain in the resting phase for most of their lives, but they can be activated depending on the hair cycle phase. Most of the concepts regarding the course and regulation of the hair cycle have been created during research on mouse models. During the hair cycle in mice, in the anagen phase, stem cells in the bulge are divided three times on average and stay within the niche, whereas cells of the germinal matrix divide intensely and differentiate, forming the growing hair stem. During the catagen phase, cells of the germinal matrix undergo apoptosis; stem cells of the bulge migrate out of it to the external hair follicle, and subsequently, at the end of the catagen phase, they form a new bulge around the hair stem and a new germinal matrix under the bulge. Stem cells in the bulge remain in the state of rest during the telogen phase, and between the telogen and anagen phases, they self-regenerate or migrate, creating a pool of germinal matrix cells which subsequently proliferate to form the hair matrix [6]. The precedence has been shown for the derivative cells in the bulge, the so-called "SC" progenitor cells of the germinal matrix, in the expression of genes that affect stem cell activation, and precedence in proliferation during the regeneration cycle, even before the cells of the bulge [8, 15, 34]. The translation of the mouse hair cycle into the human hair cycle has some limitations due to the different lengths of anagen [35, 36], asynchrony of the human cycle [35, 37], or a different reaction to the influence of hormonal factors [35, 38]. Currently, studies are conducted on human scalp skin xenografted into immunocompromised mice to establish the course of the hair cycle in vivo in humans [35].

The activity of stem cells in the bulge is controlled by the microenvironment that surrounds it, a so-called "niche." This includes daughter cells of stem cells of the bulge, which activate their self-regeneration during early and late anagen phases [39].

Stem cells are significantly affected by mesenchymal cells of the dermal papilla, which are in close contact with cells of the germinal matrix, separated only by the basal membrane [7]. They seem to be of key importance in the induction of hair growth and in signal transmission during its regeneration [8, 34]. Experiments have shown that hair regeneration is not possible after laser ablation because the hair follicle cycle stops at the telogen phase without progressing to the anagen phase [6, 7, 34, 40]. Injections of exosomes derived from DPCs to HFs have been found to accelerate the entry of anagen and catagen delay via the β-catenin and Shh pathways [41]. HFSCs are also affected by fibroblasts in the reticular and papillary layers of the dermis as well as of the subcutaneous tissue [7].

Within the niche there are also melanocyte stem cells, which are responsible for the formation of mature melanocytes that impart the colour to a growing hair. The survival and growth of MSCs depend on signals transmitted by hair follicle epithelial cells, for example, the TGF-β or the Wnt pathway [7, 39]. The extracellular matrix is another component of the microenvironment. It directly affects stem cells by the formation of the basal membrane, with which stem cells are in contact modulated, for example, by integrins [6, 8].

Stem cells of hair follicles are also affected by the macroenvironment surrounding hair follicles, for example, adipose tissue. It seems to undergo similar changes to those of the hair follicle: the thickness of the adipose tissue increases during the anagen phase, and adipocytes proliferate intensively [8, 42]. Adipocytes secrete BMP2 during the late catagen phase and early telogen phase, which favours the resting states in the niche, whereas secretion of BMP2 is reduced at the end of the telogen phase, which supports the activation of HFSCs [8, 42, 43]. Communication between adipose tissue and the epithelium runs in both directions. Mutations blocking the hair cycle have been found to inhibit adipogenesis, which suggests that epithelium cells send signals activating the proliferation of adipocytes [6, 42].

Nerve ends affect stem cells situated at the upper part of the Gli1+ bulge by a signal of the Shh pathway [6, 44]. Therefore, denervation can reduce the effect of SCs in the "isthmus" on wound healing [6, 44]. However, it seems that nerves are not indispensable components of the niche, because denervation does not impair hair follicle regeneration, which may suggest that Gli+ cells receive Shh signal from other sources [7].

The hair follicle absorbs nutrients from the surrounding microvascular network, which is transformed during the hair cycle—angiogenesis is increased during the anagen phase [6, 45]. Cells of the bulge and of the matrix can probably stimulate angiogenesis [6]. Delayed induction of angiogenesis, which accompanies impaired angiogenesis, has been observed in mice [7, 45]. It has been suggested that stem cells in general prefer a low-oxygen environment, where they secrete marker of hypoxia [6, 46]. The vascular network, especially that surrounding the "isthmus," containing venous vessels, can participate in maintaining the low-oxygen environment in the surrounding of the stem cell environment [6].

However, although the effect of the immune response has not been sufficiently elucidated, it is important that the role of maintaining the immune privilege of hair follicles, associated with decreased expression of MHC I molecules and with increased secretion of local immunosuppressors, should be maintained during the anagen phase [6, 47]. The loss of this privilege and an immune attack on cells of the matrix and the bulge are associated with alopecia [6, 48]. Dermal cells $\gamma\delta$T are known to modulate posttraumatic regeneration of hair follicles by secreting FGF9 [7, 49]. Macrophages, in turn, increase the level of Wnt7b and Wnt10a ligands during the telogen phase after undergoing apoptosis, whereby activating HFSCs [6, 7, 50]. Macrophages play an

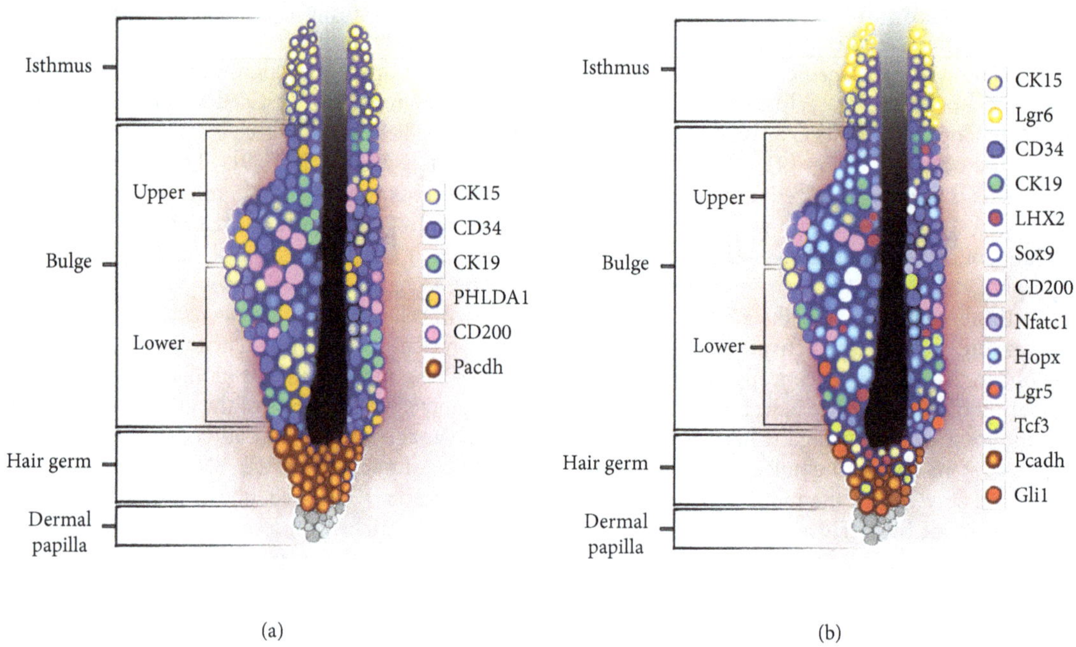

FIGURE 2: The markers of hair follicle: (a) in human, (b) in mouse.

important role in posttraumatic activation of HFSCs—arresting their recruitment into the wound delays hair growth, whereas transplantation of active macrophages is sufficient for induction of hair growth [6, 51]. Also important is the role of Treg, which presents a high level of Jag 1 from the Notch family, which affects the effective regeneration of HF [52] (Figure 2 and Table 1).

1.2. Stem Cell Use in Hair Follicle Regeneration. Hair follicles are immunologically privileged places, like the brain, eyes, and testicles, and they are under the influence of the neuroendocrine-immune network [32]. In physiological conditions, this is affected by

(1) low expression or absence of the main MHC I antigens,

(2) the presence of malfunctional Langerhans cells,

(3) local expression of immunosuppressive substances (TGF-β1 and α-melanocytes MSH) [32, 48]. Owing to this, they can be easily used in transplantation.

Multipotent stem cells can regenerate hair follicles with sebaceous glands in the skin. In the current state of knowledge, stem cells can be used to regenerate hair in several therapeutic strategies:

(1) Reversing the pathological mechanisms which contribute to hair loss (especially in androgenic alopecia)

(2) Regeneration of complete hair follicles from their parts (cells in the bulge can regenerate a whole hair)

(3) Neogenesis of hair follicles from a stem cell culture with isolated cells or tissue engineering [5, 53, 54]

1.3. Studies of Use of Autologous Stem Cell in Hair Follicle Regeneration. Hair transplant has become a conventional treatment technique in androgenic alopecia (micrografts, follicular unit transplantation (both FUT an FUE), and individual follicular group harvesting (IFGH)) [55]. Although an autologous transplant is regarded as the gold standard, its usability is limited, because of both a limited amount of material and a reduced viability of cells obtained in this way. Currently, methods are being developed which enhance the effectiveness of the use of autologous stem cells of the hair follicle.

Apart from cells of the "bulge," stem cells reside specifically in the HF mesenchyme and function to replenish the dermal papilla and connective tissue sheath. They are called self-renewing dermal stem cells (DSCs) [56, 57]. When transplanted, DSCs integrate with mesenchymal cells and they act together with epithelial stem cells, participating in creating new hair follicles [56, 57]. In cultures, they form spherical, self-regenerating colonies. However, it is labour-consuming and ineffective. Therefore, methods have been developed for their simultaneous collection, isolation, and administration *in vivo* at acceptor sites with the use of the so-called stirred suspension bioreactors. They help to obtain cells of greater uniformity; increased cell density per volume; and control of the concentration of nutrients, metabolites, and growth factors [56, 58].

The findings of the study by Agabalyan et al. have confirmed that cells can retain their phenotype and an ability to form hair follicles even after five passages in bioreactors.

Table 1: The markers of hair follicle and their role.

Author	Signal	Researched object	Conclusions
Telerman et al., 2017 [91]	Blimp1	Transgenic mouse	Ablation delayed HF morphogenesis, and growth and prevented new HF formation after wounding; role in promoting the dermal papilla inductive signaling cascade that initiates HF growth
Kobielak et al., 2007 [92]	Bmpr1a	Transgenic mouse	Ablation leads quiescent SCs to activate and to proliferate, causing an expansion of the niche and loss of slow-cycling cells; HFSCs are unable to terminally differentiate into hair
Lei et al., 2014 [93]	DKK1	Transgenic mouse	DKK reduce hair follicle enlargement and decrease proliferation; injection of DKK1 during early anagen significantly reduced the width of prospective hairs
Millar et al., 1999 [94]	Dvl2	Transgenic mouse	Overexpression in the outer root sheath causes the short-hair phenotype
Lin et al., 2015 [95]	FGF1, FGF2, FGF10	Transgenic mouse	Topical application of FGFs induced an earlier anagen phase and prolonged the mature anagen phase; FGFs promoted hair growth by inducing the anagen phase in telogenic mice
Kimura-Ueki et al., 2012 [96]	FGF18	Transgenic mouse	Ablation causes telogen to become very short, giving rise to a strikingly rapid succession of hair cycles
Higgins et al., 2014 [97]	FGF5	DNA from families with long eyelashes	FGF5 is associated with long-hair phenotype
Guo et al., 1993 [98]	FGF7	Transgenic mouse	Overexpression causes marked suppression of hair follicle morphogenesis
Petiot et al., 2003 [99]	Fgfr2	Transgenic mouse	Lack of Fgfr2 leads to a decreased number of HFs, and follicles were developmentally retarded
Öztürk et al., 2015 [100]	Gab1	Transgenic mouse	Lack of Gab1 caused HF not to enter catagen; instead HFSCs lose quiescence
Mill et al., 2003 [101]	Gli2	Transgenic mouse	Lack of Gli2 causes arrest in HF development with reduced cell proliferation and Shh-responsive gene expression, but normal epidermal differentiation
Estrach et al., 2006 [102]	Jagged-1	Transgenic mouse	Deletion of Jagged-1 results in inhibition of the hair growth cycle and conversion of hair follicles into cysts of cells undergoing interfollicular epidermal differentiation
Amalia Pasolli et al., 2014 [103]	LHX2	Transgenic mouse	Ablation of LHX2 results in cellular disorganization and HFSC polarization within the niche. LHX2 loss leads to a failure to maintain HFSC quiescence and hair anchoring and progressive transformation of the niche into a sebaceous gland
Öztürk et al., 2015 [100]	Mapk	Transgenic mouse	Activation of Mapk signaling can restore quiescence of the SCs
Du et al., 2018 [104]	miR-214	Human scalp skin tissue; in vitro	Downregulation of miR-214 promotes the proliferation and differentiation of HFSCs; overexpression of miR-214 led to decreased expression of EZH2, β-catenin, and TCF4
Horsley et al., 2008 [105]	Nfatc1	Transgenic mouse	Ablation causes stem cells to be activated prematurely, resulting in precocious follicular growth
Krieger et al., 2018 [106]	NF-κB	Transgenic mouse	Role in HF stem/progenitor cell activation during anagen induction, involvement in hair fiber morphogenesis during HF cycling

Table 1: Continued.

Author	Signal	Researched object	Conclusions
Demehri and Kopan, 2009 [107]	Notch	Transgenic mouse	Absence of Notch signaling leads bulge stem cell descendents to retain their capacity to execute the follicular differentiation program but failing to maintain it owing to their genetic deficiency
Lin et al., 2011 [108]	Pofut1	Transgenic mouse	Disruption of Pofut1 in HF resulted in aberrant telogen morphology, a decrease of bulge SC markers; HF displayed a delay in anagen reentry and dysregulation of proliferation and apoptosis during the hair cycle transition
Oro and Higgins, 2003 [109]	Ptch	Transgenic mouse	Reduced Ptch is associated with tumor formation during anagen
Hoi et al., 2010 [110]	Runx1	Transgenic mouse	Role in promoting anagen onset and HFSC proliferation
St- Jacques et al., 1998 [111]	Shh	Transgenic mouse	Shh signaling is not required for initiating hair follicle development; however, it is essential for controlling ingrowth and morphogenesis of the hair follicle
Kadaja et al., 2014 [112]	Sox9	Transgenic mouse	Sox9-deficient bulge HFSCs begin to differentiate into epidermal cells; as HFSC numbers dwindle, outer root sheath production is not sustained, and HF down-growth arrests prematurely
Foitzik et al., 2000 [113]	TGF-β1	Transgenic mouse	Injection of TGF-beta1 induced premature catagen development
Foitzik et al., 1999 [114]	TGF-β2	Transgenic mouse	Ablation causes delay of hair follicle morphogenesis, with a 50% reduced number of hair follicles
Oshimori and Fuchs, 2012 [115]	TGF-βRII	Transgenic mouse	TGF-β2 signaling antagonizes BMP signaling in HFSCs with increased telogen length
Qiu et al., 2017 [116]	TPA	Transgenic mouse	Refractory telogen hair follicles entered anagen prematurely after TPA treatment, with the enhanced proliferation of CD34-positive hair follicle stem cells
Lei et al., 2014 [93]	Wnt10b	Transgenic mouse	Prolonged overexpression increased the size of regenerated hair follicles and increased expression of CD34 in the bulge
Millar et al., 1999 [94]	Wnt3	Transgenic mouse	Overexpression causes a short-hair phenotype and cyclical balding resulting from hair shaft structural defects
Dong et al., 2017 [117]	Wnt7a	Transgenic mouse	Cultured human umbilical cord-MSCs (UC-MSCs) overexpressing Wnt7a can accelerate wound repair and induce hair regeneration via cellular communication in the wound microenvironment
Kandyba and Kobielak, 2013 [118]	Wnt7b	Transgenic mouse	Underexpression causes shorter anagen, premature catagen onset with overall shorter hair production, and diminished HF differentiation marker expression
Enshell-Seijffers et al., 2010 [119]	β-Catenin	Transgenic mouse	Inactivation in DP of HF results in reduced proliferation of the progenitors and their immediate progeny that generate the HS and premature catagen

HF: hair follicle; HS: hair shaft; DP: dermal papilla; SC: stem cell.

Moreover, the productivity is five times higher compared to static cultures [56]. This has given rise to the possibility of using this method commercially in the treatment of alopecia.

Gentile et al. [5] demonstrated the application of an innovative Rigeneracons® bioreactor (certificate CE, class I) in order to provide autologous micrografts and their immediate use in clinical practice. They proved that cells isolated from the bulge region can improve the thickness of hair in patients affected by androgenic alopecia using a new method of isolating human mature stem cells obtained from a patient self-biopsy, without culturing. Enhanced hair thickness was achieved in 11 men (aged 38 to 61 years) with androgenic alopecia even at the stage of 3–5 in the Norwood-Hamilton scale. After the biopsy and removal of unwanted remnants of fatty tissue, a medical device Rigeneracons (certificate CE, class I) was used to obtain cell suspension. The percentage of mesenchymal stem cells CD44+ from the dermal papilla was approx. 5% + 0.7% and CD200+ from the bulge was approx. 2.6% + 0.3%. After 23 weeks of therapy, after the last administration of stem cells, the average number of hairs and their thicknesses increased by 29% ± 5% compared to the baseline for the hair thickness in the treated area and by less than 1% of hair thickness increase in the placebo area [5].

Furthermore, Nilforoushzadeh et al. [59] evaluated the regeneration potential of cultured mature dermal papilla to induce the growth of a hair follicle injected to the skin of bare mice. Initially, dermal papilla cells in the culture were observed to multiply with expression of CD200, and these fusiform cells tended to form colonies after three to five days. Subsequently, after two weeks, they acquired a passaging capability and they formed an extracellular matrix after the third passaging. Histopathological examination in mice which received 1.2×10^6 of cells of dermal papilla revealed structures that transformed into hair follicles at sites of injection in the dermis [59].

Ibrahim et al. used autologous bone marrow mononuclear cells (BMMC) (including stem cells) to treat refractory patchy alopecia and androgenic alopecia, and the therapeutic effects were compared to the group treated with autologous stem cells of hair follicles. Cells were administered in a single application (1 millilitre in a density of 100,000 cell/ml was injected, using a 26-gauge needle, intradermally at per centimetre square of the treated site), and a significant improvement was observed in all patient groups under treatment [21]. Interestingly, the effect of stem cells was similar despite the fact that they had been obtained from two different sources. The effect of intradermal injection of BMMC may result from the diversity of the cell mixture: progenitor, hematopoietic stem cells, various types of inflammatory cells, and mesenchymal stem cells. BMMC can stimulate hair growth as a consequence of the ability to differentiate into various cell types, the ability to secrete bioactive molecules which stimulate angiogenesis (VEGF) and anti-inflammatory molecules with an immunomodulatory and antiapoptotic effect [21].

1.4. Studies of the Use of Adipose-Derived Stem Cells. ADSCs (adipose-derived stem cells) seem an ideal cell population for use in regenerative medicine because of the absence of immunogenic properties, their ease of obtainment, multipotential character, ease of differentiating into various cell lines, and considerable potential for angiogenesis. ADSCs have been shown to originate from mural cells located in the perivascular niche, vascular smooth muscle cells and pericytes, both involved in the formation of normal vasculature and are responsive to VEGF [60]. Naturally, hair follicles surrounded by subcutaneous adipose cells and by dermis form an interfollicular dermal macroenvironment, which is important in maintaining the proper growth of bulge and follicle cells [11, 61, 62]. ADSCs are indispensable in the activation of epidermal stem cells, which they do by secreting growth factors. The vascular endothelial growth factor (VEGF) regulates hair growth and the size of the hair follicle size by stimulation of angiogenesis. The hepatocyte growth factor (HGF) is involved in the duration of the hair cycle phases. The platelet-derived growth factor induces and maintains the anagen phase, and the insulin-like growth factor I (IGF-I) controls the hair growth cycle and hair cell differentiation [11, 63–67]. Another direction of their action is the stimulation of angiogenesis and an improvement of the blood supply to dermal papilla cells. They also have immunomodulatory and immunosuppressive properties through the direct interaction between cells and secretion of prostaglandin E2 (PGE2), leukaemia-inhibiting factor (LIF), and kynurenine [11, 62].

The paracrine activity of ADSCs is highly complex, and the factors secreted by stem cells have both a direct and an indirect effect on hair follicles. TB4 contributes to the activation of stem cells in a hair follicle, increasing their migration into the follicle and differentiation. SDF-1 acts through an increase in expression of EGR-1; it also increases the cell tropism towards the follicle and increases angiogenesis. The action of MCP-1 is less obvious; despite being an inflammatory factor, it has a proven tissue regenerative effect; also, a significant role of the microenvironment in the effect of paracrine factors in promoting the growth of the hair follicle has been emphasised [68]. Huang et al., in a study on rats, found that an addition of ADSCs to a culture of dermal papilla cells or core cells, the inner and outer sheath, enhances their viability [64]. A significant increase in the regenerative potential was recorded in a study by Huang et al., in which ADSCs were enriched with LL-37, which is an antibacterial peptide occurring naturally in wounds [64]. That study showed a significant increase in the local regenerative factors (endothelial growth factor, thymosin beta-4, monocyte chemoattractant protein-1, and stromal cell-derived factor-1). A significant promotion of the growth of hair follicles, in both *in vitro* and *in vivo* animal models, was observed [60, 69–71].

Physiologically, adipose tissue surrounding hair follicles plays an important role in extending the anagen phase. Adipocytes progenitor cells have been observed to multiply during the transition from the telogen to the anagen phase, around the hair follicle [61, 64]. The thickness of the subcutaneous layer increases significantly during the intense hair growth phase (anagen) compared to their amount in the resting phase (telogen) [11, 59]. ADSCs stimulate hair follicle cells through peroxisome proliferator-activated receptors, whose three isoforms have been found on their surface (PPARα, PPARγ, and PPARδ) [64]. Meanwhile, mature adipocytes have a negative effect on hair follicle cell proliferation and on proliferation of fibroblasts surrounding the hair follicle in simultaneous culture systems [11, 72].

Interestingly, a change in adipocyte cell line properties can cause skin and hair disorders. Lipid metabolism disorders can cause defects in the skin structure and functions. Over-expression of human apolipoprotein C1 (APOC1) with hyperlipidemia in transgenic mice causes hair growth disorders correlated with the level of expression of human APOC1 gene in the skin [11, 73].

Hypoxia, which is not toxic to mesenchymal cells, also increases the production of growth factors for ADSCs: vascular endothelial growth factor (VEGF), platelet-derived growth factor (PDGF), hepatocyte growth factor (HGF), and insulin-like growth factor II (IGF-II) [74, 75]. The effect of hypoxia on ADSCs was examined in a study conducted by Park et al. [74]. ADSCs passaged four times with CO_2 subsequently administered subcutaneously to mice to observe induction of the anagen phase and proliferation of human follicular cells of the dermal papilla and keratinocytes. Hypoxia resulted in increased secretion of insulin-like growth factor-binding protein-1 and protein-2 (IGFBP), macrophage colony stimulating factor (M-CSF), M-CSF receptor, PDGF receptor-β, and VEGF, whereas secretion of the epidermal growth factor was smaller [74].

Unfortunately, two-dimensional (2D) cultures of dermal papilla cells lose their hair formation capability in culture, which is why they require maintaining their spheroidal forms (3D) [76, 77]. It is a challenge to develop methods that mimic *in vivo* conditions, which both maintain the 3D structure of cells and contain a special medium which imitates a natural niche rich in growth factors [56, 75].

Currently, there are no known tissue regeneration protocols applied for hair transplant with the use of ADSCs. Zanzoterra et al. [78] examined the capabilities of autologous cell suspension in the Rigenera system, which were obtained by mechanical fragmentation of subcutaneous and adipose tissue from the occipital area. The cell suspension was applied in the hair transplant area, thereby increasing the amount of growth factors. Microdamage has been observed to heal more quickly and to transplant hair to grow continuously even two months after the procedure, with the telogen phase shortened [78].

An ADSC-conditioned medium (ADSC-CM) was used in patients with alopecia (both male and female) in a study by Fukuoka and Suga [63]. A commercial product containing a protein solution with ADSCs was used (AAPE, Prostemics, Seoul, Korea) with various growth factors (hepatocyte growth factor, fibroblast growth factor I, granulocyte colony-stimulating factor, granulocyte macrophage-colony-stimulating factor, IL-6, VEGF, and TGF). The preparation (0.02 ml/cm^2 of the solution) was administered intradermally every 3 to 5 weeks (4–6 sessions), and hair growth was monitored with trichograms. A significant improvement in hair thickness was achieved in patients of both sexes [63].

Shin et al. [71] used ADSC and conditioned media of ADSCs (ADSC-CM) in a retrospective, observational study in 27 women with a female pattern hair loss (FPHL). The application of ADSC-CM showed efficacy in treating FPHL after 12 weeks of therapy with increased hair density and thickness without severe adverse reactions [71]. Won et al. [79] also showed that the application of ADSC-CM enhanced proliferation of cultured human dermal papilla cells (DPCs) by up to 130% [79].

Other studies have confirmed that enriching adipose tissue with a stromal vesicular fraction (SVF) supports adipocyte viability and yields better outcomes for a hair transplant procedure when they are present in grafts [62, 80]. Lipoaspirate obtained from abdominal fat (system Puregraft LLC, Solana Beach, CA, USA) was administered to the scalp at 1.0 ml/cm^2 in a Perez-Meza study. The amount of hair was found to increase by 23% after six months of the follow-up period [80].

1.5. Studies on Using Stem Cells from Wharton's Jelly

1.5.1. The Advantage of Stem Cells from Wharton's Jelly Compared to Other Mesenchymal Cells. Wharton's jelly has become a preferential source of stem cells due to its ready availability from a large pool of donors, noninvasive and painless acquisition, no risk to the donor, no ethical limitations, weak immunogenic potential, and high multipotential differentiation capability [81, 82]. Moreover, exposure to infectious agents occurs rarely, which guarantees safety to the donor [83].

Additionally, the decellularized Wharton's jelly matrix (DWJM) (fresh jelly was subjected to two cycles of osmotic shock, alternately with a hypertonic solution of NaCl, mannitol, $MgCl_2$, and KCl with the osmolarity of approx. 1.275 mOsm/l, and centrifuged at 5000 rpm at 4°C against a hypotonic solution of 0.005% Triton X-100) can provide a natural scaffolding for stem cells as a biocompatible matrix, which supports their viability, initiating aggregation of mesenchymal cells. DWJM contains TGF-β, collagen I, fibronectin, and tenascin, which may be responsible for condensation of added WJMSC in some areas of the DWJM. Hence, DWJM is a natural biocompatible 3D matrix which ensures adhesion, penetration, growth, and proliferation of cells—both *in vitro* and *in vivo*. To conclude, this paper presents DWJM as a new and natural 3D scaffolding which can be used in tissue engineering and regenerative medicine [84].

1.5.2. Neogenesis of Hair Follicles with Stem Cell Culture on Media and Grafting Them into the Skin: In Vitro Regeneration. In 2013, two researchers, demonstrated that it is possible to obtain cells with an expression of cytokeratin 19 and hair-like structures from WJMSC in *in vitro* conditions. Cytokeratin 19 (CK19) is a marker of bulge stem cells which determines the self-regeneration potential of modified skin [85, 86].

The Korean team of Yoo et al. [87–89] examined the effect of hWJSC on the acceleration of wound healing processes along with formation of hair follicles and other skin appendages. Enriched aggregates of hWJSC cells can form new hair follicles. The addition of growth factors to the culture medium is required: hepatocyte growth factor (HGF)

Table 2: Researches on the use of stem cells in the regeneration of hair follicles.

Authors	Research object	Indication	Methods of obtaining	Results	Comments
			Usage of hair follicle stem cell		
Agabalyan et al., 2016 [56]	Sprague Dawley rats/ nude mice	Nude mice genetically mutated	Bioreactors and static cell cultures with bFGF, PGF	Inducing de novo HF formation, reconstituting the DP and connective tissue sheath	Compared with static culture, stirred suspension bioreactors were significantly reduced, but they can generate larger numbers of autologous DSCs, maintaining their regenerative function
Nilforoushzadeh et al., 2016 [59]	Human/mice	Nude mice genetically mutated	Human scalp biopsy, isolation of only papilla cells which were cultured and injected into nude mice	Evidence of hair growth in mice received epithelial and DP cells	The combination of human cultured DP and epithelial cells could induce HF in nude mice
Elmaadawi et al., 2018 [21]	Human	Alopecia areata and androgenetic alopecia	Autologous bone marrow-derived mononuclear cells compared to follicular stems cells (skin punch biopsy from unaffected areas)	Good clinical improvement in both diseases	Nonstatistically significant difference between the source of cells
Gentile et al., 2017 [5]	Human	Androgenetic alopecia	Biopsies were collected and disaggregated by Rigeneracons without culture condition, then injected to the frontal scalp	A 29% ± 5% increase in hair density for the treated area and less than 1% in hair density for the placebo area	No culture required, quick time of surgery (about 60 min)
Kalabusheva et al., 2017 [120]	Human	*In vitro* study	Human DP cells and skin epidermal keratinocytes in a hanging drop culture to develop an artificial HF germ	Aggrecan, biglycan, fibronectin, and hyaluronic acid significantly stimulated cell proliferation in a DP cell monolayer culture without any effect on DP cell identity	Most of the ECM compounds prevented the formation of cell aggregates while hyaluronic acid promoted the formation of larger organoids
Hoffman et al., 2018 [121]	Human/mice	*In vitro* study	Hair follicle-associated-pluripotent stem cells from human scalp skin and transgenic mice with nestin-driven GFP	Intensive hair growth was observed in the pieces of shaved mouse skin histocultured on Gelfoam	Model for chemotherapy-induced alopecia (observing a doxorubicin effect)
			Usage of adipose-derived stem cells		
Park et al., 2010 [74]	Human/mice	C (3)H/NeH nude mice	ADSCs in a conditioned medium injected subcutaneously induced the anagen phase from telogen and increased hair regeneration in nude mice	ADSCs in a conditioned medium increased the proliferation of human DP and human epithelial keratinocytes; the effect of hypoxia on ADSC function increased hair regrowth	The secretion of IGFBP, M-CSF receptor, PGF, and VEGF was significantly increased by hypoxia, while the secretion of EGF production was decreased

Table 2: Continued.

Authors	Research object	Indication	Methods of obtaining	Results	Comments
Zanzoterra et al., 2014 [78]	Human	Androgenic alopecia	Injection of ADSCs and growth factors	After 2 weeks, the healing of microwounds was complete and HF continued growing	Rigenera system for the automated mechanical disaggregation of cell population
Sabapathy et al., 2016 [82]	Rats	*In vitro* study	ADSCs isolated from rats were cocultured with DP spheres	A core-shell structure, outer ASCs shell, and an inner DP core exhibited superior potential to HF formation compared to a mixed sphere of ADSCs with DP cells	PPARα signal in ADSCs can induce the hair formation
Yang et al., 2016 [69]	Human/mice	C57BL/6 nude mice	Cocultured human ADSCs with LL-37 was topically applied daily on the mouse skin	The conditioned medium of ADSCs preactivated with LL-37 strongly promoted hair growth *in vivo*	LL-37 treatment significantly increased EGR-1 expression
Anderi et al., 2018 [122]	Human	Alopecia areata	Lipoaspiration, autologous ADSCs were injected into the scalp of the patient ($4–4.7 \times 10^6$ cells)	Increased hair growth and decreased pull test, 3 and 6 months after ADSCs	Significant variation was observed between men and women only for hair diameter, no differences with age
Usage of Wharton's jelly and embryo stem cells					
Yoo et al., 2010 [88]	Human	*In vitro* study	Cultivated umbilical stem cells with EGF, HGF, and NGF	Formation of aggregates similar to native DP in special media and reconstructed dermal papilla-like tissues	HGF is necessary in the differentiation step
Yoo et al., 2010 [89]	Human/mice	Athymic nude mice genetically mutated	Isolated and cultivated stem cells from bone marrow and umbilical cord, after obtaining a DP-forming medium, injected in skin of nude mice	Effect of inducing new HF in mice within 45 days	
Wu et al., 2012 [90]	Human embryo MSCs/mice	Nude mice genetically mutated	Three cultures: DP cells cocultured with hMSCs; DP cells cocultured with fibroblasts; hMSCs cultured single, next injected into skin of mice	In fibroblast injection to mice, no HF was found	The expression *in vivo* of HLA-I was confined to DP of the newly grown hair, and the survival time of hMSCs in mice is 1 month

ADSCs: adipose-derived stem cells; DP: dermal papilla; DSCs: dermal stem cells; EGF: epidermal growth factor; bFGF: basic fibroblast growth factor; HF: hair follicle; HGF: hepatocyte growth factor; HLA-I: human leucocyte antigen class I; hMSCs: human mesenchymal stem cells; IGFBP: insulin-like growth factor-binding protein; M-CSF: macrophage colony-stimulating factor; NGF: nerve growth factor; PGF: platelet-derived growth factor; VEGF: vascular endothelial growth factor.

Table 3: Current studies of stem cell use registered on ClinicalTrials.gov [122].

Number	Study	Kind of stem cells	Method	Conditions	Status	Trial institution/sponsor and country	NCT number and duration period
1	"Stem Cell Educator Therapy in Alopecia Areata"	Cord blood-derived multipotent stem cells (CB-SCs)	A closed loop system that circulates a patient's blood through a blood cell separator, briefly cocultures the patient's lymphocytes with adherent CB-SCs in vitro, and returns the educated lymphocytes (but not the CB-SCs) to the patient's circulation	Alopecia areata	UKN	The First Hospital of Hebei Medical University Shijiazhuang, Hebei, China	NCT01673789 2012-2013
2	"The Effect of Allogeneic Human Adipose Derived Stem Cell Component Extract on Androgenic Alopecia"	Allogeneic human ADSC component extract	Applying 1.2 g of allogeneic human adipose-derived stem cell component extract on their scalp for 16 weeks	Androgenic alopecia	Completed	Pusan National University Hospital, South Korea	NCT02594046 2015–2017
3	"Adipose Tissue Derived Stem Cell Based Hair Restoration Therapy for Androgenetic Alopecia"	Autologous MSC and human platelet-rich plasma	MSCs derived from adipose tissue with human platelet-rich plasma will be applied	Androgenic alopecia	Not yet recruiting	King Edward Medical University, Pakistan	NCT02865421
4	"Biocellular-Cellular Regenerative Treatment Scaring Alopecia and Alopecia Areata"	High-density platelet-rich plasma and adipose-derived tissue stromal vascular fraction (AD-tSVF)	Use of high-density platelet-rich plasma concentrates and cell-enriched emulsified adipose-derived tissue stromal vascular fraction (AD-tSVF) via intravenous infusion	Alopecia areata, scarring alopecia	Recruiting	Regeneris Medical, Global Alliance for Regenerative Medicine, Healeon Medical Inc., USA	NCT03078686 2017–2019
5	"AGA Biocellular Stem/Stromal Hair Regenerative Study"	Adipose-derived tissue stromal vascular fraction (AD-tSVF) and high-density platelet-rich plasma	Biocellular mixture of emulsified AD-tSVF and high-density platelet-rich plasma concentrate (HD-PRP) as compared with adipose-derived cell-enriched SVF (AD-cSVF)+AD-tSVF and HD-PRP using Healeon Centricyte 1000 system and intradermal injections	Androgenetic alopecia, female pattern hair loss	Recruiting	Healeon Medical Inc., Ministry of Health, Honduras Irvine, California, USA	NCT02849470 2016–2018
6	"Point-of-Care Adipose-derived Cells for Hair Growth"	Stromal vascular fraction (SVF) cells	A single injection into the scalp of autologous adipose-derived SVF cells	Androgenic alopecia	Recruiting	University of Florida Gainesville, Florida, USA	NCT02729415 2016-2017

stimulates growth of hair follicles *in vivo* and *in vitro*; basic fibroblast growth factor (bFGF) stimulates growth of dermal papilla cells *in vivo*; and vesicular endothelial growth factor (VEGF) stimulates growth of hair follicles and hair root *in vivo*. The hepatocyte growth factor (HGF) must be used at the stage of differentiation of the dermal papilla in culture, which is relatively expensive [87–89].

Moreover, Yoo et al. [88] compared effects of culturing bone marrow and umbilical cord stem cells to the spontaneous formation of dermal papilla-like tissues (DPLT). Isolated cells of the hair outer sheath were used for incubation: DPLT were recovered from 25T cell culturing plates and mixed with 1106 cells of hair sheath in 50 ml of physiological saline and injected into mice skin. The mice were examined after six weeks. Subsequently, the clinical effects of hair follicle formation in originally bare mice following their implantation in the skin were compared. No differences between the methods were observed [88].

Wu et al. (a Chinese study) [90] demonstrated the potential for differentiation of hMSC (from human embryos) to dermal papilla cells in cocultures of hMSC using dermal papilla cells previously obtained from patients. Expression of versican, CD133, SCF (stem cell factor), ET-1 (endothelin-1), and bFGF (fibroblast growth factor) was observed during the process of differentiation [90].

1.5.3. Neogenesis of Hair Follicles from Isolated Cells (Stem Cells from Wharton's Jelly): In Vivo Regeneration. Intensive studies are being conducted on the commercial use of hWJSC in alopecia treatment at the University of Kansas Innovation and Collaboration, Kansas, USA (Dr. Omar Aljitawi) (no literature data) (Tables 2 and 3).

2. Conclusion

Maintaining a pool of stem cells is necessary for tissue homeostasis and damage repair. Their divisions are not frequent in mature organisms, and most of them are in a dormant state. Therefore, it is important to understand the mechanisms of their activation, which will allow for the use of multipotent cells in regenerative medicine [33]. Their use is additionally complicated by the fact that expression of receptors on different growth factors and the effect of the microenvironment may vary. Moreover, not all target points in stem cell therapy have been identified. It requires further studies aimed not only at the use of stem cells and their various fractions and compositions with adjuvants but also at broadening of knowledge on the physiology and cytophysiology of the hair follicle [35].

References

[1] A. Adil and M. Godwin, "The effectiveness of treatments for androgenetic alopecia: a systematic review and meta-analysis," *Journal of the American Academy of Dermatology*, vol. 77, no. 1, pp. 136–141.e5, 2017.

[2] W. C. Cranwell and R. Sinclair, "Familial frontal fibrosing alopecia treated with dutasteride, minoxidil and artificial hair transplantation," *Australasian Journal of Dermatology*, vol. 58, no. 3, pp. e94–e96, 2017.

[3] S. M. Lesko, L. Rosenberg, and S. Shapiro, "A case-control study of baldness in relation to myocardial infarction in men," *Journal of the American Medical Association*, vol. 269, no. 8, pp. 998–1003, 1993.

[4] T. S. Purba, I. S. Haslam, E. Poblet et al., "Human epithelial hair follicle stem cells and their progeny: current state of knowledge, the widening gap in translational research and future challenges," *BioEssays*, vol. 36, no. 5, pp. 513–525, 2014.

[5] P. Gentile, M. G. Scioli, A. Bielli, A. Orlandi, and V. Cervelli, "Stem cells from human hair follicles: first mechanical isolation for immediate autologous clinical use in androgenetic alopecia and hair loss," *Stem Cell Investigation*, vol. 4, no. 7, p. 58, 2017.

[6] K. Turksen, *Tissue Specific Stem Cell Niche*, Springer, 2015.

[7] G. Guasch, "The epithelial stem cell niche in skin," in *Biology and engineering of stem cell niches*, A. Vishwakarma and J. Karp, Eds., pp. 127–143, Elsevier Inc., 2017.

[8] P. Rompolas and V. Greco, "Stem cell dynamics in the hair follicle niche," *Seminars in Cell and Developmental Biology*, vol. 25-26, pp. 34–42, 2014.

[9] C. Blanpain, W. E. Lowry, A. Geoghegan, L. Polak, and E. Fuchs, "Self-renewal, multipotency, and the existence of two cell populations within an epithelial stem cell niche," *Cell*, vol. 118, no. 5, pp. 635–648, 2004.

[10] H. J. Snippert, A. Haegebarth, M. Kasper et al., "Lgr6 marks stem cells in the hair follicle that generate all cell lineages of the skin," *Science*, vol. 327, no. 5971, pp. 1385–1389, 2010.

[11] P. Zhang, R. E. Kling, S. K. Ravuri et al., "A review of adipocyte lineage cells and dermal papilla cells in hair follicle regeneration," *Journal of Tissue Engineering*, vol. 5, 2014.

[12] R. R. Driskell, C. Clavel, M. Rendl, and F. M. Watt, "Hair follicle dermal papilla cells at a glance," *Journal of Cell Science*, vol. 124, no. 8, pp. 1179–1182, 2011.

[13] M. Rendl, L. Polak, and E. Fuchs, "BMP signaling in dermal papilla cells is required for their hair follicle-inductive properties," *Genes & Development*, vol. 22, no. 4, pp. 543–557, 2008.

[14] T. Matsuzaki and K. Yoshizato, "Role of hair papilla cells on induction and regeneration processes of hair follicles," *Wound Repair and Regeneration*, vol. 6, no. 6, pp. 524–530, 1998.

[15] V. Greco, T. Chen, M. Rendl et al., "A two-step mechanism for stem cell activation during hair regeneration," *Cell Stem Cell*, vol. 4, no. 2, pp. 155–169, 2009.

[16] P. Rabbani, M. Takeo, W. Chou et al., "Coordinated activation of Wnt in epithelial and melanocyte stem cells initiates pigmented hair regeneration," *Cell*, vol. 145, no. 6, pp. 941–955, 2011.

[17] C. A. B. Jahoda, C. J. Whitehouse, A. J. Reynolds, and N. Hole, "Hair follicle dermal cells differentiate into adipogenic and osteogenic lineages," *Experimental Dermatology*, vol. 12, no. 6, pp. 849–859, 2003.

[18] S. Y. Tsai, C. Clavel, S. Kim et al., "Oct4 and Klf4 reprogram dermal papilla cells into induced pluripotent stem cells," *Stem Cells*, vol. 28, no. 2, pp. 221–228, 2010.

[19] M. Ohyama, A. Terunuma, C. L. Tock et al., "Characterization and isolation of stem cell-enriched human hair follicle bulge cells," *Journal of Clinical Investigation*, vol. 116, no. 1, pp. 249–260, 2006.

[20] P. Mohammadi, K. K. Youssef, S. Abbasalizadeh, H. Baharvand, and N. Aghdami, "Human hair reconstruction: close, but yet so far," *Stem Cells and Development*, vol. 25, no. 23, pp. 1767–1779, 2016.

[21] I. H. Elmaadawi, B. M. Mohamed, Z. A. S. Ibrahim et al., "Stem cell therapy as a novel therapeutic intervention for resistant cases of alopecia areata and androgenetic alopecia," *Journal of Dermatological Treatment*, vol. 29, no. 5, pp. 431–440, 2018.

[22] A. L. Means, Y. Xu, A. Zhao, K. C. Ray, and G. Gu, "CK19^{CreERT} knockin mouse line allows for conditional DNA recombination in epithelial cells in multiple endodermal organs," *Genesis*, vol. 46, no. 6, pp. 318–323, 2008.

[23] K. Inoue, N. Aoi, T. Sato et al., "Differential expression of stem-cell-associated markers in human hair follicle epithelial cells," *Laboratory Investigation*, vol. 89, no. 8, pp. 844–856, 2009.

[24] K. Sellheyer and D. Krahl, "PHLDA1 (TDAG51) is a follicular stem cell marker and differentiates between morphoeic basal cell carcinoma and desmoplastic trichoepithelioma," *British Journal of Dermatology*, vol. 164, no. 1, pp. 141–147, 2011.

[25] V. Jaks, N. Barker, M. Kasper et al., "Lgr5 marks cycling, yet long-lived, hair follicle stem cells," *Nature Genetics*, vol. 40, no. 11, pp. 1291–1299, 2008.

[26] J. D. Hoeck, B. Biehs, A. V. Kurtova et al., "Stem cell plasticity enables hair regeneration following Lgr5+ cell loss," *Nature Cell Biology*, vol. 19, no. 6, pp. 666–676, 2017.

[27] K. B. Jensen, C. A. Collins, E. Nascimento et al., "Lrig1 expression defines a distinct multipotent stem cell population in mammalian epidermis," *Cell Stem Cell*, vol. 4, no. 5, pp. 427–439, 2009.

[28] M. Ozawa, S. Aiba, M. Kurosawa, and H. Tagami, "Ber-EP4 antigen is a marker for a cell population related to the secondary hair germ," *Experimental Dermatology*, vol. 13, no. 7, pp. 401–405, 2004.

[29] K. J. McElwee, S. Kissling, E. Wenzel, A. Huth, and R. Hoffmann, "Cultured peribulbar dermal sheath cells can induce hair follicle development and contribute to the dermal sheath and dermal papilla," *Journal of Investigative Dermatology*, vol. 121, no. 6, pp. 1267–1275, 2003.

[30] S.-H. Lee, J. Yoon, S. H. Shin et al., "Valproic acid induces hair regeneration in murine model and activates alkaline phosphatase activity in human dermal papilla cells," *PLoS One*, vol. 7, no. 4, article e34152, 2012.

[31] M. Rendl, L. Lewis, and E. Fuchs, "Molecular dissection of mesenchymal-epithelial interactions in the hair follicle," *PLoS Biology*, vol. 3, no. 11, p. e331, 2005.

[32] Y. Ito, T. S. Hamazaki, K. Ohnuma, K. Tamaki, M. Asashima, and H. Okochi, "Isolation of murine hair-inducing cells using the cell surface marker prominin-1/CD133," *Journal of Investigative Dermatology*, vol. 127, no. 5, pp. 1052–1060, 2007.

[33] J. Li, T. X. Jiang, and C. M. Chuong, "Many paths to alopecia via compromised regeneration of hair follicle stem cells," *Journal of Investigative Dermatology*, vol. 133, no. 6, pp. 1450–1452, 2013.

[34] P. Rompolas, K. R. Mesa, and V. Greco, "Spatial organization within a niche as a determinant of stem-cell fate," *Nature*, vol. 502, no. 7472, pp. 513–518, 2013.

[35] J. W. Oh, J. Kloepper, E. A. Langan et al., "A guide to studying human hair follicle cycling in vivo," *Journal of Investigative Dermatology*, vol. 136, no. 1, pp. 34–44, 2016.

[36] L. A. Garza, Y. Liu, Z. Yang et al., "Prostaglandin D2 inhibits hair growth and is elevated in bald scalp of men with androgenetic alopecia," *Science Translational Medicine*, vol. 4, no. 126, article 126ra34, 2012.

[37] J. Halloy, B. A. Bernard, G. Loussouarn, and A. Goldbeter, "Modeling the dynamics of human hair cycles by a follicular automaton," *Proceedings of the National Academy of Sciences of the United States of America*, vol. 97, no. 15, pp. 8328–8333, 2000.

[38] M. Nakamura, M. R. Schneider, R. Schmidt-Ullrich, and R. Paus, "Mutant laboratory mice with abnormalities in hair follicle morphogenesis, cycling, and/or structure: an update," *Journal of Dermatological Science*, vol. 69, no. 1, pp. 6–29, 2013.

[39] S. Tanimura, Y. Tadokoro, K. Inomata et al., "Hair follicle stem cells provide a functional niche for melanocyte stem cells," *Cell Stem Cell*, vol. 8, no. 2, pp. 177–187, 2011.

[40] E. R. Deschene, P. Myung, P. Rompolas et al., "β-catenin activation regulates tissue growth non-cell autonomously in the hair stem cell niche," *Science*, vol. 343, no. 6177, pp. 1353–1356, 2014.

[41] L. Zhou, H. Wang, J. Jing, L. Yu, X. Wu, and Z. Lu, "Regulation of hair follicle development by exosomes derived from dermal papilla cells," *Biochemical and Biophysical Research Communications*, vol. 500, no. 2, pp. 325–332, 2018.

[42] M. V. Plikus, J. A. Mayer, D. de la Cruz et al., "Cyclic dermal BMP signalling regulates stem cell activation during hair regeneration," *Nature*, vol. 451, no. 7176, pp. 340–344, 2008.

[43] R. Yi, "Concise review: mechanisms of quiescent hair follicle stem cell regulation," *Stem Cells*, vol. 35, no. 12, pp. 2323–2330, 2017.

[44] I. Brownell, E. Guevara, C. B. Bai, C. A. Loomis, and A. L. Joyner, "Nerve-derived sonic hedgehog defines a niche for hair follicle stem cells capable of becoming epidermal stem cells," *Cell Stem Cell*, vol. 8, no. 5, pp. 552–565, 2011.

[45] L. Mecklenburg, D. J. Tobin, S. Müller-Röver et al., "Active hair growth (anagen) is associated with angiogenesis," *Journal of Investigative Dermatology*, vol. 114, no. 5, pp. 909–916, 2000.

[46] A. Mohyeldin, T. Garzón-Muvdi, and A. Quiñones-Hinojosa, "Oxygen in stem cell biology: a critical component of the stem cell niche," *Cell Stem Cell*, vol. 7, no. 2, pp. 150–161, 2010.

[47] T. Christoph, S. Müller-Röver, H. Audring et al., "The human hair follicle immune system: cellular composition and immune privilege," *British Journal of Dermatology*, vol. 142, no. 5, pp. 862–873, 2000.

[48] R. PAUS, B. NICKOLOFF, and T. ITO, "A 'hairy' privilege," *Trends in Immunology*, vol. 26, no. 1, pp. 32–40, 2005.

[49] D. Gay, O. Kwon, Z. Zhang et al., "Fgf9 from dermal $\gamma\delta$ T cells induces hair follicle neogenesis after wounding," *Nature Medicine*, vol. 19, no. 7, pp. 916–923, 2013.

[50] D. Castellana, R. Paus, and M. Perez-Moreno, "Macrophages contribute to the cyclic activation of adult hair

follicle stem cells," *PLoS Biology*, vol. 12, no. 12, article e1002002, 2014.

[51] N. Osaka, T. Takahashi, S. Murakami et al., "ASK1-dependent recruitment and activation of macrophages induce hair growth in skin wounds," *The Journal of Cell Biology*, vol. 176, no. 7, pp. 903–909, 2007.

[52] N. Ali, B. Zirak, R. S. Rodriguez et al., "Regulatory T cells in skin facilitate epithelial stem cell differentiation," *Cell*, vol. 169, no. 6, pp. 1119–1129.e11, 2017.

[53] K. Asakawa, K. E. Toyoshima, N. Ishibashi et al., "Hair organ regeneration via the bioengineered hair follicular unit transplantation," *Scientific Reports*, vol. 2, no. 1, p. 424, 2012.

[54] M. E. Balañá, H. E. Charreau, and G. J. Leirós, "Epidermal stem cells and skin tissue engineering in hair follicle regeneration," *World Journal of Stem Cells*, vol. 7, no. 4, pp. 711–727, 2015.

[55] J. P. Cole, "An analysis of follicular punches, mechanics, and dynamics in follicular unit extraction," *Facial Plastic Surgery Clinics of North America*, vol. 21, no. 3, pp. 437–447, 2013.

[56] N. A. Agabalyan, B. S. Borys, H. D. Sparks et al., "Enhanced expansion and sustained inductive function of skin-derived precursor cells in computer-controlled stirred suspension bioreactors," *Stem Cells Translational Medicine*, vol. 6, no. 2, pp. 434–443, 2017.

[57] J. Biernaskie, M. Paris, O. Morozova et al., "SKPs derive from hair follicle precursors and exhibit properties of adult dermal stem cells," *Cell Stem Cell*, vol. 5, no. 6, pp. 610–623, 2009.

[58] C. A. V. Rodrigues, T. G. Fernandes, M. M. Diogo, C. L. da Silva, and J. M. S. Cabral, "Stem cell cultivation in bioreactors," *Biotechnology Advances*, vol. 29, no. 6, pp. 815–829, 2011.

[59] M. Nilforoushzadeh, E. Rahimi Jameh, F. Jaffary et al., "Hair follicle generation by injections of adult human follicular epithelial and dermal papilla cells into nude mice," *Cell Journal*, vol. 19, no. 2, pp. 259–268, 2017.

[60] M. Gaur, M. Dobke, and V. Lunyak, "Mesenchymal stem cells from adipose tissue in clinical applications for dermatological indications and skin aging," *International Journal of Molecular Sciences*, vol. 18, no. 1, 2017.

[61] E. Festa, J. Fretz, R. Berry et al., "Adipocyte lineage cells contribute to the skin stem cell niche to drive hair cycling," *Cell*, vol. 146, no. 5, pp. 761–771, 2011.

[62] M. Zhu, Z. Zhou, Y. Chen et al., "Supplementation of fat grafts with adipose-derived regenerative cells improves long-term graft retention," *Annals of Plastic Surgery*, vol. 64, no. 2, pp. 222–228, 2010.

[63] H. Fukuoka and H. Suga, "Hair regeneration treatment using adipose-derived stem cell conditioned medium: follow-up with trichograms," *Eplasty*, vol. 15, 2015.

[64] C.-F. Huang, Y.-J. Chang, Y.-Y. Hsueh et al., "Assembling composite dermal papilla spheres with adipose-derived stem cells to enhance hair follicle induction," *Science Reports*, vol. 6, no. 1, 2016.

[65] I. Hwang, K.-A. Choi, H.-S. Park et al., "Neural stem cells restore hair growth through activation of the hair follicle niche," *Cell Transplantation*, vol. 25, no. 8, pp. 1439–1451, 2016.

[66] A. Rezza, R. Sennett, M. Tanguy, C. Clavel, and M. Rendl, "PDGF signalling in the dermis and in dermal condensates is dispensable for hair follicle induction and formation," *Experimental Dermatology*, vol. 24, no. 6, pp. 468–470, 2015.

[67] K. Yano, L. F. Brown, and M. Detmar, "Control of hair growth and follicle size by VEGF-mediated angiogenesis," *The Journal of Clinical Investigation*, vol. 107, no. 4, pp. 409–417, 2001.

[68] S. Wood, V. Jayaraman, E. J. Huelsmann et al., "Pro-inflammatory chemokine CCL2 (MCP-1) promotes healing in diabetic wounds by restoring the macrophage response," *PLoS One*, vol. 9, no. 3, article e91574, 2014.

[69] Y. Yang, H. Choi, M. Seon, D. Cho, and S. I. Bang, "LL-37 stimulates the functions of adipose-derived stromal/stem cells via early growth response 1 and the MAPK pathway," *Stem Cell Research & Therapy*, vol. 7, no. 1, p. 58, 2016.

[70] H. Shin, H. H. Ryu, O. Kwon, B. S. Park, and S. J. Jo, "Clinical use of conditioned media of adipose tissue-derived stem cells in female pattern hair loss: a retrospective case series study," *International Journal of Dermatology*, vol. 54, no. 6, pp. 730–735, 2015.

[71] H. Shin, C. H. Won, W. K. Chung, and B. S. Park, "Up-to-date clinical trials of hair regeneration using conditioned media of adipose-derived stem cells in male and female pattern hair loss," *Current Stem Cell Research & Therapy*, vol. 12, no. 7, pp. 524–530, 2017.

[72] N. Misago, S. Toda, H. Sugihara, H. Kohda, and Y. Narisawa, "Proliferation and differentiation of organoid hair follicle cells co-cultured with fat cells in collagen gel matrix culture," *British Journal of Dermatology*, vol. 139, no. 1, pp. 40–48, 1998.

[73] M. C. Jong, M. J. Gijbels, V. E. Dahlmans et al., "Hyperlipidemia and cutaneous abnormalities in transgenic mice overexpressing human apolipoprotein C1," *Journal of Clinical Investigation*, vol. 101, no. 1, pp. 145–152, 1998.

[74] B.-S. Park, W.-S. Kim, J.-S. Choi et al., "Hair growth stimulated by conditioned medium of adipose-derived stem cells is enhanced by hypoxia: evidence of increased growth factor secretion," *BioMed Research International*, vol. 31, no. 1, 34 pages, 2010.

[75] S. Ramdasi and S. K. Tiwari, "Human mesenchymal stem cell-derived conditioned media for hair regeneration applications," *Journal of Stem Cells*, vol. 11, no. 4, pp. 201–211, 2016.

[76] B. M. Kang, M. H. Kwack, M. K. Kim, J. C. Kim, and Y. K. Sung, "Sphere formation increases the ability of cultured human dermal papilla cells to induce hair follicles from mouse epidermal cells in a reconstitution assay," *Journal of Investigative Dermatology*, vol. 132, no. 1, pp. 237–239, 2012.

[77] C. H. Seo, M. H. Kwack, S. H. Lee, M. K. Kim, J. C. Kim, and Y. K. Sung, "Poor capability of 3D-cultured adipose-derived stem cells to induce hair follicles in contrast to 3D-cultured dermal papilla cells," *Annals of Dermatology*, vol. 28, no. 5, pp. 662–665, 2016.

[78] F. Zanzottera, E. Lavezzari, L. Trovato, A. Icardi, and A. Graziano, "Adipose derived stem cells and growth factors applied on hair transplantation. Follow-up of clinical outcome," *Journal of Cosmetics, Dermatological Sciences and Applications*, vol. 4, no. 4, pp. 268–274, 2014.

[79] C. H. Won, H. G. Yoo, O. S. Kwon et al., "Hair growth promoting effects of adipose tissue-derived stem cells," *Journal of Dermatological Science*, vol. 57, no. 2, pp. 134–137, 2010.

[80] D. Perez-Meza, C. Ziering, M. Sforza, G. Krishnan, E. Ball, and E. Daniels, "Hair follicle growth by stromal vascular fraction-enhanced adipose transplantation in baldness,"

Stem Cells and Cloning: Advances and Applications, vol. 10, pp. 1–10, 2017.

[81] S. M. Richardson, G. Kalamegam, P. N. Pushparaj et al., "Mesenchymal stem cells in regenerative medicine: Focus on articular cartilage and intervertebral disc regeneration," *Methods*, vol. 99, pp. 69–80, 2016.

[82] V. Sabapathy, B. Sundaram, S. VM, P. Mankuzhy, and S. Kumar, "Human Wharton's jelly mesenchymal stem cells plasticity augments scar-free skin wound healing with hair growth," *PLoS One*, vol. 9, no. 4, article e93726, 2014.

[83] Q. Wang, Q. Yang, Z. Wang et al., "Comparative analysis of human mesenchymal stem cells from fetal-bone marrow, adipose tissue, and Warton's jelly as sources of cell immunomodulatory therapy," *Human Vaccines & Immunotherapeutics*, vol. 12, no. 1, pp. 85–96, 2015.

[84] S. Jadalannagari, G. Converse, C. McFall et al., "Decellularized Wharton's jelly from human umbilical cord as a novel 3D scaffolding material for tissue engineering applications," *PLoS One*, vol. 12, no. 2, article e0172098, 2017.

[85] A. G. Abdou, M. A. Wahed, A. A.-W. Saleh, D. El Sakka, M. A. W. Gaber, and W. Shehata, "Stem cell markers (cytokeratin 17 and cytokeratin 19) in scarring and nonscarring alopecia," *Journal of Cutaneous and Aesthetic Surgery*, vol. 9, no. 3, pp. 165–171, 2016.

[86] O. S. Aljitawi, Y. Xiao, D. Zhang et al., "Generating CK19-positive cells with hair-like structures from Wharton's jelly mesenchymal stromal cells," *Stem Cells and Development*, vol. 22, no. 1, pp. 18–26, 2013.

[87] B. Y. Yoo, Y. H. Shin, H. H. Yoon, Y. K. Seo, and J. K. Park, "Hair follicular cell/organ culture in tissue engineering and regenerative medicine," *Biochemical Engineering Journal*, vol. 48, no. 3, pp. 323–331, 2010.

[88] B. Y. Yoo, Y. H. Shin, H. H. Yoon, Y. K. Seo, K. Y. Song, and J. K. Park, "Application of mesenchymal stem cells derived from bone marrow and umbilical cord in human hair multiplication," *Journal of Dermatological Science*, vol. 60, no. 2, pp. 74–83, 2010.

[89] B. Y. Yoo, Y. H. Shin, H. H. Yoon, Y. K. Seo, K. Y. Song, and J. K. Park, "Optimization of the reconstruction of dermal papilla like tissues employing umbilical cord mesenchymal stem cells," *Biotechnology and Bioprocess Engineering*, vol. 15, no. 1, pp. 182–190, 2010.

[90] M. Wu, Q. Sun, X. Guo, and H. Liu, "hMSCs possess the potential to differentiate into DP cells in vivo and in vitro," *Cell Biology International Reports*, vol. 19, no. 2, pp. 37–43, 2012.

[91] S. B. Telerman, E. Rognoni, I. Sequeira et al., "Dermal Blimp1 acts downstream of epidermal TGFβ and Wnt/β-catenin to regulate hair follicle formation and growth," *Journal of Investigative Dermatology*, vol. 137, no. 11, pp. 2270–2281, 2017.

[92] K. Kobielak, N. Stokes, J. de la Cruz, L. Polak, and E. Fuchs, "Loss of a quiescent niche but not follicle stem cells in the absence of bone morphogenetic protein signaling," *Proceedings of the National Academy of Sciences of the United States of America*, vol. 104, no. 24, pp. 10063–10068, 2007.

[93] M. Lei, H. Guo, W. Qiu et al., "Modulating hair follicle size with *Wnt10b/DKK1* during hair regeneration," *Experimental Dermatology*, vol. 23, no. 6, pp. 407–413, 2014.

[94] S. E. Millar, K. Willert, P. C. Salinas et al., "WNT signaling in the control of hair growth and structure," *Developmental Biology*, vol. 207, no. 1, pp. 133–149, 1999.

[95] W. H. Lin, L. J. Xiang, H. X. Shi et al., "Fibroblast growth factors stimulate hair growth through β-catenin and Shh expression in C57BL/6 mice," *BioMed Research International*, vol. 2015, Article ID 730139, 9 pages, 2015.

[96] M. Kimura-Ueki, Y. Oda, J. Oki et al., "Hair cycle resting phase is regulated by cyclic epithelial FGF18 signaling," *Journal of Investigative Dermatology*, vol. 132, no. 5, pp. 1338–1345, 2012.

[97] C. A. Higgins, L. Petukhova, S. Harel et al., "FGF5 is a crucial regulator of hair length in humans," *Proceedings of the National Academy of Sciences*, vol. 111, no. 29, pp. 10648–10653, 2014.

[98] L. Guo, Q. C. Yu, and E. Fuchs, "Targeting expression of keratinocyte growth factor to keratinocytes elicits striking changes in epithelial differentiation in trans-genic mice," *EMBO Journal*, vol. 12, no. 3, pp. 973–986, 1993.

[99] A. Petiot, F. J. Conti, R. Grose, J. M. Revest, K. M. Hodivala-Dilke, and C. Dickson, "A crucial role for Fgfr2-IIIb signalling in epidermal development and hair follicle patterning," *Development*, vol. 130, no. 22, pp. 5493–5501, 2003.

[100] Ö. Akilli Öztürk, H. Pakula, J. Chmielowiec et al., "Gab1 and Mapk signaling are essential in the hair cycle and hair follicle stem cell quiescence," *Cell Reports*, vol. 13, no. 3, pp. 561–572, 2015.

[101] P. Mill, R. Mo, H. Fu et al., "Sonic hedgehog-dependent activation of Gli2 is essential for embryonic hair follicle development," *Genes & Development*, vol. 17, no. 2, pp. 282–294, 2003.

[102] S. Estrach, C. A. Ambler, C. L. Lo Celso, K. Hozumi, and F. M. Watt, "Jagged 1 is a β-catenin target gene required for ectopic hair follicle formation in adult epidermis," *Development*, vol. 133, no. 22, pp. 4427–4438, 2006.

[103] H. Amalia Pasolli, A. R. Folgueras, and E. Fuchs, "Architectural niche organization by LHX2 is linked to hair follicle stem cell function," *Microscopy and Microanalysis*, vol. 20, no. S3, pp. 1382-1383, 2014.

[104] K.-T. Du, J.-Q. Deng, X.-G. He, Z.-p. Liu, C. Peng, and M.-S. Zhang, "MiR-214 regulates the human hair follicle stem cell proliferation and differentiation by targeting EZH2 and Wnt/β-catenin signaling way *in vitro*," *Tissue Engineering and Regenerative Medicine*, vol. 15, no. 3, pp. 341–350, 2018.

[105] V. Horsley, A. O. Aliprantis, L. Polak, L. H. Glimcher, and E. Fuchs, "NFATc1 balances quiescence and proliferation of skin stem cells," *Cell*, vol. 132, no. 2, pp. 299–310, 2008.

[106] K. Krieger, S. E. Millar, N. Mikuda et al., "NF-κB participates in mouse hair cycle control and plays distinct roles in the various pelage hair follicle types," *Journal of Investigative Dermatology*, vol. 138, no. 2, pp. 256–264, 2018.

[107] S. Demehri and R. Kopan, "Notch signaling in bulge stem cells is not required for selection of hair follicle fate," *Development*, vol. 136, no. 6, pp. 891–896, 2009.

[108] H.-Y. Lin, C.-H. Kao, K. M.-C. Lin, V. Kaartinen, and L.-T. Yang, "Notch signaling regulates late-stage epidermal differentiation and maintains postnatal hair cycle homeostasis," *PLoS One*, vol. 6, no. 1, article e15842, 2011.

[109] A. E. Oro and K. Higgins, "Hair cycle regulation of hedgehog signal reception," *Developmental Biology*, vol. 255, no. 2, pp. 238–248, 2003.

[110] C. S. L. Hoi, S. E. Lee, S. Y. Lu et al., "Runx1 directly promotes proliferation of hair follicle stem cells and epithelial tumor

formation in mouse skin," *Molecular and Cellular Biology*, vol. 30, no. 10, pp. 2518–2536, 2010.

[111] B. St-Jacques, H. R. Dassule, I. Karavanova et al., "Sonic hedgehog signaling is essential for hair development," *Current Biology*, vol. 8, no. 19, pp. 1058–1069, 1998.

[112] M. Kadaja, B. E. Keyes, M. Lin et al., "SOX9: a stem cell transcriptional regulator of secreted niche signaling factors," *Genes & Development*, vol. 28, no. 4, pp. 328–341, 2014.

[113] K. Foitzik, G. Lindner, S. Mueller-Roever et al., "Control of murine hair follicle regression (catagen) by TGF-β1in vivo," *FASEB Journal*, vol. 14, no. 5, pp. 752–760, 2000.

[114] K. Foitzik, R. Paus, T. Doetschman, and G. Paolo Dotto, "The TGF-β2 isoform is both a required and sufficient inducer of murine hair follicle morphogenesis," *Developmental Biology*, vol. 212, no. 2, pp. 278–289, 1999.

[115] N. Oshimori and E. Fuchs, "Paracrine TGF-β signaling counterbalances BMP-mediated repression in hair follicle stem cell activation," *Cell Stem Cell*, vol. 10, no. 1, pp. 63–75, 2012.

[116] W. Qiu, M. Lei, L. Zhou et al., "Hair follicle stem cell proliferation, Akt and Wnt signaling activation in TPA-induced hair regeneration," *Histochemistry and Cell Biology*, vol. 147, no. 6, pp. 749–758, 2017.

[117] L. Dong, H. Hao, J. Liu et al., "A conditioned medium of umbilical cord mesenchymal stem cells overexpressing Wnt7a promotes wound repair and regeneration of hair follicles in mice," *Stem Cells International*, vol. 2017, Article ID 3738071, 13 pages, 2017.

[118] E. Kandyba and K. Kobielak, "Wnt7b is an important intrinsic regulator of hair follicle stem cell homeostasis and hair follicle cycling," *Stem Cells*, vol. 32, no. 4, pp. 886–901, 2014.

[119] D. Enshell-Seijffers, C. Lindon, M. Kashiwagi, and B. A. Morgan, "Beta-catenin activity in the dermal papilla regulates morphogenesis and regeneration of hair," *Developmental Cell*, vol. 18, no. 4, pp. 633–642, 2010.

[120] E. Kalabusheva, V. Terskikh, and E. Vorotelyak, "Hair germ model in vitro via human postnatal keratinocyte-dermal papilla interactions: impact of hyaluronic acid," *Stem Cells International*, vol. 2017, Article ID 9271869, 14 pages, 2017.

[121] R. M. Hoffman, L. Li, and W. Cao, "Hair-shaft growth in Gelfoam® histoculture of skin and isolated hair follicles," *Methods in Molecular Biology*, vol. 1760, pp. 133–144, 2018.

[122] R. Anderi, N. Makdissy, A. Azar, F. Rizk, and A. Hamade, "Cellular therapy with human autologous adipose-derived adult cells of stromal vascular fraction for alopecia areata," *Stem Cell Research & Therapy*, vol. 9, no. 1, p. 141, 2018.

2

Significance of Glioma Stem-Like Cells in the Tumor Periphery that Express High Levels of CD44 in Tumor Invasion, Early Progression, and Poor Prognosis in Glioblastoma

Masahiro Nishikawa ,[1] Akihiro Inoue ,[1] Takanori Ohnishi,[2] Shohei Kohno,[1] Shiro Ohue,[3] Shirabe Matsumoto,[1] Satoshi Suehiro,[1] Daisuke Yamashita,[1] Saya Ozaki,[1] Hideaki Watanabe,[1] Hajime Yano,[4] Hisaaki Takahashi,[5] Riko Kitazawa,[6] Junya Tanaka,[4] and Takeharu Kunieda[1]

[1]*Department of Neurosurgery, Ehime University Graduate School of Medicine, Toon, Ehime 791-0295, Japan*
[2]*Department of Neurosurgery, Washoukai Sadamoto Hospital, Matsuyama, Ehime 790-0052, Japan*
[3]*Department of Neurosurgery, Ehime Prefectural Central Hospital, Matsuyama, Ehime 790-0024, Japan*
[4]*Department of Molecular and Cellular Physiology, Ehime University Graduate School of Medicine, Toon, Ehime 791-0295, Japan*
[5]*Division of Pathophysiology, Faculty of Pharmaceutical Sciences, Hokuriku University, Kanazawa, Ishikawa 920-1180, Japan*
[6]*Division of Diagnostic Pathology, Ehime University Hospital, Toon, Ehime 791-0295, Japan*

Correspondence should be addressed to Akihiro Inoue; iakihiro3@gmail.com

Academic Editor: Cristina Grange

Glioblastoma multiforme (GBM) is the most aggressive malignant brain tumor and a subpopulation of glioma stem-like cells (GSCs) is likely responsible for the invariable recurrence following maximum resection and chemoradiotherapy. As most GSCs that are located in the perivascular and perinecrotic niches should be removed during tumor resection, it is very important to know where surviving GSCs are localized. Here, we investigated the existence and functions of GSCs in the tumor periphery, which is considered to constitute the invasion niche for GSCs in GBM, by analyzing expression of stem cell markers and stem cell-related molecules and measuring particular activities of cultured GSCs. In addition, the relationship between GSCs expressing particular stem cell markers and pathological features on MRI and prognosis in GBM patients was analyzed. We showed that GSCs that express high levels of CD44 are present in the tumor periphery. We also found that vascular endothelial growth factor (VEGF) is characteristically expressed at a high level in the tumor periphery. Cultured GSCs obtained from the tumor periphery were highly invasive and have enhanced migration phenotype, both of which were markedly inhibited by CD44 knockdown. Higher expression of CD44 in the tumor periphery than in the core was correlated with a highly invasive feature on MRI and was associated with early tumor progression and worse survival, whereas lower expression of CD44 in the tumor periphery corresponded to low invasion and was associated with longer survival. The low invasion type on MRI tended to show high levels of VEGF expression in the tumor periphery, thus presenting the tumor with high proliferative activity. These results imply the significance of GSCs with high levels of CD44 expression in the tumor periphery compared to the core, not only in tumor invasion but also rapid tumor progression and short survival in patients with GBM.

1. Introduction

Glioblastoma multiforme (GBM) is the most malignant type of primary brain tumor with a median survival of 15 months, even after maximum resection of the tumor followed by the current standard chemoradiotherapy [1]. The poor prognosis of this tumor type is considered to be largely due to glioma stem-like cells (GSCs), which constitute a small subpopulation of tumor cells in GBM and are responsible for early tumor progression, resistance to chemoradiotherapy, and aggressive invasion [2, 3]. After the initial treatment, most GBM tumors recur locally, arising from the periphery of the tumor cavity after resection [4, 5]. Recently, Munthe et al. reported that glioma cells in the tumor periphery of glioma patients have a stem cell phenotype [6], but the number of GBM patients in the study is very few and the role and pathophysiological functions of GSCs in the invasion zone of the tumor periphery have not been intensively investigated in GBM.

GSCs are located in a specific microenvironment called the "niche" where the stemness of the GSCs is maintained. Tumor initiation, survival, and invasion are dynamically regulated by intricate interactions between GSCs and various components of the microenvironment including host stromal cells [7, 8]. In GBM, two distinct regions, the perivascular niche and the hypoxic/perinecrotic niche, are considered specific niches where GSCs are enriched and their maintenance and survival are supported [9, 10]. GSCs located in the perivascular niche generally reside close to the endothelial cells of capillaries of the tumor neovasculature and play a central role in angiogenesis of highly disorganized vasculature to respond to a rapidly growing tumor [11, 12]. The hypoxic/perinecrotic niche, which is the hypercellular region around the necrosis, termed pseudopalisades, plays a crucial role in maintaining GSCs and promoting self-renewal of CD133-positive GSCs, thus expanding the GSC population in the entire tumor [13]. Although GSCs in these niches are thought to be critical for tumor proliferation, they are unlikely to be the main cause of tumor recurrence, particularly when the tumor is completely resected including the area of these niches.

On the other hand, the tumor invasive area at the outer edge of the tumor presents a specific microenvironment that may constitute another niche for GSCs [14, 15]. Recent genetic and molecular studies on GSCs have been performed by utilizing samples from the tumor core. Thus, little is known about the molecular features of GSCs located in the invasion niche in the tumor periphery.

In the present study, we examined the expression of stem cell markers and related molecules in tumor tissues obtained from two different sites in GBM, the core and the periphery of the tumor. By analyzing expression patterns of stem cell markers and stem cell-related molecules in the periphery compared to the core, we identified a stem cell marker and a stem cell-related molecule that were characteristically expressed at high level in the tumor periphery compared with the core. To clarify a functional role of the GSCs expressing such a specific stem cell marker at the site of the tumor periphery in tumor progression of GBM, we investigated the pathological functions of the cultured GSCs that were established by the primary cell culture of the tumor tissues obtained from the tumor periphery. In addition, to demonstrate a significant role of the GSCs expressing the specific stem cell marker in clinical aspects, we analyzed the relationship between the degree of expression of the specific marker and stem cell-related molecule in the periphery and the pathological feature on magnetic resonance imaging (MRI) and survival of GBM patients.

2. Materials and Methods

2.1. Patients and Study Design. Among 36 newly diagnosed GBM patients who underwent surgery according to the same treatment protocol at Ehime University Hospital between January 2014 and December 2016, we identified 13 patients with separate tumor samples obtained from two different sites, the core and the periphery of the tumor, with navigation-guided microsurgical techniques as described below. For the purpose of exploring stem cell markers and other molecules that were highly expressed in the tumor periphery, we first carefully analyzed the expression patterns of eight stem cell markers for GSCs (Nestin, CD133, CD15, CD44, Bmi-1, Sox2, Oct3/4, and CXCR4) and four stem cell-related molecules (HIF-1α, HIF-2α, VEGF, and transforming growth factor beta (TGF-β)) in both the core and periphery of the tumor in a small number of GBM patients (patient numbers 1 to 4 in Table 1). Next, focusing on the specific stem cell marker and stem cell-related molecule that we identified in the initial study, we investigated the pathological function of GSCs expressing the specific stem cell marker by using cultured GSCs that were established from the tumor tissue in the tumor periphery and analyzed clinical significance of GSCs expressing the specific marker in the pathological features on MRI and prognosis of patients with GBM.

2.2. Treatment and Tissue Sampling. All patients underwent craniotomy for tumor resection, followed by radiotherapy (60 Gy) and chemotherapy with temozolomide in accordance with the Stupp protocol [16]. Tumor resection was performed by multimodal navigation-guided microsurgery using fence-post catheter techniques [17]. Using the surgical techniques, tumor samples were separately obtained from the core and periphery of the tumor.

As a target for obtaining samples at the tumor periphery, we decided the position of the tip of the fence-post catheters that were placed along the tumor border using echo-linked image-guided navigation just before starting the tumor resection (Figure 1). The tumor samples at the core were obtained from the resected tumor mass. When the tumor had a large area of central necrosis (CN), tumors located outside the necrotic area were collected (Figure 1 left). The tumor samples were frozen and preserved at −80°C until use.

2.3. RNA Isolation and Quantitative Real-Time RT-PCR (qRT-PCR). Total RNA was extracted from the tissue of each tumor sample using ISOGEN (Nippon Gene, Tokyo, Japan) according to the manufacturer's instructions. cDNA was synthesized from DNase I-treated RNA (1.5 μg) by reverse transcription using M-MLV Reverse Transcriptase (Invitrogen, Tokyo, Japan) and oligo (dT) 15 primer. cDNA was diluted 1 : 3, and triplicate volumes of 1 μl were used for qRT-PCR on a MJ Mini instrument (Bio-Rad, Hercules, CA) using FastStart Universal SYBR Green Master (Roche Diagnostic Japan, Tokyo, Japan). All gene-specific mRNA expression values were presented as relative expression levels normalized to the housekeeping (reference) gene glyceraldehyde 3-phosphate dehydrogenase (GAPDH). Quantification of gene expression was performed using ΔCt values, wherein ΔCt is defined as the difference between the target and reference gene Ct values. Validity of GAPDH as an internal control was certified by additional qRT-PCR

TABLE 1: Summary of clinical features on MRI, Ki-67 SI (in the periphery), CD44, and VEGF expression values and clinical prognosis including survival and outcome in 13 patients with GBM.

Patient		Features on MRI		Ki-67 SI (P)		CD44		VEGF		Survival and outcome		
Number	Group	Intensity of invasion	Central necrosis	%	Proliferative intensity	mRNA in periphery	P/C ratio	mRNA in periphery	P/C ratio	PFS (months)	OS (months)	Status
1	II	H	–	26.1	H	0.19	76	0.041	1.75	7	10	D
2	IIIa	L	+	33.3	H	0.69	1.25	0.33	1	46	46	A
3	IIIb	L	–	68.3	H	0.053	1.9	0.076	4	43	43	A
4	I	H	+	16.8	L	0.12	14.1	0.025	1	14	17	D
5	IIIa	L	+	42	H	0.007	0.02	0.012	0.4	12	24	D
6	II	H	+	44.9	H	0.32	18.4	0.007	0.14	7	16	D
7	I	H	–	7.1	L	0.58	9.8	0.01	0.2	9	33	D
8	IIIa	L	+	42.3	H	0.13	0.65	0.043	0.23	8	26	D
9	I	H	+	13.7	L	0.31	7.48	0.18	1.3	NA	NA	D
10	I	H	+	11.6	L	0.32	32.8	0.018	0.1	9	18	D
11	I	H	–	13.2	L	0.27	18	0.009	0.8	11	14	D
12	IIIa	L	+	50.8	H	0.12	0.85	0.086	1.3	11	11	A
13	II	H	–	28	H	0.61	15.5	0.02	1.7	4	6	D

Ki-67 SI (P): Ki-67 staining index (in the tumor periphery), VEGF: vascular endothelial growth factor, P/C ratio: periphery/core ratio, PFS: progression-free survival, OS: overall survival, H: high, L: low, NA: not assessed, status: D (dead), A (alive).

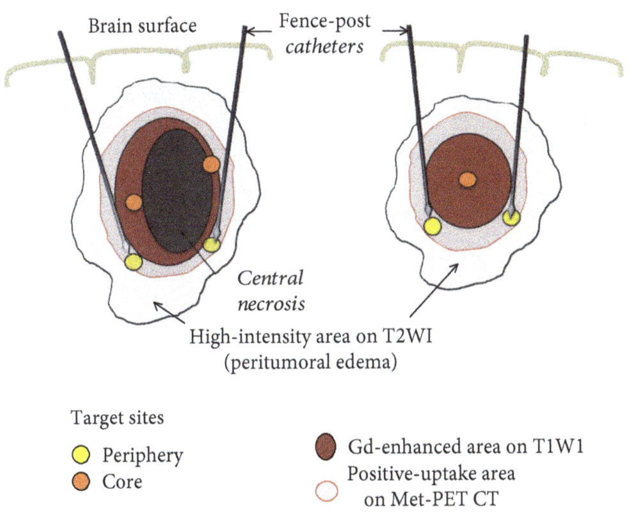

FIGURE 1: Navigation-guided surgical method for taking tumor samples from two sites, the periphery and core in GBM. The position of the tip of the fence-post catheters that are placed along the tumor border under echo-linked image-guided navigation is determined as a target for taking samples in the tumor periphery. The target area corresponds to just outside of the Gd-enhanced area and within the positive-uptake area on Met-PET. When the tumor showed a central necrosis, tumor tissues located outside the necrotic area were collected for the samples at the tumor core (left). Otherwise, the tumor samples at the core were obtained from the center of the resected tumor.

using other housekeeping genes, beta-actin (ACTB), hydroxymethylbilane synthase (HMBS), and TATA-box binding protein (TBP).

The primer sequences are listed in Suppl. Table S1.

2.4. Immunohistochemistry. Each tumor sample was fixed in formalin and embedded in paraffin. The blocks were sliced into 5 μm-thick sections, which were deparaffinized in Histo-Clear (Cosmo Bio), hydrated in a graded series of alcohol, and subjected to heat-activated antigen retrieval. After blocking endogenous peroxidase activity, the tissue was incubated with CD44 monoclonal antibody (1 : 250, Cell Signaling Technology, number 3570S) for 4 hours at room temperature. Subsequently, the sections were washed and incubated with biotinylated secondary antibody for 30 minutes at room temperature. The reaction complexes were stained with diaminobenzidine and counterstained with hematoxylin.

For double-labeling immunofluorescence, sections were incubated with a mixture of two primary antibodies to CD44 (1 : 250, Cell Signaling Technology, number 3570S) and Nestin (1 : 250, EMD Millipore, ABD69) diluted in Tris-buffered saline containing 0.02% Tween 20 (TBST) and 0.1% bovine serum albumin in a humidified chamber overnight at 4°C. After washing with TBST, sections were treated with Cy3-conjugated anti-rabbit and DyLight 488-labeled anti-mouse IgG secondary antibodies (1 : 1000; Jackson ImmunoResearch, West Grove, PA). Hoechst 33342 (Sigma-Aldrich) was used for nuclear staining. The immunostained specimens were observed with a conventional microscope (BX52; Olympus, Tokyo, Japan).

2.5. Primary Cell Culture of Tumor Tissues Obtained from the Tumor Periphery. Tumor tissues were surgically obtained from the site of the tumor periphery of four GBM patients and were mechanically minced, digested with 0.1% trypsin, and then triturated with a Pasteur pipette. Cells were passed through a 70 μm strainer (Falcon; Becton Dickinson Biosciences) and resuspended in high-glucose Dulbecco's modified Eagle's medium (DMEM) (Wako, Osaka, Japan) supplemented with 10% fetal bovine serum (FBS) and penicillin/streptomycin/amphotericin B mixture (Wako). Ability of the tumor cells in the primary cell culture to generate a sphere formation was examined by placing the cells in serum-free DMEM/Ham's F-12 (Wako) containing 10 μg/ml insulin (Wako), 10 nmol/l recombinant human basic fibroblast growth factor, 10 nmol/l recombinant human epidermal growth factor, 5 μmol/l heparin, N2 supplement (Wako), GlutaMAX supplement (GIBCO), and the penicillin/streptomycin/amphotericin B mixture (neural stem cell medium). Growth factors were purchased from PeproTech, London, UK. Primary tumor cells that were cultured in DMEM with 10% FBS, from which the sphere-forming cells (SFCs) were obtained by replacing the medium, were named as parent cells (PCs) for each SFCs.

2.6. Characterization of Sphere-Forming Cells (SFCs) as Tumor Stem Cells. To identify SFCs as cancer stem-like cells, mRNA expression of stem cell markers, Nestin, CD133, and CD44 on the SFCs was analyzed. Double-labeling immunofluorescence by using two antibodies to CD44 and Nestin was also performed as previously described. To investigate whether the SFCs had a potential for multilineage differentiation into neurons and astrocytes, the SFCs were cultured in the culture medium containing 10% FBS for 48 hours and then the immunohistochemistry using monoclonal antibodies TUJ1 (1 : 250, R&D Systems, MAB1195) and GFAP (1 : 250, Cosmo Bio, SML-ROI003) was performed. In addition, to evaluate in vivo tumorigenic activity of the SFCs, 1×10^4 of the SFCs were transplanted into the brains of NOD/SCID mice. Generation of tumors in the mice brains was confirmed by MRI and then their brains were removed, sliced into 5 μm-thick coronal sections, and the sections were stained with hematoxylin and eosin.

2.7. Cell Invasion and Migration Assays. Invasive activity of the cultured SFCs and PCs was assessed by the in vitro assay method using Falcon cell culture inserts (Becton Dickinson Biosciences, USA) and a reconstituted basement membrane, Matrigel (Becton Dickinson Biosciences), as previously described [18, 19]. Briefly, SFCs or PCs were suspended in DMEM containing 0.1% BSA and seeded onto the insert filters at a density of 5×10^4 cells/insert. The insert was placed in the lower well of the Falcon 24-well plates containing 500 μl of DMEM containing 1% FBS and incubated for 24 hours at 37°C under standard conditions.

Migration of the SFCs or PCs were assayed by the modified Boyden chamber method with 48-well microchemotaxis chambers (Nucleopore, Pleasanton, CA), as previously described [20, 21]. SFCs or PCs in DMEM containing 0.1% BSA (at a density of 1×10^4 cells/ml) were placed in the upper well and DMEM containing 1% FBS was placed in the lower well. The filter was a polyvinylpyrolidone-free polycarbonate membrane with 8 μm pores (EMD Millipore, Bedford, MA). The chamber was incubated for 6 hours at 37°C under standard conditions. In both assays, cells on the upper membrane surface were mechanically removed. Cells that had invaded or migrated to the lower side of the membrane were fixed, stained with 0.1% crystal violet, and put under a microscope (×400) to count the amount of cells in five random fields.

2.8. Treatment of Cultured SFCs with Small Interfering RNA (siRNA). To clarify the effect of CD44 on the invasion and migration of the SFCs, the silencing effects of the CD44 gene with CD44 siRNA or control siRNA on invasion and migration of the SFCs were examined. CD44 siRNA sequences are follows: sense 5′-CCUCUGCAAGGCUUUCAAUAGTT-3′ and antisense 5′-CUAUUGAAAGCCUUGCAGAGGTT-3′. As a control for CD44 siRNA, we used a corresponding random siRNA sequence (5′-GCGCGCUUUGUAGGAUUCG dTdT). SFCs were transfected with CD44 siRNA using Lipofectamine 3000 Reagent (Invitrogen, Grand Island, United States) according to the manufacturer's instructions. After 24 hours' incubation of SFCs transfected with CD44 siRNA, invasion and migration assays were performed.

2.9. Analysis of Pathological Features of the Tumor Periphery on MRI. We evaluated the degree of invasiveness of the tumor in the periphery based on the findings of MRI. To make certain the features on MRI, we referred to the findings of 11C-methionine (Met) positron emission tomography (PET) studies and/or intraoperative 5-aminolevulinic acid-(5-ALA-) derived protoporphyrin IX (PpIX) fluorescence analysis for detecting the infiltrated tumor.

"High invasion" on MRI was defined as a tumor image that presented the findings of more than two features of the following three features. These included tumors with (1) an irregular or unclear margin, (2) extensive or diffusely surrounded peritumoral edema, and (3) extension to the contralateral side through the commissural fibers. Tumors presenting only one feature were evaluated for invasiveness through the Met-PET study, demonstrating that the tumor showing a much larger Met-uptake area than the Gd-enhanced area was highly invasive [22, 23] or had a higher fluorescence intensity of PpIX of the brain in the resection cavity. Tumors with a demarcated margin and with focal or scant edema were defined as "low invasion" on MRI. The degree of invasion was presented as high or low (Table 1).

This study was approved by the institutional review board of the Ethics Committee for Clinical Research of Ehime University Hospital, and written informed consent was obtained from each patient and/or a family member before initiating the study.

The mouse experiments were performed according to protocols approved by the Animal Care and Use Committees of Ehime University. The study protocol was approved by the Animal Care and Use Committees of Ehime University (permit number: 1708013).

2.10. Statistical Analysis. Parametric data were expressed as means ± standard deviations and compared using the Student's t-test. Nonparametric data were expressed as median values (interquartile range) and compared using the Mann–Whitney U test. Receiver operating characteristic curve analysis was used to determine a cutoff value for predicting the highly invasive type on MRI based on the periphery/core (P/C) ratio of CD44 expression. Kaplan-Meier plots, in which survival was expressed as a function of the time after surgery, were generated to estimate progression-free survival (PFS) and overall survival (OS) for each group, and the log-rank test was performed to determine statistically significant differences between groups.

3. Results

3.1. Clinical Features. The median age of the 13 patients identified in the present study was 66 years (range 44–79 years), and they presented with a median Karnofsky performance status (KPS) score of 70 (range 60–90). All patients underwent image-guided microsurgical resection followed by chemotherapy and radiation therapy. All tumors had a histopathologically confirmed diagnosis of GBM according to the World Health Organization classification system, and all tumors had no mutation in *IDH1*. Expression of O(6)-methylguanine-DNA methyltransferase (MGMT) and the Ki-67 SI in the core of the tumors in the 13 patients are summarized in Suppl. Table S2. The extent of resection (EOR) was evaluated by volumetric analysis on MRI before and after surgery as previously described [24]. Gross total resection (GTR: 100% resection of the tumor volume), subtotal resection (95 to 100% resection), and partial resection (<95% resection) were achieved in 10 (76.9%), 2 (15.4%), and 1 patient (7.7%), respectively. After the initial standard therapy was completed, nine patients developed progression of the tumor, of whom seven patients showed local recurrence and two developed cerebrospinal fluid dissemination. One patient died of a sudden onset of pulmonary embolism 7 days after surgery. Three patients are alive and in good health without tumor recurrence. The surviving time of these patients is presented as overall survival (OS) in Table 1.

3.2. Expression of Stem Cell Markers and Stem Cell-Related Molecules in Two Different Sites, the Periphery and Core of the Tumor, in Four Patients. We analyzed the mRNA expression of eight stem cell markers (CD133, CD15, CD44, Nestin, Bmi-1, Sox2, Oct-3/4, and CXCR4) and four stem cell-related molecules (HIF-1α, HIF-2α, VEGF, and TGF-β) in two different sites of tumors in four patients. Most stem cell markers were expressed at only a low level in the both core and periphery of the tumor, except for Sox2 and CD44, which showed high expression in both sites, and CXCR4, which showed slightly higher expression in the periphery (Figure 2(a)). Regarding the stem cell-related molecules, VEGF and TGF-β were expressed at a relatively high level, with slightly higher expression of VEGF in both the core and periphery than TGF-β (Figure 2(a)). To identify specific stem cell markers that may play an important role in the tumor periphery, we analyzed expression patterns of the stem cell markers by evaluating the intensity and patterns of the ratio of expression of these markers in the periphery to expression in the core (P/C ratio). Among eight stem cell markers, CD44 showed the highest P/C ratio in two patients, in marked contrast to two other patients who had a low P/C ratio (Figure 2(b)). Although CD133 also showed a high P/C ratio in the same patients as those with a high CD44 P/C ratio, the expression of CD133 mRNA was too low in all patients. Thus, we focused on CD44 as a stem cell marker for further analysis.

The P/C ratios for stem cell-related molecules other than VEGF showed various values among patients (Figure 2(c)). TGF-β showed high P/C ratios in two patients (numbers 1 and 3), but immunohistochemical analysis showed that the expression was partly derived from tumor-associated macrophages (data not shown). Unlike stem cell markers expressed on glioma stem cells, it is considered that these molecules closely participate in not only regulating the biological function of the stem cells but also modifying the condition of the microenvironment. So, we put much focus on the molecule that was expressed in the highest quantity. As a result, we selected VEGF for further investigation in the present study.

3.3. Immunohistochemical Study. To confirm the expression of CD44 at the cellular level, immunohistochemical expression of CD44 in the core and the periphery of the tumors was examined. CD44 showed positive immunostaining that was much stronger in the tumor cells in the periphery than in the core in patients with much higher CD44 mRNA expression in the periphery than in the core (patients with a high P/C ratio). However, the difference in the degree of positive staining for CD44 between the periphery and the core was not remarkable in the patients with slightly higher CD44 mRNA expression in the periphery compared to the core (patients with a low P/C ratio) (Figure 3(a)). Double-labeling immunofluorescence disclosed that about a half of the CD44-positive cells in the periphery in patients with a high P/C ratio also expressed Nestin, but coexpression of CD44 and Nestin was not observed in most tumor cells in the periphery in the patients with a low P/C ratio (Figure 3(b)).

3.4. Identification of SFCs as Glioma Stem-Like Cells. In the primary cell culture of the tumor tissues obtained from the tumor periphery of four GBM patients, we obtained two SFCs (SFC-1 and SFC-2), both of which expressed much higher amounts of mRNA of neural stem cell markers CD133, Nestin, and CD44 than each PCs (Figure 4(a)). The expression level of CD44 in SFC-1 was higher than that in SFC-2. Double-labeling immunofluorescence demonstrated colocalization of CD44 and Nestin in both SFCs (Figure 4(b)). When these SFCs were cultured in the serum-containing medium, they were positively stained for TUJI and GFAP antibodies (Figure 4(c)). In addition, transplanted SFCs in the brains of NOD/SCID mice generated a highly invasive tumor whose invasion front was positively stained for CD44 (Figure 4(d)).

3.5. Invasive and Migratory Activities of Cultured SFCs and Inhibitory Effects of CD44 Knockdown on These Activities. In vitro invasion and migration studies disclosed that both SFC-1 and SFC-2 had much higher invasive and migratory activities than their PCs (PC-1 and PC-2) (Figures 5(a) and 5(b)). SFC-1 showed much stronger activity than SFC-2 in both invasion and migration. These high activities

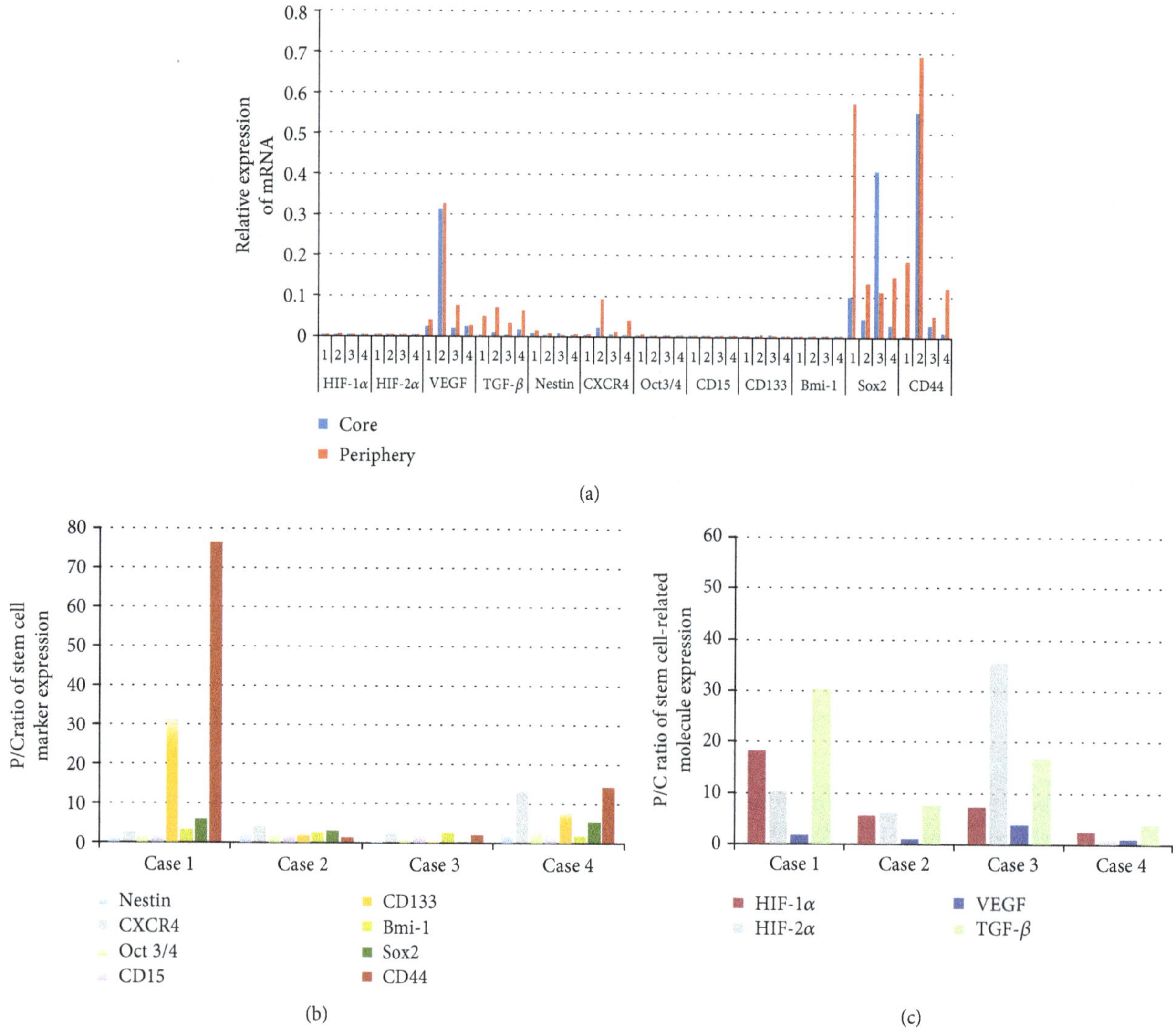

Figure 2: Expression of stem cell markers and stem cell-related molecules in the core and the periphery of the tumor in four glioblastoma (GBM) patients. (a) mRNA expression of eight stem cell markers (Nestin, CXCR4, Oct3/4, CD15, CD133, Bmi-1, Sox2, and CD44) and four stem cell-related molecules (HIF-1α, HIF-2α, VEGF, and TGF-β) in the core and the periphery was determined with qRT-PCR. The values are relative expression of mRNA of stem cell markers and molecules normalized to the GAPDH. (b) Expression of eight stem cell markers shown as the P/C expression ratio for each marker in each patient. The P/C ratios for the marker were calculated by dividing the amount of mRNA expression of the marker in the tumor periphery by that in the core for each patient. (c) Expression of four stem cell-related molecules shown as the P/C expression ratio for each molecule in each patient. The P/C ratios for the molecule were calculated as described for the stem cell markers. The numbers on the x-axis are the patient numbers.

of invasion and migration of both SFC-1 and SFC-2 were significantly inhibited by CD44 knockdown with the siRNA (Figures 5(a) and 5(b)).

3.6. Expression of CD44 and VEGF in the Core and the Periphery of the Tumor in 13 GBM Patients. We extensively investigated the expression of CD44 and VEGF in both the core and periphery of the tumor in 13 patients. Ten of 13 patients showed higher expression of CD44 in the periphery than in the core (Figure 6(a)). Among them, eight patients had very high P/C ratio values (>7.48; Figure 6(b)). On the other hand, three patients presented with higher expression of CD44 in the core than in the periphery.

Six patients showed higher expression of VEGF in the periphery than in the core (Figure 6(c)). However, because the difference in the amount of VEGF expression between the periphery and the core was low, no significant difference in the P/C ratio among the patients was found (Figure 6(d)).

3.7. Evaluation of Invasive Feature on MRI in the Periphery of GBM. We evaluated the degree of invasiveness of the tumor in the periphery by analyzing characteristic features on MRI in 13 patients. Five patients who showed almost the same findings on MRI of an irregular tumor margin with necrosis and diffuse peritumoral edema (Group I) were judged as the high invasion (Hi-I) type. All Hi-I type tumors

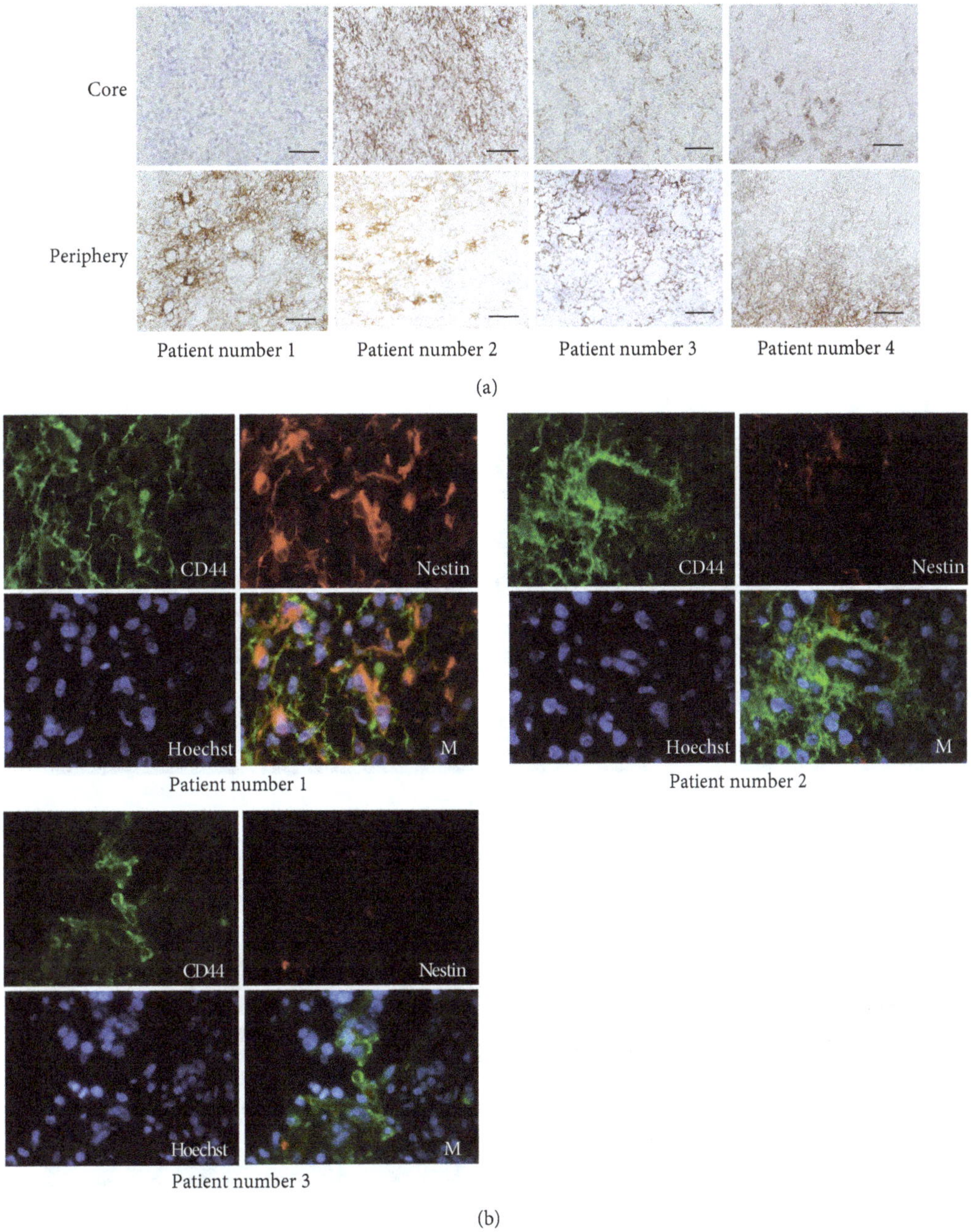

FIGURE 3: Immunohistochemical expression of the stem cell markers CD44 and Nestin. (a) Immunostaining for CD44 in the core and the periphery of the tumor in four GBM patients. The number of tumor cells showing positive staining for CD44 in the periphery was much higher than that in the core in tumors with a high P/C ratio for CD44 expression (patient numbers 1 and 4) (scale bar: 100 μm) (×400). (b) Double-labeling immunofluorescence. CD44 (green) and Nestin (red) were colocalized (M: merge) at the cell membrane in some GBM cells in the tumor periphery. Nuclei were labeled with Hoechst (blue).

showed low Ki-67 SI (12.5 ± 3.6%) in the tumor periphery. Three patients with extensive, diffuse edema and various configurations of a Gd-enhanced tumor (Group II) were considered the Hi-I type with high proliferative activity (Ki-67 SI (33 ± 10.4%)) in the tumor periphery. Four patients whose tumor showed large central necrosis (CN) with a ring-like enhanced wall with a relatively smooth margin and was accompanied by only focal edema on MRI (Group IIIa) were considered the low invasion (Lo-I) type, and they all presented with high proliferative activity (Ki-67 SI (42.1 ± 7.2%)) in the tumor periphery. One patient with a solid tumor mass and a clear margin without CN and with slight, focal edema (Group IIIb) was also considered the Lo-I type but with much higher proliferation (Ki-67 SI (68%)). Representative MR and PET scan images of each group are shown in Figure 7. Table 1 shows the intensity of tumor invasion as seen on MRI, the proliferative activity shown by Ki-67 SI in the tumor periphery, CD44 and VEGF expression values presented as both mRNA in the periphery and the P/C ratio, and the clinical outcome including PFS and OS in 13 patients.

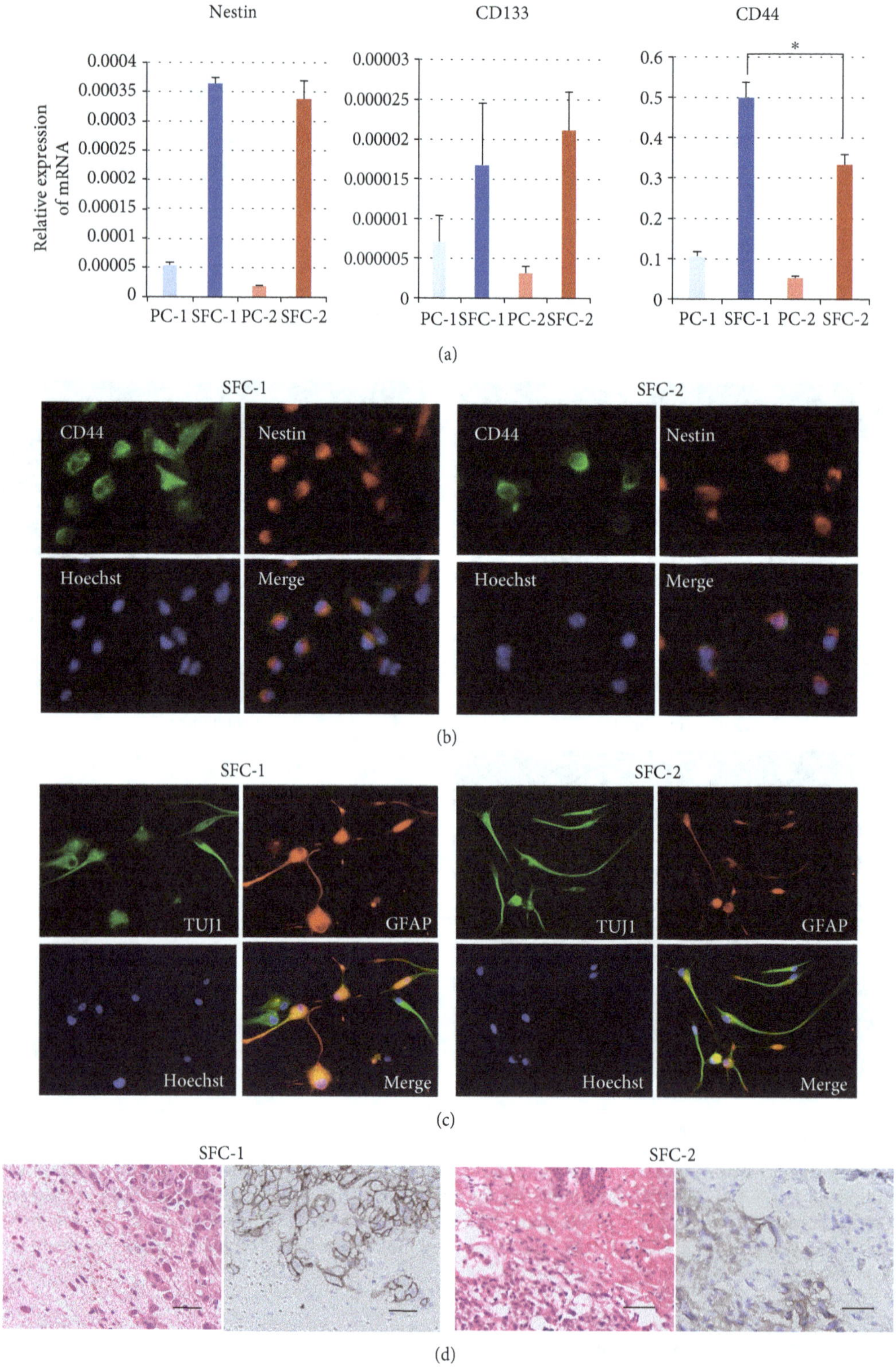

Figure 4: Characterization of sphere-forming cells (SFCs) as glioma stem-like cells. (a) Both SFC-1 and SFC-2 expressed much more CD133 and Nestin mRNA than those parent cells (PC-1 and PC-2). SFC-1 expressed CD44 at a significantly higher level than SFC-2. $^{*}p < 0.01$. (b) CD44 (green) and Nestin (red) were colocalized at the cell membrane in both SFC-1 and SFC-2. (c) Both SFC-1 and SFC-2 showed the capacity for multilineage differentiation into neurons (TUJ1; green) and astrocytes (GFAP; red). The nuclei are labeled with Hoechst (blue). (d) Both SFCs transplanted in the mouse brain generated invasive tumors (HE × 400), in which tumor cells in the periphery were positively stained for CD44 (bar 100 μm) (×400).

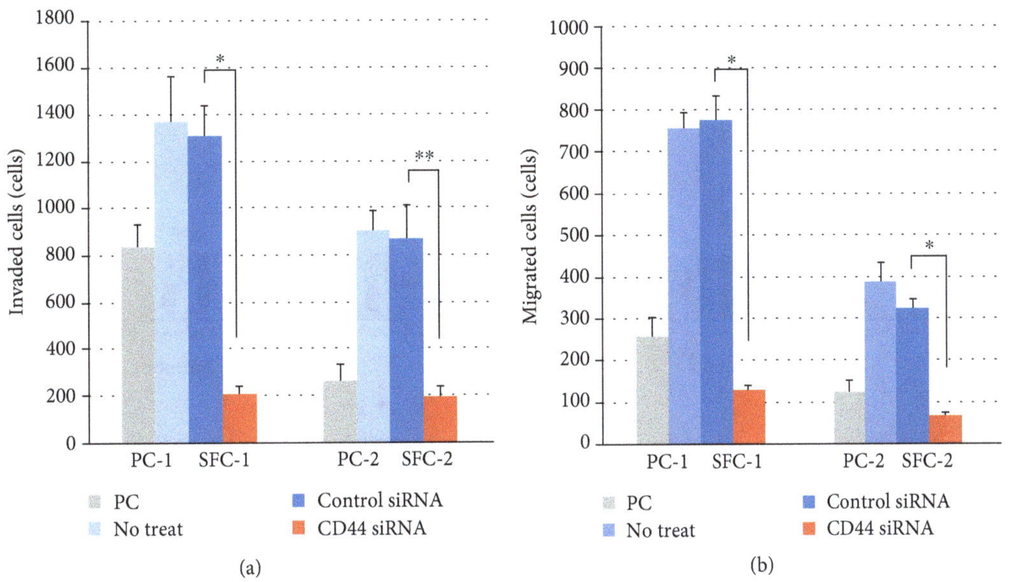

Figure 5: Invasive and migratory activities of cultured SFCs and PCs and inhibitory effect of CD44 knockdown with CD44 siRNA on their activities. In both invasion (a) and migration (b), cultured SFCs (SFC-1 and SFC-2) showed much higher activity than each PCs (PC-1 and PC-2). These high activities of invasion and migration of SFCs were significantly inhibited by knockdown of CD44 with the siRNA. $^{*}p < 0.001$ and $^{**}p < 0.005$.

3.8. Relationship between CD44 and VEGF Expression in the Tumor Periphery and Pathological Features on MRI and the Clinical Outcome. We next analyzed the relationship between the degree of CD44 and VEGF expression in the tumor periphery and pathological features on MRI and clinical outcomes.

As presented in Table 1, all eight patients with a high P/C ratio for CD44 expression showed the Hi-I type on MRI (Groups I and II), whereas all five patients with a low P/C ratio for CD44 showed the Lo-I type (Groups IIIa and IIIb). The difference in the P/C ratio for CD44 expression between Hi-I and Lo-I types on MRI was statistically significant (Hi-I (24.0 ± 22.31) versus Lo-I (0.93 ± 0.7), $p = 0.0441$) (Figure 8(a)). On the other hand, we found no significant difference in the level of CD44 mRNA expression in the tumor periphery between the two types (Hi-I (33.93 ± 17.22) versus Lo-I (20.03 ± 27.84), $p = 0.285$) (Figure 8(b)). The Lo-I type on MRI tended to show higher amounts of VEGF expression in the periphery (Lo-I (10.84 ± 12.5) versus Hi-I (3.92 ± 5.85), $p = 0.201$) (Figure 8(c)).

To evaluate the relationship between the degree of CD44 expression in the tumor periphery and prognostic outcome, Kaplan-Meier survival plots were generated for two groups of patients: those with a high P/C ratio for CD44 and those with a low P/C ratio for CD44. PFS and OS in each group were statistically analyzed (Figures 8(d) and 8(e)). Patients with a high P/C ratio for CD44 had significantly earlier tumor progression and a worse outcome than those with a low P/C ratio for CD44 (PFS: 9 ± 4.24 months (high P/C ratio) versus not available (NA) (low P/C ratio), $p = 0.0359$; OS: 16 ± 3.78 months (high P/C ratio) versus 26 ± 5.22 months (low P/C ratio), $p = 0.0215$). No significant differences were found in age, KPS score, immunostaining for MGMT, or Ki-67 SI (C) between the two groups with high and low P/C ratios for CD44 expression. Patients with high VEGF expression in the tumor periphery tended to have longer survival without tumor progression than those with low VEGF in the tumor periphery.

4. Discussion

In the present study, we demonstrated that GSCs with high expression of the stem cell marker, CD44, were present in the periphery of GBM. The periphery is a border area between the outer edge of the tumor and the normal brain, constituting the tumor-border (invasion) niche. Several stem cell markers, including eight markers examined in this study, have been identified as GSC markers, and the expression of these markers in tumor tissue and primary culture of GBM has been investigated. Bien-Möller et al. [25] analyzed the expression of seven stem cell markers as well as differentiation and microglia markers and demonstrated that CD44, ELF4, Nanog, and Nestin were elevated at both mRNA and protein levels in GBM, but only CD133 and Nestin were associated with survival rates. However, no marker has been established as a universal GSC marker [26], even CD133 still remains controversial [27, 28]. In addition, most of these studies were based on tumor samples obtained from the core of the GBM tumor.

Consequently, to explore the possible importance of stem cell markers with characteristically high expression in the tumor periphery, we analyzed the expression pattern of eight stem cell markers in both the core and periphery of the tumor in GBM patients. Expression of the eight stem cell markers was represented as the P/C ratio to illustrate expression in the tumor periphery compared to the core.

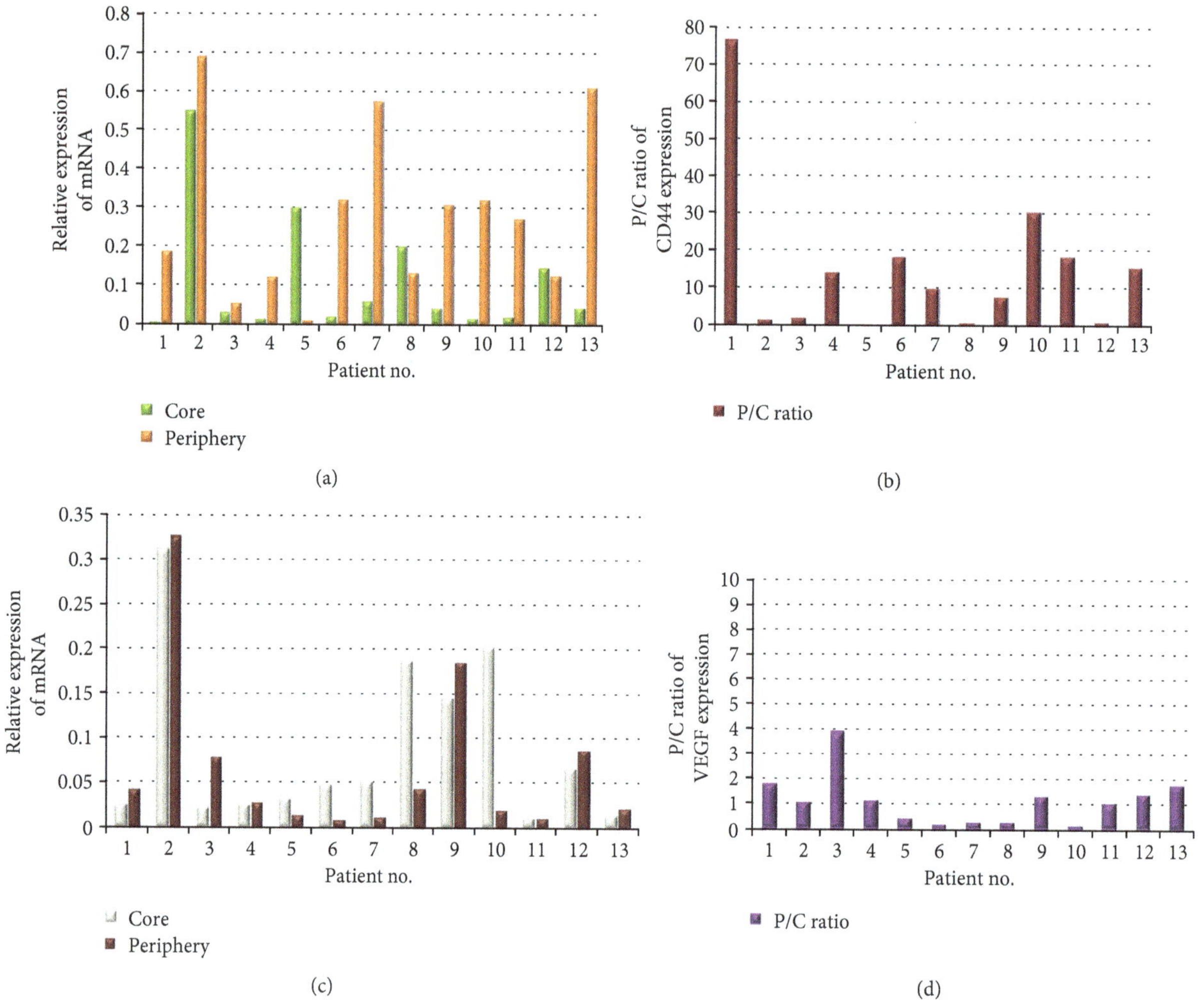

FIGURE 6: Expression of the stem cell marker, CD44, and the stem cell-related molecule, VEGF, in 13 GBM patients. (a) mRNA expression of CD44 in the tumor core and periphery was determined with qRT-PCR. The values are relative expression of mRNA normalized to the GAPDH. (b) Expression of CD44 represented by the P/C ratio. The P/C ratios for CD44 were calculated by dividing the amount of mRNA expression of CD44 in the tumor periphery by that in the core for each patient. (c) mRNA expression of VEGF in the tumor core and periphery. The expression and the level were determined as described for CD44. (d) Expression of VEGF represented by the P/C ratio. The P/C ratios for VEGF were determined as described for CD44.

Most markers except CD44 and CD133 showed almost the same values, with a P/C ratio of about 2.0 in all patients. This result suggests that stem-like cells with the same function as GSCs in the tumor core also exist in the periphery. The present double immunostaining study showed that CD44 and Nestin were colocalized at the cell membrane of the tumor cells in the tumor periphery, demonstrating existence of stem cells expressing CD44 in the invasion area. Guadagno et al. [29] reported that coexpression of CD44 and Nestin in GBM is specifically observed at the cell membrane in undifferentiated stem-like cells. Our immunohistochemical study, showing that the tumors with a high P/C ratio for CD44 contained much more GSCs expressing CD44 in the tumor periphery compared with those with a low P/C ratio for CD44, may suggest that there are many more GSCs in the microenvironment with upregulating CD44 expression on GSCs than those in the microenvironment without stimulation for CD44 expression. This may be a reason we could not obtain sphere-forming cells by the primary cell culture of the tumor tissues expressing a low P/C ratio for CD44. To investigate the existence and biological functions of GSCs expressing CD44 in the tumor periphery of GBM, we tried to establish stem-like cells by placing the cells in primary culture from the tumor tissues in the tumor periphery in neural stem cell culture medium. Among the cell cultures from four tumor tissues, we obtained two SFCs (SFC-1 and SFC-2), both expressing stem cell markers CD133 and Nestin at almost the same levels. On the other hand, SFC-1 expressed much more highly CD44 than SFC-2. These SFCs had abilities to show multilineage differentiation to neurons and astrocytes and make a rapid tumorigenesis by the mouse xenograft model, thus demonstrating that these SFCs were identified as GSCs. In vitro invasion and migration studies disclosed that these cultured GSCs had high invasive and migratory activity, and GSC-1 expressing more CD44 had much stronger activities in both invasion

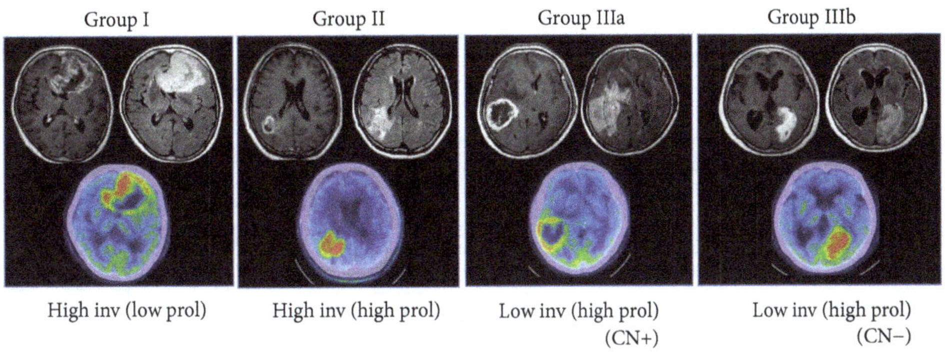

Group	I ($n = 5$)	III ($n = 3$)	IIIb ($n = 4$)	IIIb ($n = 1$)
P/C ratio of CD44	16.4 ± 10.0	33.6 ± 34.1	0.69 ± 0.51	1.9
Ki-67 SI (P) (%)	12.5 ± 3.6	33.0 ± 10.4	42.8 ± 7.2	68.0

FIGURE 7: Representative combined images of MRI and PET-computed tomography for four groups of features with different intensities representing invasion and proliferation in the tumor periphery. Inv: invasion, prol: proliferation, CN: central necrosis. In all images, the upper left is T1-Gd, the upper right is a fluid-attenuated inversion recovery image, and the lower image is Met-PET. Values at the bottom are the mean ± SD of the P/C ratio for CD44 expression (upper row) and the Ki-67 SI in the tumor periphery (lower row). n: number of patients.

and migration than GSC-2 expressing less CD44. In addition, the fact that their activities were significantly decreased by knockdown of the CD44 gene strongly indicates that CD44 has an essential activity of enhancing invasion and migration of the GSCs. These results indicate that GSCs with a higher expression of CD44 in the tumor periphery than the core are actually present in the tumor-border niche in GBM and they have high invasive and migratory activities that are promoted by CD44.

CD44 is a cell membrane glycoprotein that is involved in various cellular processes including cell motility, proliferation, apoptosis, and angiogenesis [30, 31]. CD44 is expressed in many cancers, including lung, breast, colon, prostate, and brain cancer [32–34]. In particular, CD44 expression in GBM enhances the invasion of GBM by promoting tumor cell migration through cell-extracellular matrix interactions [35]. Ariza et al. [36] described that GBM expressing CD44 showed high invasiveness, but meningioma lacking the CD44 expression could not infiltrate the brain extracellular matrix. Recent studies have described CD44 as a marker of GBM cancer stem cells, also known as glioma-initiating cells or GSCs, and CD44 expression is enriched in GSCs [37]. In addition to the invasive activity that is based on the interaction of the extracellular domain of CD44 with the extracellular matrix, CD44 can act as an intracellular signaling molecule by enhancing the expression of the CD44 intracellular domain to maintain and increase the stemness of these stem-like cells [38].

Little is known about the clinical significance of the GSCs highly expressing CD44 with such multifunctional activities, particularly, in the tumor progression of GBM. To clarify the role of the GSCs that highly expressed CD44 in the tumor progression, we investigated the possible association between the degree of expression of CD44 in the tumor periphery and imaging features on MRI and survival in GBM patients.

From our analysis of CD44 expression in 13 patients, we found that patients with a high P/C ratio for CD44 expression showed the Hi-I phenotype as seen on MRI and vice versa. These results indicate that the presence of GSCs that express higher levels of CD44 in the tumor-border zone than in the core may contribute to the invasive nature of the tumor as the GSCs highly expressing CD44 showed high invasive activity in in vitro studies. In particular, among Hi-I tumors, those of the high proliferation type in the periphery (Group II) showed much earlier progression. This group showed very high values in not only the P/C ratios for CD44 but also the relative amounts of CD44 mRNA; they also showed relatively low amounts of VEGF expression in the tumor periphery. The reason why some Hi-I type of GSCs expressing high levels of CD44 also show strong tumor proliferation is not clear. In our first study, the tumor with high invasion and high Ki-67 SI expressed CD133 at a distinctly high level (Figure 2(b)). As Brown et al. [39] reported, the worst type of GBM may result from alteration of the intratumor equilibrium of CD44+ and CD133+ subpopulations of GSCs, which may be influenced by environmental factors, resulting in a shift in the balance from CD44+ to CD133+ and hence, high proliferative activity.

A high P/C ratio for CD44 expression in GSCs was also strongly associated with not only early tumor progression but also worse survival. We found no significant difference in age, KPS score, MGMT immunostaining, or Ki-67 SI in the tumor core between the two groups with a high or low P/C ratio for CD44 expression. We also found no significant difference in OS between patients younger than 65 years and those who were older, patients with a KPS less than or equal to 70 and those with a KPS greater than or equal to 80,

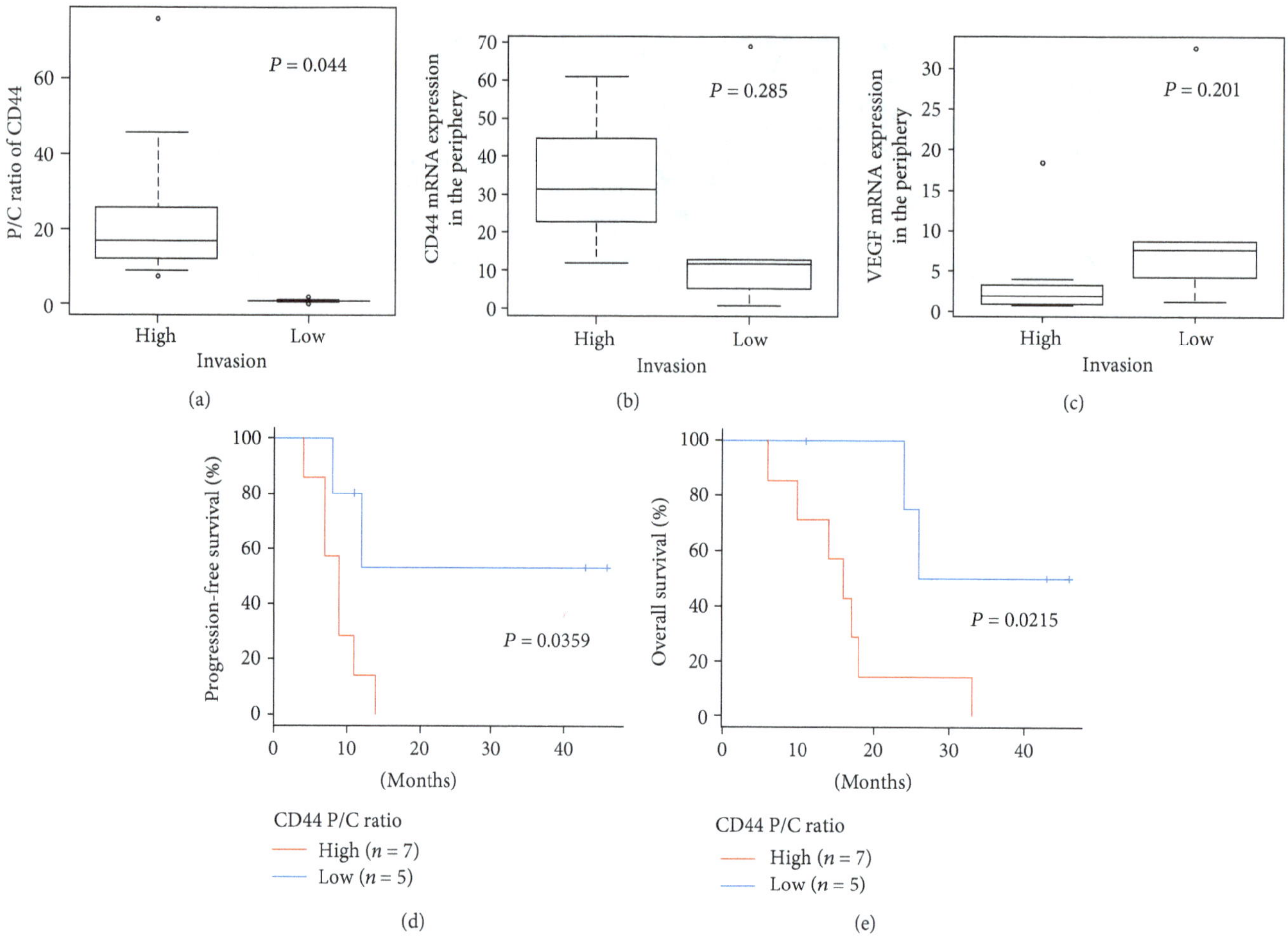

Figure 8: (a) Relationship between the P/C ratio for CD44 expression and tumor invasiveness as seen on MRI. Patients with a high P/C ratio showed a significant, more highly invasive type on MRI than those with a low P/C ratio ($p = 0.0441$, t-test). (b) Relationship between the level of CD44 mRNA expression in the tumor periphery and tumor invasiveness as seen on MRI. The level of CD44 mRNA expression in the tumor periphery did not correlate with invasiveness on MRI ($p = 0.285$, t-test). (c) Relationship between the level of VEGF mRNA expression in the tumor periphery and tumor invasiveness as seen on MRI. The low invasive type on MRI tended to have higher amounts of VEGF expression in the tumor periphery ($p = 0.201$, t-test). (d, e) Kaplan-Meier survival curves for the P/C ratio for CD44 expression predicting PFS (d) and OS (e). Patients with a high P/C ratio for CD44 expression showed significantly earlier tumor progression and worse survival than those with a low P/C ratio ($p = 0.0359$ and 0.0215, respectively, log-rank test).

patients with an EOR of GTR and those with non-GTR (subtotal resection and partial resection), or patients with positive and those with negative MGMT staining. Consequently, a high P/C ratio for CD44 with a cutoff value of 7.48 for high invasiveness on imaging may also be a novel marker for poor prognosis.

CD44 is highly expressed in the mesenchymal subtype of GBM [40], and expression of CD44 has been indicated to be correlated with poor survival [41]. However, Pietras et al. reported that CD44 expression only in the perivascular niche of the proneural subtype of GBM is correlated with aggressive growth and poor prognosis [38]. On the other hand, gene coexpression analysis demonstrated that tumors with a CD133 coexpression module signature (CD133-CMS) are enriched for the proneural GBM subtype, which shows enhanced proliferation, and those with the CD44 coexpression module signature (CD44-CMS) are enriched for the mesenchymal subtype and show enhanced invasion. However, the study showed no long-term survival difference between CD44-CMS and CD133-CMS patients [42]. This result may be due to evaluation of the expression of markers using tissue samples obtained from the core of the tumor. In this context, Bhat et al. [43] demonstrated that NF-κB-induced mesenchymal differentiation (transition) from the proneural subtype of GBM to the mesenchymal subtype was associated with increases of CD44 subpopulations and radio resistance, resulting in shorter survival in GBM patients. Taken together, it is strongly suggested that increased expression of CD44 may become a predictor for poor survival in GBM.

In addition to CD44, VEGF was the most highly expressed molecule, not only in the tumor periphery but also in the core. VEGF promotes angiogenesis, which is a key process of vascular formation by GSCs. In our study, although a high level of VEGF expression in the tumor periphery was not always associated with increased proliferative activity of the tumor in the periphery, we demonstrated that GBMs with the Lo-I phenotype as seen on MRI tended to show the high proliferative activity. These tumors also expressed high levels of VEGF in the periphery. The data in the present study also showed that Hi-I and high proliferative tumors expressed HIF-1α and CD133 most strongly, whereas Lo-I and high proliferative tumors expressed much more HIF-2α than HIF-1α (Figure 2(c)). These data suggest that the microenvironment around GSCs with the Hi-I type is much more hypoxic than the tumor with high proliferative activity. These phenomena may resemble the pathophysiology of the migration/proliferation dichotomy or the "Go or Grow" theory [44, 45].

The present study demonstrates the existence of GSCs in the tumor periphery of GBM, corresponding to the tumor-border (invasion) niche where the blood-brain barrier is not disrupted and thus, a much more hypoxic microenvironment is present compared with the peripheral contrast-enhancing layer of GBM [46]. In highly invasive GBM, GSCs located in such an invasion niche are thought to promote tumor invasion by increasing the expression of CD44, resulting in early tumor progression or dissemination. On the other hand, a high level of VEGF in the tumor periphery may suppress the invasive activity of CD44.

The relatively small number of patients, in whom the tumors are accurately taken from two different sites, is a critical limitation for particularly performing statistical analysis in the clinical study that should be mentioned. More extensive analysis with an increased number of patients would be required to obtain a definite conclusion and before application to clinical practice.

5. Conclusions

We demonstrated that GSCs highly expressing CD44 exist in the invasion niche at the tumor periphery of GBM. The cultured GSCs with a high expression of CD44 obtained from the tumor periphery had a high invasive activity that is enhanced by CD44. The higher expression of CD44 in the tumor periphery compared to the tumor core (high P/C ratio for CD44 expression) was correlated to early tumor progression and short survival of GBM patients. On the other hand, the stem cell-related molecule, VEGF, in the tumor periphery was highly expressed in the low invasive type of tumors, thus being considered to have a role in tumor proliferation in the tumor periphery. In the future, not only clarification of the predominant expression of CD44 in the tumor-border zone but also functional analysis of CD44 at the molecular level may enable researchers and clinicians to present the specific treatment strategy for each patient, more exactly predict the clinical prognosis, and develop a novel targeted therapy for GSCs with a high expression of CD44 to eradicate the tumor.

Acknowledgments

The authors would like to express their gratitude to Taichi Furumochi and Yasuhiro Shiraishi of the Department of Neurology, and Satsuki Myoga of the Department of Pathology, Ehime University Hospital, and Takeshi Kiyoi of the Advanced Research Support Center, Ehime University, Japan, for their help with radiological image and pathological acquisition.

References

[1] R. Stupp, M. E. Hegi, W. P. Mason et al., "Effects of radiotherapy with concomitant and adjuvant temozolomide versus radiotherapy alone on survival in glioblastoma in a randomised phase III study: 5-year analysis of the EORTC-NCIC trial," *The Lancet Oncology*, vol. 10, no. 5, pp. 459–466, 2009.

[2] S. K. Singh, C. Hawkins, I. D. Clarke et al., "Identification of human brain tumour initiating cells," *Nature*, vol. 432, no. 7015, pp. 396–401, 2004.

[3] R. Galli, E. Binda, U. Orfanelli et al., "Isolation and characterization of tumorigenic, stem-like neural precursors from human glioblastoma," *Cancer Research*, vol. 64, no. 19, pp. 7011–7021, 2004.

[4] A. Giese, T. Kucinski, U. Knopp et al., "Pattern of recurrence following local chemotherapy with biodegradable carmustine (BCNU) implants in patients with glioblastoma," *Journal of Neuro-Oncology*, vol. 66, no. 3, pp. 351–360, 2004.

[5] J. Oh, A. Sahgal, P. Sanghera et al., "Glioblastoma: patterns of recurrence and efficacy of salvage treatments," *The Canadian Journal of Neurological Sciences*, vol. 38, no. 4, pp. 621–625, 2011.

[6] S. Munthe, S. A. Petterson, R. H. Dahlrot, F. R. Poulsen, S. Hansen, and B. W. Kristensen, "Glioma cells in the tumor periphery have a stem cell phenotype," *PloS One*, vol. 11, no. 5, article e0155106, 2016.

[7] J. D. Lathia, J. Gallagher, J. T. Myers et al., "Direct in vivo evidence for tumor propagation by glioblastoma cancer stem cells," *PloS One*, vol. 6, no. 9, article e24807, 2011.

[8] L. Cheng, Z. Huang, W. Zhou et al., "Glioblastoma stem cells generate vascular pericytes to support vessel function and tumor growth," *Cell*, vol. 153, no. 1, pp. 139–152, 2013.

[9] C. Calabrese, H. Poppleton, M. Kocak et al., "A perivascular niche for brain tumor stem cells," *Cancer Cell*, vol. 11, no. 1, pp. 69–82, 2007.

[10] Z. Li, S. Bao, Q. Wu et al., "Hypoxia-inducible factors regulate tumorigenic capacity of glioma stem cells," *Cancer Cell*, vol. 15, no. 6, pp. 501–513, 2009.

[11] R. Wang, K. Chadalavada, J. Wilshire et al., "Glioblastoma stem-like cells give rise to tumour endothelium," *Nature*, vol. 468, no. 7325, pp. 829–833, 2010.

[12] B. Campos, L. Zeng, P. H. DaoTrong et al., "Expression and regulation of AC133 and CD133 in glioblastoma," *Glia*, vol. 59, no. 12, pp. 1974–1986, 2011.

[13] A. M. McCord, M. Jamal, U. T. Shankavarum, F. F. Lang, K. Camphausen, and P. J. Tofilon, "Physiologic oxygen concentration enhances the stem-like properties of $CD133^+$ human glioblastoma cells in vitro," *Molecular Cancer Research*, vol. 7, no. 4, pp. 489–497, 2009.

[14] D. Hambardzumyan and G. Bergers, "Glioblastoma: defining tumor niches," *Trends in Cancer*, vol. 1, no. 4, pp. 252–265, 2015.

[15] S. J. Sundar, J. K. Hsieh, S. Manjila, J. D. Lathia, and A. Sloan,

"The role of cancer stem cells in glioblastoma," *Neurosurgical Focus*, vol. 37, no. 6, article E6, 2014.

[16] R. Stupp, W. P. Mason, M. J. van den Bent et al., "Radiotherapy plus concomitant and adjuvant temozolomide for glioblastoma," *The New England Journal of Medicine*, vol. 352, no. 10, pp. 987–996, 2005.

[17] S. Ohue, S. Kohno, A. Inoue et al., "Accuracy of diffusion tensor magnetic resonance imaging-based tractography for surgery of gliomas near the pyramidal tract: a significant correlation between subcortical electrical stimulation and postoperative tractography," *Neurosurgery*, vol. 70, no. 2, pp. 283–294, 2012.

[18] A. Albini, Y. Iwamoto, H. K. Kleinman et al., "A rapid in vitro assay for quantitating the invasive potential of tumor cells," *Cancer Research*, vol. 47, no. 12, pp. 3239–3245, 1987.

[19] T. Ohnishi, N. Arita, T. Hayakawa, K. Kawahara, K. Kato, and A. Kakinuma, "Purification of motility factor (GMF) from human malignant glioma cells and its biological significance in tumor invasion," *Biochemical and Biophysical Research Communications*, vol. 193, no. 2, pp. 518–525, 1993.

[20] T. Ohnishi, N. Arita, T. Hayakawa, S. Izumoto, T. Taki, and H. Yamamoto, "Motility factor produced by malignant glioma cells: role in tumor invasion," *Journal of Neurosurgery*, vol. 73, no. 6, pp. 881–888, 1990.

[21] T. Ohnishi, N. Arita, S. Hiraga et al., "Fibronectin-mediated cell migration promotes glioma cell invasion through chemokinetic activity," *Clinical & Experimental Metastasis*, vol. 15, no. 5, pp. 538–546, 1997.

[22] K. Miwa, J. Shinoda, H. Yano et al., "Discrepancy between lesion distributions on methionine PET and MR images in patients with glioblastoma multiforme: insight from a PET and MR fusion image study," *Journal of Neurology, Neurosurgery, and Psychiatry*, vol. 75, no. 10, pp. 1457–1462, 2004.

[23] N. Galldiks, R. Ullrich, M. Schroeter, G. R. Fink, A. H. Jacobs, and L. W. Kracht, "Volumetry of [^{11}C]-methionine PET uptake and MRI contrast enhancement in patients with recurrent glioblastoma multiforme," *European Journal of Nuclear Medicine and Molecular Imaging*, vol. 37, no. 1, pp. 84–92, 2010.

[24] S. Ohue, S. Kohno, A. Inoue et al., "Surgical results of tumor resection using tractography-integrated navigation-guided fence-post catheter techniques and motor-evoked potentials for preservation of motor function in patients with glioblastomas near the pyramidal tracts," *Neurosurgical Review*, vol. 38, no. 2, pp. 293–307, 2015.

[25] S. Bien-Möller, E. Balz, S. Herzog et al., "Association of glioblastoma multiforme stem cell characteristics, differentiation, and microglia marker genes with patient survival," *Stem Cells International*, vol. 2018, Article ID 9628289, 19 pages, 2018.

[26] D. L. Schonberg, D. Lubelski, T. E. Miller, and J. N. Rich, "Brain tumor stem cells: molecular characteristics and their impact on therapy," *Molecular Aspects of Medicine*, vol. 39, pp. 82–101, 2014.

[27] D. Beier, P. Hau, M. Proescholdt et al., "CD133^{+} and CD133^{-}glioblastoma-derived cancer stem cells show differential growth characteristics and molecular profiles," *Cancer Research*, vol. 67, no. 9, pp. 4010–4015, 2007.

[28] F. Gambelli, F. Sasdelli, I. Manini et al., "Identification of cancer stem cells from human glioblastomas: growth and differentiation capabilities and CD133/prominin-1 expression," *Cell Biology International*, vol. 36, no. 1, pp. 29–38, 2012.

[29] E. Guadagno, G. Borrelli, M. Califano, G. Calì, D. Solari, and M. del Basso de Caro, "Immunohistochemical expression of stem cell markers CD44 and nestin in glioblastomas: evaluation of their prognostic significance," *Pathology-Research and Practice*, vol. 212, no. 9, pp. 825–832, 2016.

[30] D. Naor, S. Nedvetzki, I. Golan, L. Melnik, and Y. Faitelson, "CD44 in cancer," *Critical Reviews in Clinical Laboratory Sciences*, vol. 39, no. 6, pp. 527–579, 2008.

[31] D. Naor, S. B. Wallach-Dayan, M. A. Zahalka, and R. V. Sionov, "Involvement of CD44, a molecule with a thousand faces, in cancer dissemination," *Seminars in Cancer Biology*, vol. 18, no. 4, pp. 260–267, 2008.

[32] M. Al-Hajj, M. S. Wicha, A. Benito-Hernandez, S. J. Morrison, and M. F. Clarke, "Prospective identification of tumorigenic breast cancer cells," *Proceedings of the National Academy of Sciences of the United States of America*, vol. 100, no. 7, pp. 3983–3988, 2003.

[33] P. Dalerba, S. J. Dylla, I. K. Park et al., "Phenotypic characterization of human colorectal cancer stem cells," *Proceedings of the National Academy of Sciences of the United States of America*, vol. 104, no. 24, pp. 10158–10163, 2007.

[34] J. B. Park, H. J. Kwak, and S. H. Lee, "Role of hyaluronan in glioma invasion," *Cell Adhesion & Migration*, vol. 2, no. 3, pp. 202–207, 2014.

[35] A. Merzak, S. Koocheckpour, and G. J. Pilkington, "CD44 mediates human glioma cell adhesion and invasion *in vitro*," *Cancer Research*, vol. 54, no. 15, pp. 3988–3992, 1994.

[36] A. Ariza, D. López, J. L. Mate et al., "Role of CD44 in the invasiveness of glioblastoma multiforme and the noninvasiveness of meningioma: an immunohistochemistry study," *Human Pathology*, vol. 26, no. 10, pp. 1144–1147, 1995.

[37] J. Anido, A. Sáez-Borderías, A. Gonzàlez-Juncà et al., "TGF-β receptor inhibitors target the CD44^{high}/Id1^{high} glioma-initiating cell population in human glioblastoma," *Cancer Cell*, vol. 18, no. 6, pp. 655–668, 2010.

[38] A. Pietras, A. M. Katz, E. J. Ekström et al., "Osteopontin-CD44 signaling in the glioma perivascular niche enhances cancer stem cell phenotypes and promotes aggressive tumor growth," *Cell Stem Cell*, vol. 14, no. 3, pp. 357–369, 2014.

[39] D. V. Brown, G. Filiz, P. M. Daniel et al., "Expression of CD133 and CD44 in glioblastoma stem cells correlates with cell proliferation, phenotype stability and intra-tumor heterogeneity," *PloS One*, vol. 12, no. 2, article e0172791, 2017.

[40] H. S. Phillips, S. Kharbanda, R. Chen et al., "Molecular subclasses of high-grade glioma predict prognosis, delineate a pattern of disease progression, and resemble stages in neurogenesis," *Cancer Cell*, vol. 9, no. 3, pp. 157–173, 2006.

[41] M. Jijiwa, H. Demir, S. Gupta et al., "CD44v6 regulates growth of brain tumor stem cells partially through the AKT-mediated pathway," *PloS One*, vol. 6, no. 9, article e24217, 2011.

[42] D. V. Brown, P. M. Daniel, G. M. D'Abaco et al., "Coexpression analysis of CD133 and CD44 identifies proneural and mesenchymal subtypes of glioblastoma multiforme," *Oncotarget*, vol. 6, no. 8, pp. 6267–6280, 2015.

[43] K. P. L. Bhat, V. Balasubramaniyan, B. Vaillant et al., "Mesenchymal differentiation mediated by NF-κB promotes radiation resistance in glioblastoma," *Cancer Cell*, vol. 24, no. 3, pp. 331–346, 2013.

[44] H. Hatzikirou, D. Basanta, M. Simon, K. Schaller, and A. Deutsch, ""Go or grow": the key to the emergence of invasion in tumour progression?," *Mathematical Medicine and*

Biology: A Journal of the IMA, vol. 29, no. 1, pp. 49–65, 2012.

[45] A. Giese, M. A. Loo, N. Tran, D. Haskett, S. W. Coons, and M. E. Berens, "Dichotomy of astrocytoma migration and proliferation," *International Journal of Cancer*, vol. 67, no. 2, pp. 275–282, 1996.

[46] L. Persano, E. Rampazzo, A. Della Puppa, F. Pistollato, and G. Basso, "The three-layer concentric model of glioblastoma: cancer stem cells, microenvironmental regulation, and therapeutic implications," *Scientific World Journal*, vol. 11, pp. 1829–1841, 2011.

3

Osteogenic Induction of Wharton's Jelly-Derived Mesenchymal Stem Cell for Bone Regeneration

Ayu Suraya Ansari,[1] Muhammad Dain Yazid,[2] Nur Qisya Afifah Veronica Sainik,[1] Rabiatul Adawiyah Razali,[1] Aminuddin Bin Saim,[3] and Ruszymah Bt Hj Idrus[1]

[1]*Department of Physiology, Faculty of Medicine, Universiti Kebangsaan Malaysia Medical Centre, Jalan Yaacob Latif, 56000 Cheras, Kuala Lumpur, Malaysia*
[2]*Tissue Engineering Centre, Universiti Kebangsaan Malaysia Medical Centre, Jalan Yaacob Latif, 56000 Cheras, Kuala Lumpur, Malaysia*
[3]*Ear, Nose & Throat Consultant Clinic, Ampang Puteri Specialist Hospital, 68000 Ampang, Selangor, Malaysia*

Correspondence should be addressed to Ruszymah Bt Hj Idrus; ruszyidrus@gmail.com

Academic Editor: Jeong-Chae Lee

Wharton's jelly-derived mesenchymal stem cells (WJ-MSCs) are emerging as a promising source for bone regeneration in the treatment of bone defects. Previous studies have reported the ability of WJ-MSCs to be induced into the osteogenic lineage. The purpose of this review was to systematically assess the potential of WJ-MSC differentiation into the osteogenic lineage. A comprehensive search was conducted in Medline via Ebscohost and Scopus, where relevant studies published between 1961 and 2018 were selected. The main inclusion criteria were that articles must be primary studies published in English evaluating osteogenic induction of WJ-MSCs. The literature search identified 92 related articles, but only 18 articles met the inclusion criteria. These include two animal studies, three articles containing both *in vitro* and *in vivo* assessments, and 13 articles on *in vitro* studies, all of which are discussed in this review. There were two types of osteogenic induction used in these studies, either chemical or physical. The studies demonstrate that WJ-MSCs are able to differentiate into osteogenic lineage and promote osteogenesis. In light of these observations, it is suggested that WJ-MSCs can be a potential source of stem cells for osteogenic induction, as an alternative to bone marrow-derived mesenchymal stem cells.

1. Introduction

1.1. Human Umbilical Cord. About 25 years ago, the umbilical cord was considered to be a type of medical waste, until it was found to be a rich source of stem cells [1]. The abundance of stem cells and the ease of isolation have become deciding factors while choosing the source of adult stem cells. The human umbilical cord (HUC) is approximately 65 cm in length and 1.5 cm in diameter [2, 3]; it connects the fetus to the mother and supplies nourishment. The cord is covered by single or multiple layer of squamous cubic epithelial cells derived from the developing amnion [4–6]. The HUC contains two arteries and one vein, which are surrounded by a mucoid connective tissue known as Wharton's jelly (WJ) [7]. This mucous connective tissue is made up of mucopolysaccharides that are hyaluronic acid and chondroitin sulphate [8]. Basically, WJ can be divided into 4 layers with the outer layer being the amniotic epithelium followed by cord lining WJ and intermediate WJ. The inner layer of WJ is also known as perivascular WJ which contains arteries and vein [7] (Figure 1).

It has been reported that WJ also contains myofibroblast-like stromal cells, collagen fibers, proteoglycans, fibroblasts, and macrophages. WJ has garnered interest due to its availability, the noninvasive method of collection, and high cell yields. It has been demonstrated that mesenchymal stem cells (MSCs) isolated from the umbilical cord express matrix receptors (CD44 and CD105) and integrins (CD29 and CD51), but not hematopoietic lineage markers (CD34 and

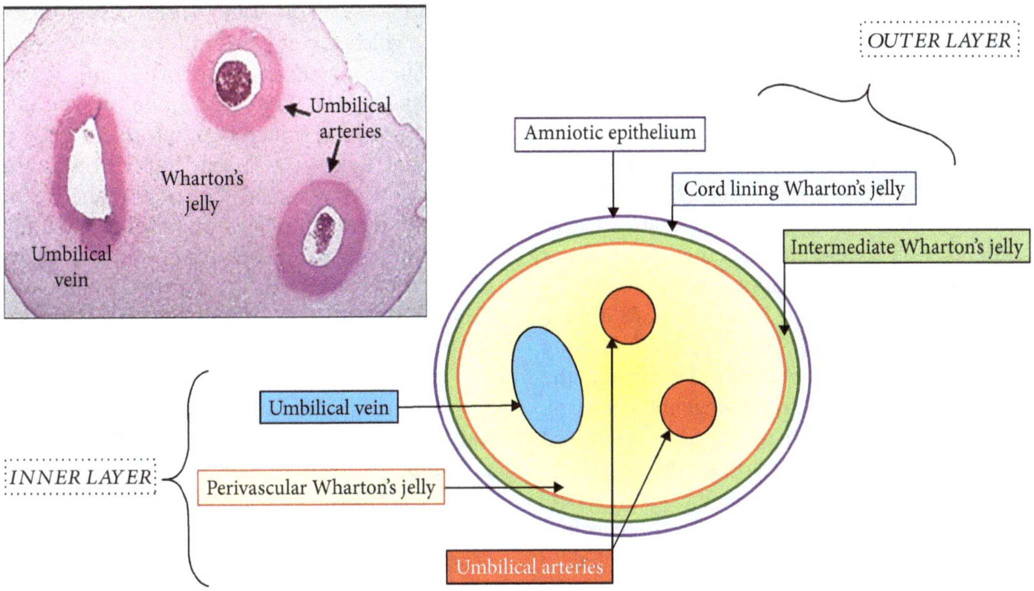

FIGURE 1: Anatomical compartment of Wharton's jelly mesenchymal stem cell.

CD45) [9]. These cells exhibit a phenotype similar to that of mesenchymal stem cells from other tissue sources [10]. According to the International Society for Cellular Therapy (ISCT), stem cells should demonstrate plastic adherence, not expressing hematopoietic markers, and be able to commit to the adipogenic, osteogenic, and chondrogenic lineage [11]. WJ-MSCs have a huge advantage where the phenotype and stemness are remained despite being in a long-term culture. This enables a mass production of cells which is usually required for regenerative medicine [12].

1.2. WJ-MSCs and Their Potential in the Treatment of Diseases. WJ, also known as *substantia gelatinea funiculi umbilicalis*, consists of fibroblast-like cells and mast cells that are embedded in proteoglycans, mainly hyaluronic acid. The cells are thought to be trapped in WJ during the early stage of embryogenesis, when they migrate from the aortic gonadotropin mesonephric region to the fetal liver through the umbilical cord [13]. WJ-MSCs have many advantages over other types of stem cells, including higher proliferation rates and broader multipotency. WJ-MSCs are able to differentiate into many cell types such as adipocytes [14, 15], osteoblasts [14, 16], hepatocytes [17], chondrocytes [18], and neural cells [19, 20]. Interestingly, it has also been demonstrated in a three-dimensional model that WJ-MSCs are able to differentiate *in vitro* into cornea epithelial-like cells, which may offer a solution for patients with limbus stem cell deficiency [21].

Cui and colleagues have successfully improved cognitive function in a mouse model of Alzheimer's disease using intravenously delivered WJ-MSCs, which reduced oxidative stress and promoted hippocampal neurogenesis [20]. In a clinical trial conducted by Hu and colleagues, an intravenous infusion of WJ-MSCs in type 2 diabetes mellitus patients improved the function of islet β-cells and reduced the incidence of diabetic complications [22]. Additionally, WJ-MSC therapy is now used to treat corneal epithelial, stromal, and endothelial disorders apart from the conventional intervention such as surgery, ionizing radiation, or drug treatment [23, 24].

1.3. Immunomodulatory Aspect of WJ-MSCs and BM-MSCs. WJ harbours MSCs that possess a similar phenotype as harvested from the bone marrow and other sources. WJ-MSCs do not express HLA-DR and costimulatory molecules CD40, CD80, and CD86 which are essential for the activation of T-cells [1, 2, 9, 25–27]. WJ-MSCs have been proven to have lower immunogenicity than BM-MSCs as depicted by Weiss et al. [1] who conducted an experiment using mixed lymphocyte reaction (MCR) assay [26]. In a study conducted by Prasanna et al. and Deuse et al., both consistently showed low HLA-DR expression compared to BM-MSCs after stimulation with IFN-γ and proinflammatory cytokines [28, 29]. In normal culture conditions, HLA-DR is not expressed; hence, the activation of T-cell is inhibited, reducing the risk of allograft rejection which potentially makes it safe for human transplantation.

It is documented that BM-MSCs harbour viruses, which is a major drawback in clinical application. There are reports from patients who undergo BM-MSC transplant who are infected with viral infection as a complication of the cell-based therapy [9]. Interestingly, the virus can escape from detection therefore increasing the morbidity and mortality [30]. Moreover, there are various diseases such as aplastic anemia, leukaemia, and bone marrow failure that impedes the application of BM-MSCs in therapy [31].

1.4. WJ-MSC Homing and Migration for Bone Healing. Generally, MSCs are known to migrate towards the injury site and help the healing process. The migration process, known as homing, is defined as the arrest of MSCs within the vasculature of a tissue before it crosses over the endothelium [24, 32]. As for now, the mechanism of MSC homing is still vague and BM-MSCs are postulated to have a mechanism similar to leukocyte homing. The mechanism is initiated when MSCs collide with the endothelium rolling, causing a slackening of cells in the blood flow. The G-protein-coupled receptors activated the cells and activated integrin mediation, causing activation-dependent arrest. The process is completed with the transmigration of the cells through the endothelium and the underlying basement membrane [33]. There are several factors that contribute to the homing mechanism which are growth factor expression as well as chemokine and extracellular matrix receptors on the MSCs' surfaces [34].

In a study conducted by Granero-Moltó et al., MSCs are migrated to the fracture site via the CXCR4 receptor causing improvement of biomechanical properties and increasing the cartilage and bone of the callus [24]. Zwingenberger et al. demonstrated that the combination of the SDF-1 released and bone morphogenetic protein 2 contributes to the migration of the stem cell [35]. This occurrence markedly boosts bone regeneration. Apart from that, MSCs are also recruited towards wear-particle-related osteolysis which is indicated by the inflammatory macrophage that is also the chemokine CC receptor (CCR) 1 of MSCs [30, 36]. The MSCs are demonstrated to increase bone mineral density and decrease the osteolytic process [37].

1.5. Cellular Mechanism of Bone Remodelling for Bone Regeneration. Bone repair or bone regeneration is characterized by a series of tissue transformation mechanisms including resorption and formation of hard and soft tissue. Therefore, mineralized tissue remodelling is required for the involvement of various cell types including osteoclast and osteoblast. Osteoblasts are bone-forming cells that can be found at the surface of bone, while osteoclasts are multinucleated bone-resorbing cells derived from bone marrow stem cells [38]. Bone remodelling is a cyclical process in which bone undergoes consistent renewal to ensure the replacement of primary bone, to maintain calcium homeostasis, and especially to heal ischemic and microfractured bone [7, 20, 32–34, 39]. This process requires a correct balance of bone resorption and bone formation and thus involves osteoclasts and osteoblasts, respectively.

Bone remodelling consists of five consecutive phases: (1) the resorption phase, where osteoclasts break down the bone tissue, resulting in mineral release; (2) the reversal phase, where mononuclear cells appear on the bone surface; (3) the formation phase, where osteoblasts trapped in the bone matrix become osteocytes; (4) the mineralization phase, where osteocytes produce type I collagen and other substances that make up the bone extracellular matrix; and (5) the termination phase [38, 40]. Resorption is initiated by osteoclast progenitors that are recruited and disseminated into the bloodstream. These cells proliferate and differentiate into mature osteoclasts, aided by osteoblast stromal cells via cell-to-cell interactions. These osteoblasts express two cytokines, i.e., receptor activator of NF-κB ligand (RANKL) and osteoprotegrin (OPG), involved in osteoclast progenitor cell differentiation. Under parathyroid hormone (PTH) stimulation, RANKL will bind to RANK, a cytoplasmic membrane receptor on osteoclast progenitor cells, to stimulate their fusion, differentiation, and activation. In contrast, OPG binds to RANKL to counterbalance the effect of RANKL-RANK, which thereby determines the extent of bone resorption. These events are important in maintaining bone homeostasis [41] (Figure 2). Bone resorption is terminated when osteoclasts undergo apoptosis and the reversal phase is initiated. Reversal cells may thus represent the missing link necessary to understand the coupling between bone resorption and formation. Researchers have found that reversal cells colonizing the resorbed bone surface are immature osteoblastic cells that gradually mature into bone-forming osteoblasts during the reversal phase and prepare the bone surface for bone formation [42].

1.6. Molecular Mechanism of Bone Remodelling for Bone Regeneration. The differentiation of MSCs depends on which signalling pathway is activated. Apart from osteoblasts, WJ-MSCs have also been demonstrated to differentiate into other mesenchymal cell lineages such as hepatocytes [43], chondrocytes [18, 44], and adipocytes [14, 15]. The markers for osteogenic differentiation are alkaline phosphatase (ALP), an early marker of osteogenic differentiation and mineralization, and RUNX2, a runt domain-containing transcription factor that is crucial for osteogenic differentiation and bone formation. The activation of RUNX2 triggers COL1 (collagen type 1), osteopontin (OPN), and osteocalcin (OC), which are osteoblast-specific markers. OPN is expressed later in the differentiation stage [45, 46]. Both OPN and COL1 are synthesized by osteoblasts. OC is also expressed later and is important for maintaining bone resorption. Osterix (Osx) is a downstream factor of Runx2 that binds to activated NFAT2 in bone development [47]. A study by Zhou et al. explored the function of Osx where it regulates bone homeostasis after birth for bone and cartilage formation [26].

In osteoblasts, lineage-specific gene expression control by specific transcription factors, i.e., Cbfa-1/RUNX2, acts to regulate osteoblastic specific gene expression [48]. Cbfa-1/RUNX2 is required for osteoblast differentiation, since Cbfa-1 knockout mice display impaired or even absent bone formation [49, 50]. This transcription factor contains a runt DNA-binding domain, which can bind to DNA as a monomer or as a subunit of a monomeric complex. It binds to various enhancers and promoters, including those for the genes encoding osteocalcin, osteopontin, bone sialoprotein, and GM-CSF. The expression of these proteins contributes to the bone matrix, leading to the maturation of osteoblasts. These genes can also be used as markers for different stages of osteoblast development [51–53].

The expression of transcription factors is controlled by several pathways that are activated by growth factors (GFs) that bind to a specific receptor. These growth factors include fibroblast growth factor (FGF), transforming growth factor-β (TGF-β), insulin-like growth factor (IGF), platelet-derived growth factor (PDGF), and vascular endothelial growth factor (VEGF) [54]. It has been reported that these GFs are responsible for regulating the expression of Cbfa-1/RUNX2 via the MAPK [55], ERK [52], and PI3K-Akt pathways [54, 56]. GF binding to its receptor tyrosine kinase (RTK) activates a downstream signaling cascade. The activated RTK activates class I phosphatidylinositol 3-kinase (PI3K) or

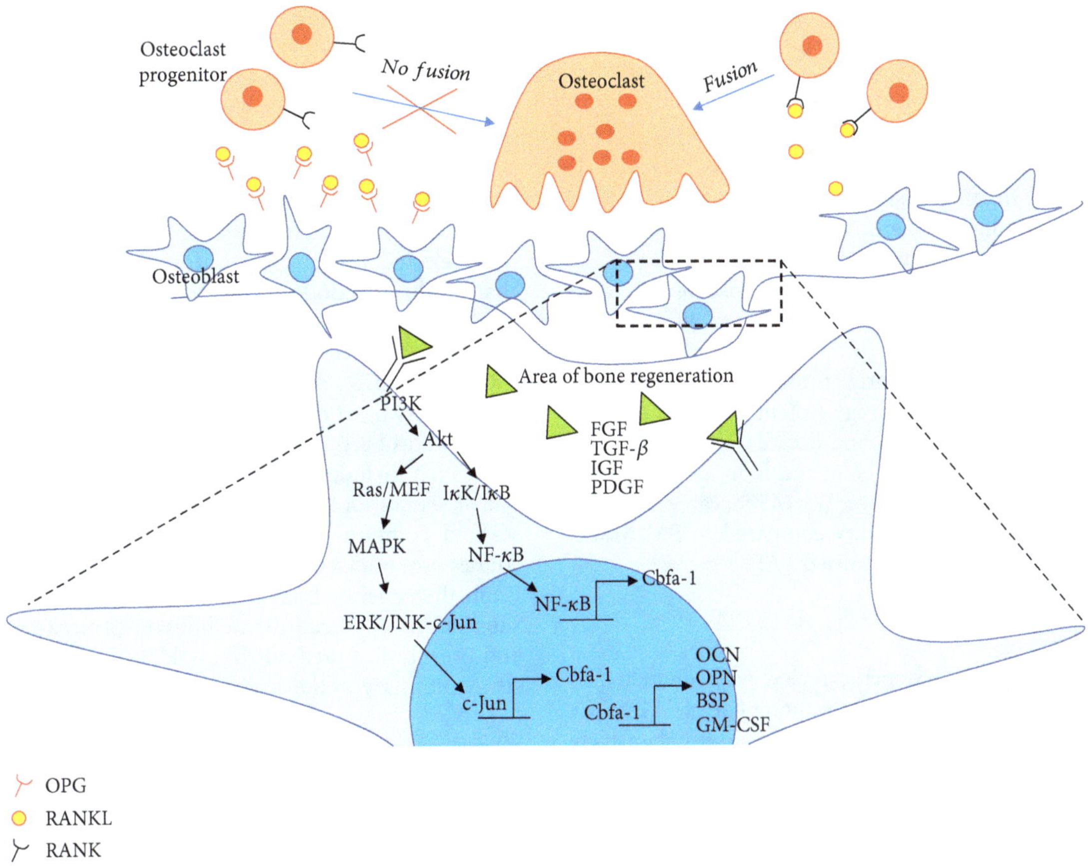

Figure 2: Mechanism of bone regeneration and activation of signaling pathways.

guanosine nucleotide-binding protein (Ras) and propagates the signal through direct binding or tyrosine phosphorylation. This then activates Akt/PKB, IκK/IκB, or Raf/MEK, which then activates NF-κB or MAPK, accordingly. Activated NF-κB and MAPK act through direct binding to phosphorylate ERK/JNK-cJun, which then activate Cbfal/RUNX2 gene expression. TGF-β plays important roles in osteoblast precursor recruitment, FGF enhances osteoblast recruitment and proliferation, IGF is involved in the regulation of bone matrix synthesis and migration, VEGF regulates osteoblast differentiation, and PDGF is involved in osteoprogenitor migration [51, 52]. Cumulatively, the osteogenic differentiation capability owned by WJ-MSCs supplemented with specific GF is postulated to have a high potential for bone regeneration.

1.7. WJ-MSCs for Bone Regeneration. Albeit many have used WJ-MSCs in the studies, the safety and efficacy of its application are indecisive particularly in bone regeneration. There are several aspects that need to be considered prior to using WJ-MSCs that may influence the yield and its stemness potency. Different parts of the umbilical cord generated diverse frequencies of MSCs and cell populations [6–8, 57–59]. It is known that Runx2 plays a pivotal role in osteoblast differentiation. In a previous study, it has shown that WJ-MSCs have lower capability to differentiate due to the high level of RUNX2 but lower ALP expression. ALP is important for matrix maturation [60, 61]. WJ-MSCs also exhibited higher expression of pluripotent markers, OCT 4, SOX 2, and NANOG than in other parts of the umbilical cord [62]. From those findings, it can be postulated that regulation of Runx2 and pluripotent impedes ALP expression, thus needing a specific modulator that can serve as a molecular switch of WJ-MSCs' fate. Current study by Bustos and colleagues have demonstrated that JARID1B (Jumonji AT-rich interactive domain 1B) histone demethylase represses Runx2 in undifferentiated WJ-MSCs. In JARID1B knockdown murine, it can be seen that Runx2 is highly expressed and ready for osteogenic commitment indicating that this molecular mechanism is relevant to modulating osteoblastic lineage commitment [63].

1.8. Clinical Application of WJ-MSCs in Bone Regeneration. The current standard commonly used for bone tissue replacement is bone grafting obtained from patients themselves (autograft) or from other individuals (allograft). However, this has raised various effects including immunoreactivity and infection as well as procedure. WJ-MSCs have proved its capability to help in bone regeneration for clinical application. Qu et al. treated 36 patients with nonunion bone fracture with WJ-MSCs cultured with platelet-rich plasma (PRP) resulting in a faster recovery with no infection recorded compared to the other 36 patients with autoiliac treatment [64]. In another study, the intravenous injection of 3–5 million WJ-MSCs alleviated the condition of Becker muscular dystrophy patients with increased muscle strength, improved appetite, and also improved patient's gait [65]. Recently, a patient in Indonesia with infected nonunion bone is able to walk with no pain and no postoperative complications recorded after local implantation of 5 million cells supplemented with BMP-2 and hydroxyapatite [66]. A transplantation of autologous BM-MSCs and allogeneic WJ-MSCs in treating osteonecrosis of femoral head showed improvement where it relieved the pain and improved the joint function [67].

To this date, there are many various positive outcomes upon WJ-MSC treatment in clinical trials for different disorders including neurology [67], hematology [68], liver diseases [69], and particularly musculoskeletal diseases [65, 70]. WJ-MSCs have a huge potential to be used as an alternative treatment for bone disorders as it does not require ethical issues to obtain and it is alleviating patients' morbidities [71]. Since WJ-MSCs can retain the stemness and phenotypic stability compared to BM-MSCs, it has potency to be commercialised [72].

2. Methods

2.1. Search Strategy. A systematic review was conducted to systematically assess articles on the potential of WJ-MSCs for bone regeneration. Two databases were comprehensively used to search for relevant studies, i.e., Medline via Ebscohost and Scopus. For search term keywords, the combination of words used was "Wharton's jelly" AND "osteo*" OR "bone".

2.2. Selection Criteria. The year limit for searches was from 1961 to 2018, and only studies published in English were considered. The search outcomes identified all articles containing the words Wharton's jelly, umbilical cord, osteogenesis, osteogenic, and bone. Databases were searched individually to ensure all relevant studies were considered. The titles and abstracts were carefully screened for eligibility related to the topic of interest. Primary studies related to bone formation or bone regeneration were included. Review articles, news articles, letters, editorials, and case studies were excluded from the search.

2.3. Data Extraction and Management. Data were extracted from each eligible article by two reviewers. The selected papers were screened in several phases prior to inclusion. First, the titles that were not relevant to the topic were excluded. Next, the abstracts of the papers were screened, and unrelated studies were excluded. All duplicates were removed. The following data were summarized from the selected studies: (1) authors, (2) type of study, (3) subject/sample, (4) induction factor, (5) methodology, (6) results, and (7) conclusions.

3. Results

3.1. Search Results. The primary searches identified 386 articles: 41 articles came from Medline and 345 articles were found in Scopus. To minimize bias and improve the strength of the related articles, two reviewers independently assessed the articles according to the inclusion and exclusion criteria. There were 244 articles removed as they were unrelated to either Wharton's jelly or osteogenesis/bone. A joint discussion was conducted to achieve consensus where differences emerged during the assessment. From the 142 remaining articles, 50 duplicates were removed before full articles were retrieved. From 92 articles, 74 articles were rejected based on the inclusion criteria as the articles were not primary studies, were not related to Wharton's jelly or osteogenesis, or were not available as full articles. Finally, a total of 18 studies were selected for data extraction in this review. The flow chart of the selection process is shown in Figure 3.

3.2. Study Characteristics. All studies were published between 1961 and 2018. An article reported on animal studies (in vivo), two articles on both *in vitro* and *in vivo* assessments, and 14 articles on *in vitro* studies. There were six articles which included scaffold fabrication in the study. Three out of six scaffold studies involved the optimization of the scaffold component for better bone regeneration. Eleven studies proposed a different type of tissue as the MSC source. From the generated data, we classified the articles into two subgroups: (1) chemical methods to promote osteogenesis and (2) physical methods (scaffolds) to promote osteogenesis. A summary of the studies is provided in Table 1.

4. Discussion

The database search provided 18 articles related to Wharton's jelly, umbilical cord, osteogenesis, osteogenic lineage, and bone. From these articles, various tissue sources were assessed for potential MSCs. Each of these sources was examined regarding MSC differentiation capacities into the adipogenic, chondrogenic, and osteogenic lineages. This review assessed the osteogenic potential of WJ-MSCs, which may have remarkable potential for bone regeneration in the clinic.

4.1. Mesenchymal Stem Cells: Potential Sources. Mesenchymal stem cells (MSCs) have attracted attention because of their unique plasticity and ability to differentiate into multiple cell lineages, i.e., osteoblasts, chondrocytes, and adipocytes, with potential for clinical usage. The bone marrow is a primary source of MSCs. However, it has been reported that the frequency as well as the differentiation potential of BM-derived MSCs (BM-MSCs) decline with increasing age [73]. Therefore, alternative sources of MSCs are needed, especially those that can be obtained noninvasively. Currently, various tissues are under consideration for MSC isolation, including adipose tissue, muscle, amniotic fluid, menstrual blood [74, 75], fetal blood [76], and periodontal ligaments (PDL) [61]. The human umbilical cord is a promising source of MSCs, as MSCs can be isolated either from the whole umbilical cord [16, 77], the umbilical vein subendothelium [78], or WJ [14, 19, 74]. One group of researchers divided the umbilical cord into three anatomical segments, i.e., the maternal, middle, and fetal segments [79]. They demonstrated that MSCs from the maternal and fetal segments displayed greater viability, possessed significantly higher proliferation rates, and underwent more complete osteogenic differentiation, showing that these segments are a good source of MSCs for bone tissue engineering [79].

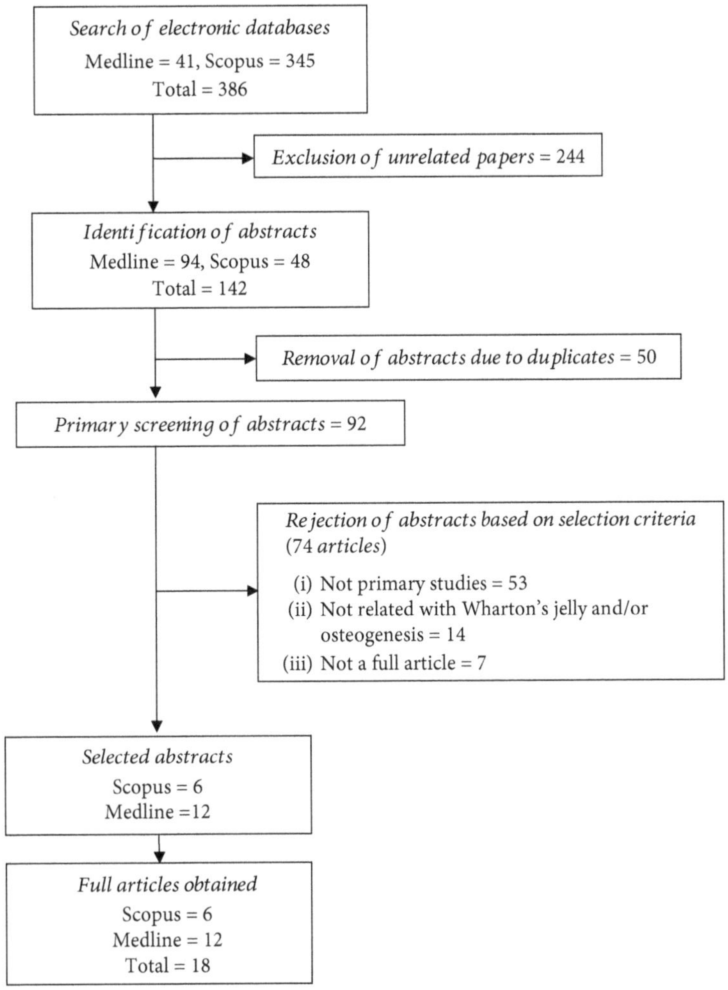

FIGURE 3: Flow chart of the article selection process using the Scopus and MEDLINE databases.

It is important to characterize cells derived from tissues to determine the type of cell population that exists in the preparation. A heterogeneous population could influence the differentiation properties, specifically the osteogenic potential of MSCs for bone regeneration. There are a few surface markers that are commonly reported for MSCs such as CD13, CD29, CD44, CD73, CD90, CD105, and CD166. MSCs do not express CD31, CD144, and CD309 (endothelial cell markers) or CD14, CD34, CD45, CD117, and CD133 (hematopoietic cell markers) [61, 79].

4.2. Wharton's Jelly Mesenchymal Stem Cells Undergo Osteogenic Differentiation. WJ-MSCs have been shown to have good potential for osteogenic differentiation. These cells display all features of functional osteocytes/osteoblasts based on osteogenic gene expression, extracellular matrix (ECM) mineralization, and the ability to adhere to a fabricated scaffold [80, 81]. Although WJ-MSCs have been broadly investigated, there are still problems when it comes to transplantation, as an immune response and rejection could occur [82]. In the database search, we only found one article that used autoserum for WJ-MSCs *in vitro* as a substitute for FBS to reduce the rejection rate. Autoserum is serum obtained from the umbilical cord blood. Baba et al. reported that the cell culture medium using autologous serum is superior in quality to medium using FBS. WJ-MSCs cultured in autologous serum exhibited successful osteoblastic and adipogenic differentiation. The WJ-MSCs were then transplanted subcutaneously into nude mice, and their potential to form bone was proven [16].

4.2.1. Chemical Induction. Seven studies out of 18 selected articles used chemical factors to promote osteogenesis in WJ-MSCs. Batsali et al. [83] demonstrated that WJ-MSCs are able to differentiate into the osteogenic lineage, although this was inferior compared to BM-MSCs. They demonstrated that WISP1, a canonical Wnt pathway target protein, was able to promote better osteogenic differentiation in WJ-MSCs [83]. A study by Szepesi et al. [61] showed that adipose tissue-derived mesenchymal stem cells (AT-MSCs) and periodontal ligament-derived mesenchymal stem cells (PDL-MSCs) have excellent potential for bone replacement applications and better endothelial differentiation ability as compared to WJ-MSCs [61]. The high degree of calcification in AT-MSCs and PDL-MSCs demonstrates that calcium deposition was better as compared to WJ-MSCs for generating vascularized bone grafts [61]. Similar findings were reported by [84] where AD-

Table 1: Summary and classification of the 18 articles selected from the database search.

No.	Author and year	Type of study	Subject/sample	Induction factor	WJ-MSC isolation method	Results	Conclusion
1.	Fu et al. 2018 [91]	*In vitro* and *in vivo*	(i) Human umbilical cord-derived mesenchymal stem cells (UC-MSCs) (ii) Sprague-Dawley's osteoblast (iii) Sprague-Dawley's osteoclast	Differentiation medium Osteogenic medium: (1) High-glucose DMEM (2) 10% serum (3) 10^{-8} M dexamethasone (4) 50 ng/mL L-ascorbic acid (5) 10 mM β-glycerophosphate Osteoclast differentiation (1) 10 or 100 ng RANKL	(i) Enzymatic digestion (ii) Part of UC: not mentioned	(1) MicroCT result showed that transplantation of UC-MSCs increased bone mass in the distal condyle of normal rat femur compared to other groups (2) Goldner's staining indicated that compact arrangement of collagen with less trabecular thickness in the group undergoes implantation with UC-MSCs. A trabeculae-like structure containing lamellae was detected, but there are no cell arrangements found in the area (3) Osteocalcin (OC) staining showed increased osteocalcin level in OVX-receiving UC-MSCs (4) Antihuman-specific nuclei antigen showed engrafted UC-MSCs had differentiated into osteoblasts (5) RT PCR: (i) Human osteocalcin and abundant osterix (OSX) was detected in ovx-receiving UC-MSCs (6) *In vitro* coculture system showed more expression of alkaline phosphatase (ALP) if the osteoblast is cocultured with UC-MSCs	UC-MSCs able to be differentiated into osteoblast and are safe for transplantation in bone disease treatment.
2.	Al Jofi et al. 2018 [92]	*In vitro*	(i) Wharton's jelly mesenchymal stem cells (WJ-MSCs)	(i) 10 μmol/L metformin (antidiabetic drug)	(i) Commercial UC-MSCs (ii) Part of UC: not mentioned	Metformin-treated UC-MSCs increased in mineralization stained through Alizarin Red Staining. But in OCT-1- (organic cation transporter-) siRNA-transfected cells, a significant decrease in calcium-rich nodule formation was observed.	OCT-expressing WJ-MSCs have the ability to be differentiated into osteoblasts when induced with metformin.
3.	Bharti et al. (2018) [44]	*In vitro*	(i) Wharton's jelly mesenchymal stem cells (WJ-MSCs)	(i) Osteogenic medium (1) ADMEM (2) 0.1 mM dexamethasone (3) 50 mM ascorbic acid (4) 10 mM glycerol-2-phosphate (ii) Adipogenic medium: (1) ADMEM (2) 500 mM isobutyl methylxanthine (3) 1 mM dexamethasone (4) Insulin (5) 100 mM indomethacin (6) 10 mM insulin (iii) Chondrogenic medium using comer (1) StemPro1Osteocyte/ Chondrocyte Differentiation Basal Medium; StemPro1 Chondrogenesis supplement; Gibco). (2) Hepatocyte (3) ADMEM (4) 2% FBS (5) 10 ng/ml of oncostatin M (6) 10 nmol/L dexamethasone (7) 1% insulin transferrin-selenium	(i) Explant method (ii) Part of UC: maternal, middle and fetal segments	(1) Bone nodules: formed by cells from all segments (2) Chondrogenic potential: occurred in cells from all segments	WJ-MSCs are a good cell source for autologous/ allogeneic stem cell source.
4.	Batsali et al. 2017 [83]	*In vitro*	(i) Bone marrow mesenchymal stem cell (BM-MSCs) (ii) Wharton's jelly	Differentiation medium: Osteogenic medium: (1) High-glucose DMEM (2) 10% serum (3) 10^{-7} M dexamethasone	(i) Explant method (ii) Part of UC: maternal, middle, and fetal segments	(1) Osteogenic differentiation (Alizarin Red and von Kossa staining): WJ-MSCs showed similar staining potential as BM-MSC (2) Real-time- (RT-) PCR: (i) Osteocyte-related gene expression: higher expression of Runt-related transcription factor 2 (RUNX2), distal-less homeobox protein 5 (DLX5),	The osteogenic differentiation potential of WJ-MSCs is regulated by WISP1 and sFRP4, respectively.

Table 1: Continued.

No.	Author and year	Type of study	Subject/sample	Induction factor	WJ-MSC isolation method	Results	Conclusion
			mesenchymal stem cells (WJ-MSCs)	(4) 25 μg/mL L-ascorbic acid (5) 3 mM NaH_2PO_4		osteocalcin (OCN), and alkaline phosphatase (ALP) by BM-MSCs (3) Differential expression of WNT ligands; sFRP4 (*secreted frizzled-related protein 4*) and WISP1 (WNT1-inducible signalling pathway protein 1) were significantly reduced in WJ-MSCs (4) WISP1 implicated in osteogenic differentiation; RUNX2, ALP, and OSC were significantly upregulated	
5.	Zajdel et al. 2017 [84]	*In vitro*	(i) Adipose tissue (AT-MSCs) (ii) WJ-MSCs	Osteogenic medium (Lonza): (1) Dexamethasone (2) Ascorbic acid (3) β-Glycerophosphate	(i) Commercial AT-MSCs and UC-MSCs (ii) Part of UC: not mentioned	(1) Calcium deposition by Alizarin Red staining (i) Calcium deposition was greater in AT-MSCs when compared to WJ-MSCs (2) ALP activity (i) ALP activity was higher in AT-MSCs when compared to WJ-MSCs (3) Osteoprotogerin (OPG) secretion (i) Both osteo-induced cell types showed high OPG secretion when compared to control (4) Osteocalcin (OC) secretion (i) OC secretion was higher in WJ-MSCs when compared to AT-MSCs	WJ-MSCs have the ability to differentiate into the osteogenic lineage.
6.	Mechiche Alami et al. 2017 [88]	*In vitro*	(i) WJ-MSCs	Calcium phosphate (CaP) substrate build-up (without osteogenic induction	(i) Commercial UC-MSCs (ii) Part of UC: not mentioned	(1) Gene expression analysis (i) Day 7: Runt-related transcription factor 2 (RUNX2) and secreted phosphoprotein 1 (SPP-1) were upregulated (ii) Day 14: collagen type 1 Alpha 1 (COL1A1) and ALP were upregulated (iii) Day 21: bone gamma-carboxyglutamic acid-containing protein (BGLP) and ALP were upregulated (2) Nodule characterization (i) Hematoxylin-eosin-saffron (HES) staining revealed continuous layers of cells at the surface of the nodule with randomly distributed cells embedded within fibrous tissues (ii) Masson's trichrome staining showed the presence of green-stained fibrous tissue composed of newly formed collagen	Excellent osteogenic potential of sprayed CaP and WJ-MSCs in bone tissue engineering
7.	Szepesi et al. 2016 [61]	*In vitro*	(i) WJ-MSCs (ii) AT-MSCs (iii) Periodontal ligament MSCs (PDL-MSCs)	Differentiation medium: (i) StemPro Osteogenesis Differentiation kit (ii) StemPro Chondrogenesis Differentiation kit (iii) StemPro Adipogenesis Differentiation kit (iv) Endothelial Cell Growth Medium	(i) Enzymatic digestion UC-MSCs (ii) Part of UC: not mentioned	(1) Osteogenic differentiation: AT-MSCs and PDL-MSCs showed greater calcium deposition (2) Osteogenic differentiation assessed via RT-PCR: (i) Runt-related transcription factor 2 (RUNX2): all cell types showed high expression after induction (ii) Alkaline phosphatase (ALP): AT-MSCs and PDL-MSCs showed increased expression, but ALP was significantly lower in WJ-MSCs (iii) Calcium deposition: AT-MSCs and PDL-MSCs showed greater calcium deposition as compared to WJ-MSCs (3) There was a significant correlation between CD90 expression and the levels of calcium deposition in different MSC isolates	WJ-MSCs have osteogenic potential and are good cell sources for bone regeneration.
8.	Lim et al. 2016 [79]	*In vitro*	Human WJ-MSCs (i) Fetal segment (ii) Maternal segment (iii) Middle segment	(i) Osteogenic medium (1) Alpha-MEM (2) Dexamethasone (3) Ascorbic acid (4) β-Glycerol phosphate (ii) Adipogenic medium: (1) DMEM/F12 (2) 3-Isobutyl-3-methylxanthine (3) Dexamethasone (4) Insulin (iii) Chondrogenic medium (1) Alpha-MEM	(i) Enzymatic digestion (ii) Maternal, middle, and fetal segments	Bone nodules: formed by cells from all segments	WJ-MSCs are a good cell source for bone regeneration.

Table 1: Continued.

No.	Author and year	Type of study	Subject/sample	Induction factor	WJ-MSC isolation method	Results	Conclusion
				(2) Transforming growth factor 3 (TGF-β3)			
9.	Kargozar et al. 2018 [80]	*In vitro* and *in vivo*	(i) BM-MSCs (ii) AT-MSCs (iii) UC-MSCs	(i) Nanocomposite scaffolds (3D bioactive glass/gelatin scaffolds (BaG/Gel) consisting of SiO_2-P_2O_5-CaO (64% SiO_2, 5% P_2O_5, and 31% CaO).	(i) Enzymatic digestion (ii) Part of UC: not mentioned	*In vitro* study (1) Cell viability: (i) Scaffold had no significant inhibitory effect on MSC proliferation over time (ii) MSC proliferation gradually increased with incubation time *In vivo* study (1) Histological observations: (i) H&E staining: all MSC-seeded scaffolds successfully generated new bone and demonstrated an ongoing healing process at 4 and 12 weeks after transplantation. The UC-MSC-seeded scaffold showed significantly increased neovascularization compared to the others (ii) IHC staining: increased expression of OCN and ALP in the BM-MSC-seeded scaffold. Vascular endothelial growth factor (VEGF) expressed in all the groups of treated cell/scaffold. Increased neovascularization with the UC-MSC-seeded scaffold (iii) Histomorphometry: BM-MSC-seeded scaffolds showed more bone regeneration at 4 and 12 weeks	BM-MSCs, grown on BaG/Gel nanocomposite scaffolds, are possible sources for bone regeneration.
10.	Todeschi et al. 2015 [81]	*In vivo*	(i) UC-MSCs (ii) BM-MSCs	(i) Ceramic scaffolds (Skelite; 4 × 4 × 4 mm cubes of 33% hydroxyapatite and 67% silicon-stabilized tricalcium phosphate, Si-TCP) (ii) Platelet-rich plasma (PRP) (iii) Conditioned medium (CM)	(i) Explant method (ii) Part of UC: not mentioned	(1) Histological assessment revealed the formation an immature bone-like structures and compact fibrous tissue in UC-MSC-seeded constructs (2) Polarized light examination revealed less organized collagen fibers in the UC-MSC-seeded scaffolds. The immature bone-like matrix in UC-MSC-seeded scaffolds was mostly filled with a loose connective tissue (3) Histological evaluation in an orthotopic mouse model showed that none of the bone defects had completely closed. However, gold MTC staining indicated the presence of red blood cells in blood vessel-like structures which is significant in the UC-MSC-transplanted group (4) Osteocytes were clearly detectable in the BMMSC-seeded scaffolds (5) However, human ALU sequences were not detected in osteocytes within the newly formed bone in the UC-MSC implants and nonseeded implants	UC-MSCs promote bone regeneration.
11.	Karadas et al. 2014 [74]	*In vitro*	(i) WJ-MSCs (ii) BM-MSCs (iii) Menstrual blood mesenchymal stem cells (MBMSCs)	(i) Collagen scaffolds with *in situ* calcium phosphate (CaP) (ii) Differentiation medium: (1) High-glucose DMEM (2) 10 nM dexamethasone (3) 50 μg/mL ascorbic acid (4) 10 mM β-glycerophosphate (5) 10% FBS (6) 100 units/mL penicillin (7) 100 μg/mL streptomycin	(i) Explant method (ii) Part of UC: not mentioned	(1) Cell proliferation assays: (i) WJ-MSCs on tissue culture polystyrene (TCPS) and collagen without CaP treatment increased proliferation (2) Cell attachment (fluorescence staining): (i) Good attachment of both cell types to the scaffold (ii) Confocal micrographs showed that the cells were able to penetrate into the pores (3) Osteogenic differentiation: (i) ALP assay: (a) WJ-MSCs showed better differentiation on untreated and CaP-containing foams than in growth medium (b) ALP levels were higher in WJ-MSCs grown on CaP-free foams than on TCPS (c) ALP activity was significantly higher in cells grown on collagen with CaP crystals formed in situ for both WJ-MSCs and MBMSCs (days 14 and 21) von Kossa staining: (1) WJ-MSCs had higher ALP activity and denser mineral deposition compared to MBMSCs	Collagen foam with the use of CaP crystals formed *in situ* enhances the osteogenic induction of WJ-MSCs.

TABLE 1: Continued.

No.	Author and year	Type of study	Subject/sample	Induction factor	WJ-MSC isolation method	Results	Conclusion
12.	Ramesh et al. 2014 [93]	*In vitro*	(i) WJ-MSCs	(i) Hydrogel alginate microspheres (ii) Osteogenic differentiation media: (1) Basal medium (2) 10 mM β-glycerophosphate (3) 1 mM dexamethasone (4) 5 mg/mL ascorbic acid	(i) Explant method (ii) Part of UC: not mentioned	(1) Characterization of osteodifferentiated WJ-MSCs via: (i) Bradford assay: calcium deposition increased in 2% alginate (ii) Alizarin Red staining: excellent matrix mineralization in WJ-MSCs immobilized on 2% alginate (iii) Immunocytochemical analysis (osteocalcin): significant expression of osteocalcin in WJ-MSC aggregates in 1.5% and 2% alginate at day 21 (2) Genotypic analysis of encapsulated WJ-MSCs showed that OCN and Runx2 were upregulated in 1.5% and 2% alginate	WJ-MSCs encapsulated in hydrogel alginate microspheres have osteogenic potential for stem cell-based tissue engineering.
13.	Baba et al. 2012 [16]	*In vivo* & *in vitro*	Human umbilical cord mesenchymal stem cells (hUC-MSCs)	Differentiation medium: (i) NH OsteoDiff Medium (ii) NH AdipoDiff Medium (iii) rhBMP2 (iv) Scaffold	(i) Enzymatic digestion (ii) Part of UC: not mentioned	(3) Osteogenic differentiation: strong calcium deposition Adipogenic differentiation: lipid droplet production (4) H&E staining: positive for bone tissue producing osteocalcin (OCN) (5) RT-PCR: high expression of RUNX2, ALP, and OCN as compared to undifferentiated cells	UC-MSCs supplemented with growth factors and serum have osteogenic differentiation potential for bone regeneration.
14.	Penolazzi et al. 2012 [89]	*In vitro*	(i) WJ-MSCs	(i) Porcine urinary bladder matrix (pUBM)	(i) Enzymatic digestion (ii) Part of UC: not mentioned	(1) Proliferation assays showed (i) pUBM did not have an effect on cells in suspension conditions but affected cells cultured in adherent conditions (ii) Viable cells were homogenously distributed over the entire scaffold (2) TUNEL assays showed (i) No apoptosis in hWJ-MSCs cultured in agarose-coated wells with increasing amounts of pUBM (ii) The scaffold upregulated cyclin D1 (iii) Matrix metanoproteinase (MMPI3) was lower but this did not affect β-catenin (3) Morphological characterization: (i) Scanning electron microscope (SEM) analysis showed (a) There was a significant interaction between the cells and the biomaterial (b) WJ-MSCs completely were enveloped in pUBM particles to form smooth spheroids, displaying an ECM network covering the surface (c) The cells and the biomaterial formed a dense structure (ii) X-ray energy-dispersive spectroscopy (EDX) showed that spheroids in osteogenic medium contained high amounts of calcium and phosphorous (high degree of mineralization) (iii) Transmission electron microscopy (TEM) showed the presence of focal contacts between cells and the pUBM scaffold (4) RT-PCR: (i) RUNX2 expression was not affected by pUBM, but increased upon osteoinduction (ii) WJ-MSCs seeded on pUBM were able to produce Col IAI and OPN after 21 days in osteogenic medium (iii) WJ-MSCs showed increased ALP activity and ability to deposit mineralized matrix (iv) OPN expression was higher in cells grown on pUBM scaffolds in osteogenic medium than in osteogenic medium alone	The combination of WJ-MSCs and pUBM shows the promise of scaffolds for bone regeneration.
15.	Wang et al. 2011 [94]	*In vitro*	(i) UC-MSCs	(i) Poly-L-lactic acid (PLLA) scaffold (ii) Osteogenic induction medium: (1) Low-glucose DMEM (2) 10% FBS (3) 1% penicillin/streptomycin (4) 100 nM dexamethasone, (5) 10 mM sodium β-glycerophosphate,	(i) Enzymatic digestion (ii) Part of UC: not mentioned	(1) Biochemical assays were performed to assess (i) DNA content: osteogenic parts of the C-cell-O composites had higher DNA contents than the O-O composites and the osteogenic parts of the C-O composites (ii) Glycosaminoglycan (GAG) content: all osteogenic groups had similar GAG contents (iii) Hydroxyproline (HYP) content: osteogenic groups had a significantly higher HYP content	WJ-MSCs are a suitable cell source for a sandwich approach strategy in osteochondral tissue engineering.

TABLE 1: Continued.

No.	Author and year	Type of study	Subject/sample	Induction factor	WJ-MSC isolation method	Results	Conclusion
				(6) 50 μg/mL ascorbic acid 2-phosphate (AA2P) (7) 10 nM 1α,25-dihydroxyvitamin D3 (i) Chondrogenic induction medium: (1) High-glucose DMEM (DMEM-HG) (2) 1% nonessential amino acids (NEAA) (3) 1x sodium pyruvate (4) 1x insulin-transferrin-selenium premix (ITS) (5) 50 μg/mL (AA2P) (6) 40 μg/mL L-proline (7) 100 nM dexamethasone (8) 10 ng/mL TGF-β1		(iv) Calcium content: osteogenic groups showed significantly increased calcium levels over time (2) Histological analyses: positive Alizarin Red staining in the osteogenic group (3) RT-PCR: (i) Collagen type II (ColII): not expressed in the osteogenic group (ii) Collagen type I (ColI): upregulated in all groups (iii) RUNX2: increased in the osteogenic group (iv) Aggrecan: increased significantly in chondrogenic group	
16.	Schneider et al. 2010 [85]	*In vitro*	Human mesenchymal stem cells (hMSC): (i) UC-MSCs (ii) BM-MSCs	(i) Scaffold: 3D collagen gel (ii) Osteogenic induction medium: (1) Low-glucose DMEM (2) 10% FCS (3) 100 nM dexamethasone (4) 10 mM sodium β-glycerophosphate (5) 0.05 mM/L-ascorbic acid 2-phosphate (iii) Adipogenic induction medium: (1) DMEM high glucose (2) 1 μM dexamethasone (3) 0.2 mM indomethacin (4) 0.01 mg/mL insulin (5) 0.5 mM 3-isobutyl-1-methylxanthine (6) 10% FCS	(i) Enzymatic digestion (ii) Part of UC: not mentioned	(1) Scaffold: (i) 3D collagen gel underwent progressive contraction (ii) After osteogenic differentiation, collagen gels were stronger and harder with BM-MSCs and UC-MSCs (2) Characterization of BM-MSCs and UC-MSCs by (i) Osteogenic differentiation: UC-MSCs showed increased extracellular matrix (ECM) deposition by Alizarin Red (AR) staining (ii) Adipogenic differentiation: UC-MSCs showed a limited number of small lipid vacuoles stained by Oil Red O (ORO) (iii) Immunofluorescence: positive expression of collagen IV and laminin in UC-MSCs after 21 days of osteogenic differentiation on collagen gels (iv) Immunohistochemistry analyses: positive expression of osteopontin (OPN) and bisphosphonate [2-(2-pyridinyl) ethylidene-BP] (PEBP) in the collagen gel (3) TEM analysis: (i) Osteogenic differentiation: contraction of the collagenous matrix on the UC-MSC-seeded collagen surface (ii) Adipogenic differentiation: UC-MSC-derived lipid vacuoles were small and stained with toluidine blue (4) RT-PCR: UC-MSCs expressed collagen I, collagen III, collagen IV, and laminin (5) Cell migration: migrating UC-MSCs appeared as spindle-shaped cells with elongated cytoplasmic processes	UC-MSCs have a significant therapeutic impact in bone tissue engineering in the future.
17.	Hsieh et al. 2010 [14]	(i) *In vitro*	(i) WJ-MSCs (ii) BM-MSCs	Osteogenic differentiation medium: (1) DMEM (2) 10% FBS (3) 0.1 mM dexamethasone (4) 10 mM β-glycerophosphate (5) 50 mM ascorbic acid	(i) Enzymatic digestion (ii) Part of UC: not mentioned	(1) Array data showed that both BM-MSCs and WJ-MSCs expressed multilineage differentiation properties. (2) Real-time-PCR: BM-MSCs > WJ-MSCs in terms of (i) Adipocytic marker expression: *lipoprotein lipase* (LPL), leptin, peroxisome proliferator-activated receptor gamma (PPARγ), and fatty acid-binding protein 4 (FABP4) (ii) Lipid accumulation (3) Osteogenic differentiation potential (i) BM-MSCs > WJ-MSCs when cultured in defined MesenCult (ii) Expressed higher levels of ALP, SPP-1, and RUNX2	WJ-MSCs are capable of differentiating into the osteogenic lineage, but BM-MSCs are superior.

Table 1: Continued.

No.	Author and year	Type of study	Subject/sample	Induction factor	WJ-MSC isolation method	Results	Conclusion
						(iii) BM-MSCs > WJ-MSCs when cultured in defined cultured in 10% FBS: (a) Expressed higher levels of ALP, osteopontin, and RUNX2 (4) ALP staining (better osteogenic ability)	
18.	Hou et al. 2009 [15]	(i) *In vitro*	(i) hUC-MSCs (ii) BM-MSCs	(i) BMP-2 treatment: (a) Bone morphogenetic protein 2-blocking antibodies (BMP2 Ab) (b) Recombinant human BMP2 (rhBMP2) (c) Noggin (ii) Osteogenic differentiation medium: (1) DMEM/F12 (2) 10% FBS (3) Dexamethasone (4) Ascorbic acid (AsA) 2-phosphate (5) β-Glycerophosphate (iii) Adipogenic differentiation medium: (1) DMEM/F12 (2) 1% FBS (3) 100 nM dexamethasone (4) 1 nM insulin (iv) Chondrogenic differentiation medium: (1) DMEM/F12 (2) Dexamethasone (3) AsA (4) TGF-β1 (5) ITS$^+$ Premix	(i) Enzymatic digestion (ii) Part of UC: not mentioned	(1) Trilineage differentiation (i) Osteogenesis: osteonectin, ALP, and RUNX2 were expressed (ii) Chondrogenesis: COL II, collagen type X (COL X), and aggrecan were expressed (iii) Adipogenesis: adipsin, PPARγ, and lipoprotein lipase (2) ALP activity was significantly increased in BMP2-induced UC-MSCs (i) Western blot revealed activation of the BMP2 signaling pathway in both cell types via SMADs, p38, and extracellular regulated kinase activation	BMP2-induced UC-MSCs have good osteogenic differentiation (indicated by the activation of BMP2 signaling) and may be used in tissue-engineered bone.

MSCs were found to be superior to WJ-MSCs in terms of differentiating into the osteogenic lineage after 21 days compared. In a different study by Lim and colleagues, MSCs derived from different parts of the umbilical cord, i.e., the fetal, middle, and maternal segments, have the ability to differentiate into osteogenic lineage cells using the osteogenic medium consisting of dexamethasone, ascorbic acid, and β-glycerophosphate. The fetal part was shown to have the best differentiation potential [79]. A study by Hsieh et al. [14] showed that BM-MSCs express more osteogenic genes compared to WJ-MSCs; conversely, WJ-MSCs are more responsible for angiogenesis [66]. Bone morphogenetic protein 2 (BMP-2) was used in a study by Hou et al. to promote osteogenic differentiation in WJ-MSCs [15].

4.2.2. Physical Induction. It is noteworthy that the microenvironment influences cell behaviour and leads to the production of a specific chemical composition that builds the ECM. Therefore, fabricated scaffolds have been actively investigated to find better materials and to produce the best structure of ECM-like components. From the database search, eight out of 18 articles investigated the fabrication of various scaffolds to test the potential of WJ-MSCs to promote complex bone regeneration. Various biomaterials were used to construct these scaffolds, ranging from collagen hydrogels [85] to bioactive glass [80]. 3D scaffolds have been documented as one of the best carriers for cell delivery in bone regeneration. The ideal scaffold should be osteoconductive, biocompatible, and bioresorbable; possess interconnected porosity; and promote cell binding/attachment [82, 86].

The first phase in scaffold development used collagen as the main organic component in bone tissue for bone grafting [85]. Collagen type I can be isolated from Sprague-Dawley rat tails after processing and pelleting. Genipin has been selectively used for crosslinking collagen scaffolds to improve the stability and mechanical strength of the scaffolds in the culture medium [74]. Other crosslinkers have also been used, such as glutaraldehyde and formaldehyde. However, those have been reported to have some cytotoxic effects [87]. Calcium phosphate is another major constituent in bone that has been widely studied as a scaffold material for bone tissue engineering [88]. A study by Karadas et al. [74] produced an in situ mineralized collagen scaffold whereby, after crosslinking with genipin, the scaffold was immersed in a calcium and phosphate solution. As a result, highly integrated calcium phosphate minerals were successfully formed [74]. The combination of collagen I and III has also been reported to resemble the native ECM, where umbilical cord MSCs (UC-MSCs) were found to have better osteogenic potential compared to BM-MSCs [85]. In addition, porcine ECM, derived from the urinary bladder, has also been used as a biomaterial for scaffold preparation as it contains collagen, glycoproteins, glycosaminoglycans, and GFs [89].

Scaffold design then moved to the second phase, in which bioactive glass has been used as a scaffold in bone tissue engineering [80]. Kargozar and colleagues used a combination of bioactive glass/gelatin (BaG/Gel) scaffolds, aiming for a highly porous structure, which is considered ideal for bone substitution. A comprehensive physiochemical analysis showed that the structure had an intact, 3D porous microstructure with interconnected pores. It was also shown that the properties were very close to those of natural spongy bone [80]. They demonstrated that neovascularization was significantly better in the UC-MSC-seeded scaffold when compared to the BM-MSC-seeded scaffold, indicating that the BaG/Gel scaffold is MSC type-dependent. A study by Todeschi and colleagues used hydroxyapatite (HA), beta-tricalcium phosphate (β-TCP), or a mixture of the two [81] as the scaffold. They showed that a significantly higher number of blood vessels were present in the UC-MSC-seeded implants [81].

5. Conclusion

WJ-MSCs were first isolated by Mitchell et al. in 2003. During embryogenesis, totipotent cells such as primordial germ cells and hematopoietic stem cells migrate from the yolk sac through this region to populate target tissues in the embryo and fetus [90]. Characterization indicated that these cells are stem cells, as they express c-kit and can differentiate into neural cells. WJ-MSCs have similar proliferation and differentiation capacity and have multilineage differentiation potential [77], including osteogenesis. This review demonstrates that WJ-MSCs are capable of differentiation into osteoblasts, which may be useful for more effective bone fracture healing as these cells have been shown to migrate into and colonize a collagenous matrix. With the aid of 3D scaffolds, cell proliferation and survival are improved as these scaffolds provide structural stability similar to that of bone. However, MSCs have to be compatible with the scaffold prior to integration and incorporation into engineered bone.

Acknowledgments

The research was carried out with the financial support of Universiti Kebangsaan Malaysia and AMRUS Medik Sdn. Bhd. through research grant numbers FF-2017-482 and FF-2017-020, respectively.

References

[1] M. L. Weiss and D. L. Troyer, "Stem cells in the umbilical cord," *Stem Cell Reviews*, vol. 2, no. 2, pp. 155–162, 2006.

[2] L. Raio, F. Ghezzi, E. di Naro et al., "Prenatal diagnosis of a lean umbilical cord: a simple marker for the fetus at risk of being small for gestational age at birth," *Ultrasound in Obstetrics & Gynecology*, vol. 13, no. 3, pp. 176–180, 1999.

[3] E. Di Naro, F. Ghezzi, L. Raio, M. Franchi, and V. D'Addario, "Umbilical cord morphology and pregnancy outcome," *European Journal of Obstetrics & Gynecology and Reproductive Biology*, vol. 96, no. 2, pp. 150–157, 2001.

[4] F. A. Meyer, Z. Laver-Rudich, and R. Tanenbaum, "Evidence for a mechanical coupling of glycoprotein microfibrils with collagen fibrils in Wharton's jelly," *Biochimica et Biophysica Acta (BBA) - General Subjects*, vol. 755, no. 3, pp. 376–387, 1983.

[5] I. B. Copland, S. L. Adamson, M. Post, S. J. Lye, and I. Caniggia, "TGF-β3 expression during umbilical cord development and its alteration in pre-eclampsia," *Placenta*, vol. 23, no. 4, pp. 311–321, 2002.

[6] M. Mizoguchi, Y. Suga, B. Sanmano, S. Ikeda, and H. Ogawa, "Organotypic culture and surface plantation using umbilical cord epithelial cells: morphogenesis and expression of differentiation markers mimicking cutaneous epidermis," *Journal of Dermatological Science*, vol. 35, no. 3, pp. 199–206, 2004.

[7] J. E. Davies, J. T. Walker, and A. Keating, "Concise review: Wharton's jelly: the rich, but enigmatic, source of mesenchymal stromal cells," *Stem Cells Translational Medicine*, vol. 6, no. 7, pp. 1620–1630, 2017.

[8] K. Sobolewski, E. Bańkowski, L. Chyczewski, and S. Jaworski, "Collagen and glycosaminoglycans of Wharton's jelly," *Neonatology*, vol. 71, no. 1, pp. 11–21, 1997.

[9] H.-S. Wang, et al.S.-C. Hung, S.-T. Peng et al., "Mesenchymal stem cells in the Wharton's jelly of the human umbilical cord," *Stem Cells*, vol. 22, no. 7, pp. 1330–1337, 2004.

[10] I. Kalaszczynska and K. Ferdyn, "Wharton's jelly derived mesenchymal stem cells: future of regenerative medicine? Recent findings and clinical significance," *BioMed Research International*, vol. 2015, Article ID 430847, 11 pages, 2015.

[11] M. Dominici, K. le Blanc, I. Mueller et al., "Minimal criteria for defining multipotent mesenchymal stromal cells. The International Society for Cellular Therapy position statement," *Cytotherapy*, vol. 8, no. 4, pp. 315–317, 2006.

[12] S. Tipnis, C. Viswanathan, and A. S. Majumdar, "Immunosuppressive properties of human umbilical cord-derived mesenchymal stem cells: role of B7-H1 and IDO," *Immunology & Cell Biology*, vol. 88, no. 8, pp. 795–806, 2010.

[13] X. Y. Wang, Y. Lan, W. Y. He et al., "Identification of mesenchymal stem cells in aorta-gonad-mesonephros and yolk sac of human embryos," *Blood*, vol. 111, no. 4, pp. 2436–2443, 2008.

[14] J.-Y. Hsieh, Y.-S. Fu, S.-J. Chang, Y.-H. Tsuang, and H.-W. Wang, "Functional module analysis reveals differential osteogenic and stemness potentials in human mesenchymal stem cells from bone marrow and Wharton's jelly of umbilical cord," *Stem Cells and Development*, vol. 19, no. 12, pp. 1895–1910, 2010.

[15] T. Hou, J. Xu, X. Wu et al., "Umbilical cord Wharton's jelly: a new potential cell source of mesenchymal stromal cells for bone tissue engineering," *Tissue Engineering Part A*, vol. 15, no. 9, pp. 2325–2334, 2009.

[16] K. Baba, Y. Yamazaki, S. Ikemoto, K. Aoyagi, A. Takeda, and E. Uchinuma, "Osteogenic potential of human umbilical cord-derived mesenchymal stromal cells cultured with umbilical cord blood-derived autoserum," *Journal of Cranio-Maxillofacial Surgery*, vol. 40, no. 8, pp. 768–772, 2012.

[17] G. la Rocca, M. Lo Iacono, T. Corsello, S. Corrao, F. Farina, and R. Anzalone, "Human Wharton's jelly mesenchymal stem cells maintain the expression of key immunomodulatory molecules when subjected to osteogenic, adipogenic and chondrogenic differentiation in vitro: new perspectives for cellular therapy," *Current Stem Cell Research & Therapy*, vol. 8, no. 1, pp. 100–113, 2013.

[18] M. Esposito, A. Lucariello, C. Costanzo et al., "Differentiation of human umbilical cord-derived mesenchymal stem cells, *WJ-MSCs*, into chondrogenic cells in the presence of pulsed electromagnetic fields," *In Vivo*, vol. 27, no. 4, pp. 495–500, 2013.

[19] M. Messerli, A. Wagner, R. Sager et al., "Stem cells from umbilical cord Wharton's jelly from preterm birth have neuroglial differentiation potential," *Reproductive Sciences*, vol. 20, no. 12, pp. 1455–1464, 2013.

[20] Y. B. Cui, S. S. Ma, C. Y. Zhang et al., "Human umbilical cord mesenchymal stem cells transplantation improves cognitive function in Alzheimer's disease mice by decreasing oxidative stress and promoting hippocampal neurogenesis," *Behavioural Brain Research*, vol. 320, pp. 291–301, 2017.

[21] I. Garzón, M. A. Martín-Piedra, C. Alfonso-Rodríguez et al., "Generation of a biomimetic human artificial cornea model using wharton's jelly mesenchymal stem cells," *Investigative Opthalmology & Visual Science*, vol. 55, no. 7, pp. 4073–4083, 2014.

[22] J. Hu, Y. Wang, H. Gong et al., "Long term effect and safety of Wharton's jelly-derived mesenchymal stem cells on type 2 diabetes," *Experimental and Therapeutic Medicine*, vol. 12, no. 3, pp. 1857–1866, 2016.

[23] M. L. Weiss, et al.C. Anderson, S. Medicetty et al., "Immune properties of human umbilical cord Wharton's jelly-derived cells," *Stem Cells*, vol. 26, no. 11, pp. 2865–2874, 2008.

[24] F. Granero-Moltó, J. A. Weis, M. I. Miga et al., "Regenerative effects of transplanted mesenchymal stem cells in fracture healing," *Stem Cells*, vol. 27, no. 8, pp. 1887–1898, 2009.

[25] H. Kaneki, R. Guo, D. Chen et al., "Tumor necrosis factor promotes Runx2 degradation through up-regulation of Smurf1 and Smurf2 in osteoblasts," *Journal of Biological Chemistry*, vol. 281, no. 7, pp. 4326–4333, 2006.

[26] X. Zhou, et al.Z. Zhang, J. Q. Feng et al., "Multiple functions of Osterix are required for bone growth and homeostasis in postnatal mice," *Proceedings of the National Academy of Sciences of the United States of America*, vol. 107, no. 29, pp. 12919–12924, 2010.

[27] Y.-i. Kawabe, Y. X. Wang, I. W. McKinnell, M. T. Bedford, and M. A. Rudnicki, "Carm1 regulates Pax7 transcriptional activity through MLL1/2 recruitment during asymmetric satellite stem cell divisions," *Cell Stem Cell*, vol. 11, no. 3, pp. 333–345, 2012.

[28] S. J. Prasanna, D. Gopalakrishnan, S. R. Shankar, and A. B. Vasandan, "Pro-inflammatory cytokines, IFNγ and TNFα, influence immune properties of human bone marrow and Wharton jelly mesenchymal stem cells differentially," *PLoS One*, vol. 5, no. 2, article e9016, 2010.

[29] T. Deuse, M. Stubbendorff, K. Tang-Quan et al., "Immunogenicity and immunomodulatory properties of umbilical cord lining mesenchymal stem cells," *Cell Transplantation*, vol. 20, no. 5, pp. 655–667, 2011.

[30] R. Sarugaser, D. Lickorish, D. Baksh, M. M. Hosseini, and J. E. Davies, "Human umbilical cord perivascular (HUCPV) cells: a source of mesenchymal progenitors," *Stem Cells*, vol. 23, no. 2, pp. 220–229, 2005.

[31] S. B. Goodman, P. Huie, Y. Song et al., "Cellular profile and cytokine production at prosthetic interfaces: study of tissues retrieved from revised hip and knee replacements," *The Journal of Bone and Joint Surgery*, vol. 80, no. 3, pp. 531–539, 1998.

[32] N. M. Moll and R. M. Ransohoff, "CXCL12 and CXCR4 in bone marrow physiology," *Expert Review of Hematology*, vol. 3, no. 3, pp. 315–322, 2010.

[33] E. C. Butcher and L. J. Picker, "Lymphocyte homing and homeostasis," *Science*, vol. 272, no. 5258, pp. 60–67, 1996.

[34] L. da Silva Meirelles, A. M. Fontes, D. T. Covas, and A. I. Caplan, "Mechanisms involved in the therapeutic properties of mesenchymal stem cells," *Cytokine & Growth Factor Reviews*, vol. 20, no. 5-6, pp. 419–427, 2009.

[35] S. Zwingenberger, Z. Yao, A. Jacobi et al., "Enhancement of BMP-2 induced bone regeneration by SDF-1α mediated stem cell recruitment," *Tissue Engineering Part A*, vol. 20, no. 3-4, pp. 810–818, 2014.

[36] I. Majore, P. Moretti, F. Stahl, R. Hass, and C. Kasper, "Growth and differentiation properties of mesenchymal stromal cell populations derived from whole human umbilical cord," *Stem Cell Reviews and Reports*, vol. 7, no. 1, pp. 17–31, 2011.

[37] S. Karahuseyinoglu, O. Cinar, E. Kilic et al., "Biology of stem cells in human umbilical cord stroma: in situ and in vitro surveys," *Stem Cells*, vol. 25, no. 2, pp. 319–331, 2007.

[38] D. J. Hadjidakis and I. I. Androulakis, *Bone Remodeling*, Annals of the New York Academy of Sciences, 2006.

[39] U. Kini and B. N. Nandeesh, "Physiology of bone formation, remodeling, and metabolism," in *Radionuclide and Hybrid Bone Imaging*, pp. 29–57, Springer, Berlin, Heidelberg, 2012.

[40] L. J. Raggatt and N. C. Partridge, "Cellular and molecular mechanisms of bone remodeling," *Journal of Biological Chemistry*, vol. 285, no. 33, pp. 25103–25108, 2010.

[41] S. Kohli and V. Kohli, "Role of RANKL-RANK/osteoprotegerin molecular complex in bone remodeling and its immunopathologic implications," *Indian Journal of Endocrinology and Metabolism*, vol. 15, no. 3, pp. 175–181, 2011.

[42] T. L. Andersen, M. E. Abdelgawad, H. B. Kristensen et al., "Understanding coupling between bone resorption and formation," *The American Journal of Pathology*, vol. 183, no. 1, pp. 235–246, 2013.

[43] M. Borhani-Haghighi, T. Talaei-Khozani, M. Ayatollahi, and Z. Vojdani, "Wharton's jelly-derived mesenchymal stem cells can differentiate into hepatocyte-like cells by HepG2 cell line extract," *Iranian Journal of Medical Sciences*, vol. 40, no. 2, pp. 143–151, 2015.

[44] D. Bharti, S. B. Shivakumar, J.-K. Park et al., "Comparative analysis of human Wharton's jelly mesenchymal stem cells derived from different parts of the same umbilical cord," *Cell and Tissue Research*, vol. 372, no. 1, pp. 51–65, 2018.

[45] D. T. Denhardt and M. Noda, "Osteopontin expression and function: role in bone remodeling," *Journal of Cellular Biochemistry*, vol. 72, no. S30-S31, pp. 92–102, 1998.

[46] J. Klein-Nulend, J. Roelofsen, C. M. Semeins, A. L. J. J. Bronckers, and E. H. Burger, "Mechanical stimulation of osteopontin mRNA expression and synthesis in bone cell cultures," *Journal of Cellular Physiology*, vol. 170, no. 2, pp. 174–181, 1997.

[47] T. M. Liu and E. H. Lee, "Transcriptional regulatory cascades in Runx2-dependent bone development," *Tissue Engineering Part B: Reviews*, vol. 19, no. 3, pp. 254–263, 2013.

[48] T. Komori, "Signaling networks in RUNX2-dependent bone development," *Journal of Cellular Biochemistry*, vol. 112, no. 3, pp. 750–755, 2011.

[49] T. Komori, H. Yagi, S. Nomura et al., "Targeted disruption of *Cbfa1* results in a complete lack of bone formation owing to maturational arrest of osteoblasts," *Cell*, vol. 89, no. 5, pp. 755–764, 1997.

[50] Q. Tu, J. Zhang, L. James et al., "Cbfa1/Runx2-deficiency delays bone wound healing and locally delivered Cbfa1/Runx2 promotes bone repair in animal models," *Wound Repair and Regeneration*, vol. 15, no. 3, pp. 404–412, 2007.

[51] J. H. Jonason, G. Xiao, M. Zhang, L. Xing, and D. Chen, "Post-translational regulation of Runx2 in bone and cartilage," *Journal of Dental Research*, vol. 88, no. 8, pp. 693–703, 2009.

[52] R. T. Franceschi, G. Xiao, D. Jiang, R. Gopalakrishnan, S. Yang, and E. Reith, "Multiple signaling pathways converge on the Cbfa1/Runx2 transcription factor to regulate osteoblast differentiation," *Connective Tissue Research*, vol. 44, no. 1, pp. 109–116, 2003.

[53] M. D. Yazid, S. H. Z. Ariffin, S. Senafi, M. A. Razak, and R. M. A. Wahab, "Determination of the differentiation capacities of murines' primary mononucleated cells and MC3T3-E1 cells," *Cancer Cell International*, vol. 10, no. 1, p. 42, 2010.

[54] F. Ng, S. Boucher, S. Koh et al., "PDGF, TGF-β, and FGF signaling is important for differentiation and growth of mesenchymal stem cells (MSCs): transcriptional profiling can identify markers and signaling pathways important in differentiation of MSCs into adipogenic, chondrogenic, and osteogenic lineages," *Blood*, vol. 112, no. 2, pp. 295–307, 2008.

[55] G. Xiao, D. Jiang, P. Thomas et al., "MAPK pathways activate and phosphorylate the osteoblast-specific transcription factor, Cbfa1," *Journal of Biological Chemistry*, vol. 275, no. 6, pp. 4453–4459, 2000.

[56] N. Rucci, "Molecular biology of bone remodelling," *Clinical Cases in Mineral and Bone Metabolism*, vol. 5, no. 1, pp. 49–56, 2008.

[57] L. F. Bonewald and G. R. Mundy, "Role of transforming growth factor-beta in bone remodeling," *Clinical Orthopaedics and Related Research*, no. 250, pp. 261–276, 1990.

[58] J. M. Hock, M. Centrella, and E. Canalis, "Insulin-like growth factor I has independent effects on bone matrix formation and cell replication," *Endocrinology*, vol. 122, no. 1, pp. 254–260, 1988.

[59] R. M. Locklin, R. O. Oreffo, and J. T. Triffitt, "Effects of TGFβ and BFGF on the differentiation of human bone marrow stromal fibroblasts," *Cell Biology International*, vol. 23, no. 3, pp. 185–194, 1999.

[60] E. Torreggiani, G. Lisignoli, C. Manferdini et al., "Role of slug transcription factor in human mesenchymal stem cells," *Journal of Cellular and Molecular Medicine*, vol. 16, no. 4, pp. 740–751, 2012.

[61] Á. Szepesi, Z. Matula, A. Szigeti et al., "In vitro characterization of human mesenchymal stem cells isolated from different tissues with a potential to promote complex bone regeneration," *Stem Cells International*, vol. 2016, Article ID 3595941, 9 pages, 2016.

[62] A. Subramanian, C. Y. Fong, A. Biswas, and A. Bongso, "Comparative characterization of cells from the various compartments of the human umbilical cord shows that the Wharton's jelly compartment provides the best source of clinically utilizable mesenchymal stem cells," *PLoS One*, vol. 10, no. 6, article e0127992, 2015.

[63] F. Bustos, H. Sepúlveda, C. P. Prieto et al., "Runt-related transcription factor 2 induction during differentiation of Wharton's jelly mesenchymal stem cells to osteoblasts is regulated by Jumonji AT-rich interactive domain 1B histone demethylase," *Stem Cells*, vol. 35, no. 12, pp. 2430–2441, 2017.

[64] Z. Qu, S. Mi, and G. Fang, "Clinical study on treatment of bone nonunion with MSCs derived from human umbilical cord,"

Zhongguo Xiu Fu Chong Jian Wai Ke Za Zhi, vol. 23, no. 3, pp. 345–347, 2009.

[65] P. Li, K. Cui, B. Zhang et al., "Transplantation of human umbilical cord-derived mesenchymal stems cells for the treatment of Becker muscular dystrophy in affected pedigree members," *International Journal of Molecular Medicine*, vol. 35, no. 4, pp. 1051–1057, 2015.

[66] I. H. Dilogo, M. R. A. Primaputra, J. A. Pawitan, and I. K. Liem, "Modified Masquelet technique using allogeneic umbilical cord-derived mesenchymal stem cells for infected non-union femoral shaft fracture with a 12 cm bone defect: a case report," *International Journal of Surgery Case Reports*, vol. 34, pp. 11–16, 2017.

[67] J. Cai, Z. Wu, L. Huang et al., "Cotransplantation of bone marrow mononuclear cells and umbilical cord mesenchymal stem cells in avascular necrosis of the femoral head," *Transplantation Proceedings*, vol. 46, no. 1, pp. 151–155, 2014.

[68] M. Shi, S. Yu, R. Xu, and F. S. Wang, "Human mesenchymal stem cell therapy is feasible for liver cirrhosis associated with HBV infection," *Hepatology International*, vol. 10, no. 1, pp. S341–S342, 2016.

[69] N. Morishima, K. Nakanishi, K. Tsuchiya, T. Shibata, and E. Seiwa, "Translocation of Bim to the endoplasmic reticulum (ER) mediates ER stress signaling for activation of caspase-12 during ER stress-induced apoptosis," *Journal of Biological Chemistry*, vol. 279, no. 48, pp. 50375–50381, 2004.

[70] A. Patel and N. Riordan, "Allogeneic transplantation of human umbilical cord mesenchymal stem cells (UC-MSC) for a single male patient with duchenne muscular dystrophy (DMD)," *Cytotherapy*, vol. 17, no. 6, article S46, 2015.

[71] D.-W. Kim, M. Staples, K. Shinozuka, P. Pantcheva, S.-D. Kang, and C. Borlongan, "Wharton's jelly-derived mesenchymal stem cells: phenotypic characterization and optimizing their therapeutic potential for clinical applications," *International Journal of Molecular Sciences*, vol. 14, no. 6, pp. 11692–11712, 2013.

[72] A. Can, F. T. Celikkan, and O. Cinar, "Umbilical cord mesenchymal stromal cell transplantations: a systemic analysis of clinical trials," *Cytotherapy*, vol. 19, no. 12, pp. 1351–1382, 2017.

[73] M. S. Choudhery, M. Badowski, A. Muise, J. Pierce, and D. T. Harris, "Donor age negatively impacts adipose tissue-derived mesenchymal stem cell expansion and differentiation," *Journal of Translational Medicine*, vol. 12, no. 1, p. 8, 2014.

[74] O. Karadas, D. Yucel, H. Kenar, G. Torun Kose, and V. Hasirci, "Collagen scaffolds with in situ-grown calcium phosphate for osteogenic differentiation of Wharton's jelly and menstrual blood stem cells," *Journal of Tissue Engineering and Regenerative Medicine*, vol. 8, no. 7, pp. 534–545, 2014.

[75] M. Torkaman, M. Ghollasi, M. Mohammadnia-Afrouzi, A. Salimi, and A. Amari, "The effect of transplanted human Wharton's jelly mesenchymal stem cells treated with IFN-γ on experimental autoimmune encephalomyelitis mice," *Cellular Immunology*, vol. 311, pp. 1–12, 2017.

[76] K. O'Donoghue, M. Choolani, J. Chan et al., "Identification of fetal mesenchymal stem cells in maternal blood: implications for non-invasive prenatal diagnosis," *Molecular Human Reproduction*, vol. 9, no. 8, pp. 497–502, 2003.

[77] D. Baksh, R. Yao, and R. S. Tuan, "Comparison of proliferative and multilineage differentiation potential of human mesenchymal stem cells derived from umbilical cord and bone marrow," *Stem Cells*, vol. 25, no. 6, pp. 1384–1392, 2007.

[78] I. Arutyunyan, A. Elchaninov, A. Makarov, and T. Fatkhudinov, "Umbilical cord as prospective source for mesenchymal stem cell-based therapy," *Stem Cells International*, vol. 2016, Article ID 6901286, 17 pages, 2016.

[79] J. Lim, Z. R. M. Razi, J. Law, A. M. Nawi, R. B. H. Idrus, and M. H. Ng, "MSCs can be differentially isolated from maternal, middle and fetal segments of the human umbilical cord," *Cytotherapy*, vol. 18, no. 12, pp. 1493–1502, 2016.

[80] S. Kargozar, M. Mozafari, S. J. Hashemian et al., "Osteogenic potential of stem cells-seeded bioactive nanocomposite scaffolds: a comparative study between human mesenchymal stem cells derived from bone, umbilical cord Wharton's jelly, and adipose tissue," *Journal of Biomedical Materials Research Part B: Applied Biomaterials*, vol. 106, no. 1, pp. 61–72, 2018.

[81] M. R. Todeschi, R. el Backly, C. Capelli et al., "Transplanted umbilical cord mesenchymal stem cells modify the in vivo microenvironment enhancing angiogenesis and leading to bone regeneration," *Stem Cells and Development*, vol. 24, no. 13, pp. 1570–1581, 2015.

[82] L. Polo-Corrales, M. Latorre-Esteves, and J. E. Ramirez-Vick, "Scaffold design for bone regeneration," *Journal of Nanoscience and Nanotechnology*, vol. 14, no. 1, pp. 15–56, 2014.

[83] A. K. Batsali, C. Pontikoglou, D. Koutroulakis et al., "Differential expression of cell cycle and WNT pathway-related genes accounts for differences in the growth and differentiation potential of Wharton's jelly and bone marrow-derived mesenchymal stem cells," *Stem Cell Research & Therapy*, vol. 8, no. 1, p. 102, 2017.

[84] A. Zajdel, M. Kałucka, E. Kokoszka-Mikołaj, and A. Wilczok, "Osteogenic differentiation of human mesenchymal stem cells from adipose tissue and Wharton's jelly of the umbilical cord," *Acta Biochimica Polonica*, vol. 64, no. 2, pp. 365–369, 2017.

[85] R. K. Schneider, A. Puellen, R. Kramann et al., "The osteogenic differentiation of adult bone marrow and perinatal umbilical mesenchymal stem cells and matrix remodelling in three-dimensional collagen scaffolds," *Biomaterials*, vol. 31, no. 3, pp. 467–480, 2010.

[86] S. Bose, M. Roy, and A. Bandyopadhyay, "Recent advances in bone tissue engineering scaffolds," *Trends in Biotechnology*, vol. 30, no. 10, pp. 546–554, 2012.

[87] H. W. Sun, R. J. Feigal, and H. H. Messer, "Cytotoxicity of glutaraldehyde and formaldehyde in relation to time of exposure and concentration," *Pediatric Dentistry*, vol. 12, no. 5, pp. 303–307, 1990.

[88] S. Mechiche Alami, H. Rammal, C. Boulagnon-Rombi et al., "Harnessing Wharton's jelly stem cell differentiation into bone-*like* nodule on calcium phosphate substrate without osteoinductive factors," *Acta Biomaterialia*, vol. 49, pp. 575–589, 2017.

[89] L. Penolazzi, S. Mazzitelli, R. Vecchiatini et al., "Human mesenchymal stem cells seeded on extracellular matrix-scaffold: viability and osteogenic potential," *Journal of Cellular Physiology*, vol. 227, no. 2, pp. 857–866, 2012.

[90] K. E. Mitchell, M. L. Weiss, B. M. Mitchell et al., "Matrix cells from Wharton's jelly form neurons and glia," *Stem Cells*, vol. 21, no. 1, pp. 50–60, 2003.

[91] Y. S. Fu, C. H. Lu, K. A. Chu et al., "Xenograft of human umbilical mesenchymal stem cells from Wharton's jelly differentiating into osteocytes and reducing osteoclast activity reverses osteoporosis in ovariectomized rats," *Cell Transplantation*, vol. 27, no. 1, pp. 194–208, 2018.

[92] F. E. Al Jofi, T. Ma, D. Guo et al., "Functional organic cation transporters mediate osteogenic response to metformin in human umbilical cord mesenchymal stromal cells," *Cytotherapy*, vol. 20, no. 5, pp. 650–659, 2018.

[93] A. Ramesh, M. M. Kanafi, and R. R. Bhonde, "Modulus-dependent characteristics of Wharton's jelly mesenchymal stem cells (WJMSC) encapsulated in hydrogel microspheres," *Journal of Biomaterials Science, Polymer Edition*, vol. 25, no. 17, pp. 1946–1961, 2014.

[94] L. Wang, L. Zhao, and M. S. Detamore, "Human umbilical cord mesenchymal stromal cells in a sandwich approach for osteochondral tissue engineering," *Journal of Tissue Engineering and Regenerative Medicine*, vol. 5, no. 9, pp. 712–721, 2011.

4

Chimeric RNA in Cancer and Stem Cell Differentiation

Justin Elfman[1] **and Hui Li**[1,2]

[1]*Department of Biochemistry and Molecular Genetics, University of Virginia, 22903, USA*
[2]*Department of Pathology, University of Virginia, 22903, USA*

Correspondence should be addressed to Hui Li; hl9r@virginia.edu

Academic Editor: Jacob H. Hanna

Gene fusions are considered hallmarks of cancer which can be produced by chromosomal rearrangements. These DNA-level fusion events may result in the expression of chimeric RNAs; however, chimeric RNAs can be also produced by intergenic splicing events. Chimeric transcripts created by the latter mechanism are regulated at the transcriptional level and thus present additional modes of action and regulation. They have demonstrated importance in normal cell physiology, and their dysregulation can induce oncogenesis and impact cell differentiation. In this review, we outline proven mechanisms through which intergenically spliced chimeric RNAs are involved in carcinogenesis. We highlight their similarity to canonical chimeric RNAs resulting from gene fusions as well as their unique qualities. Additionally, we review known roles of chimeric RNA in cell differentiation and propose means through which chimeric RNAs may be valuable as stage-specific markers or as targets for expression profiling.

1. Introduction

Chimeric RNAs are transcripts comprising the nucleotide sequence from different parental genes [1–5]. These transcripts are known to not only be produced by gene fusion but can also be formed via intergenic splicing events. Intergenically spliced chimeric RNAs have been shown to occur via *cis*-splicing of adjacent genes (*cis*-SAGe) as well as long-range intrachromosomal and interchromosomal *trans*-splicing events [3, 5, 6]. While specific mechanisms for intergenically spliced chimeric RNA generation are unclear, some recurring patterns have emerged. For instance, in *cis*-SAGe chimeras, most transcripts follow the 2-2 rule, where the penultimate exon of the $5'$ gene is spliced to the second exon of the $3'$ gene [7, 8], and several occurrences of intergenic *trans*-splicing have been found to occur between neighboring genes on opposite strands [9–12]. Both patterns suggest potential importance of parental gene proximity in chimeric RNA production. Despite their mysterious origin, intergenically spliced chimeric RNAs are found across tissue types and have proven importance in normal cell states [2, 3, 5, 8] as well as demonstrated roles in both oncogenesis and cell differentiation. While similar in concept to chimeric transcripts created by gene fusion, transcription-level processing presents additional functionality and nuanced regulation unique to intergenically spliced chimeras. In this review, we present several examples of similarities between both sources of chimeric RNA as well as these differences. We also present examples of chimeric RNAs involved in oncogenesis and cell differentiation as well as further possible mechanisms for the role of chimeric RNA in these events. Finally, we highlight the potential of chimeric RNA to serve as a cell type and stage-specific marker for expression profiling.

2. Gene Fusion and Fusion Transcripts

In this manuscript, we refer to chimeric RNAs generated by gene fusions as *fusion transcripts*. These transcripts are typically transcribed from abnormal genomic regions created by chromosomal rearrangement rather than by intergenic splicing. Gene fusions are often distinctive features of particular cancer types and generate cytogenetic

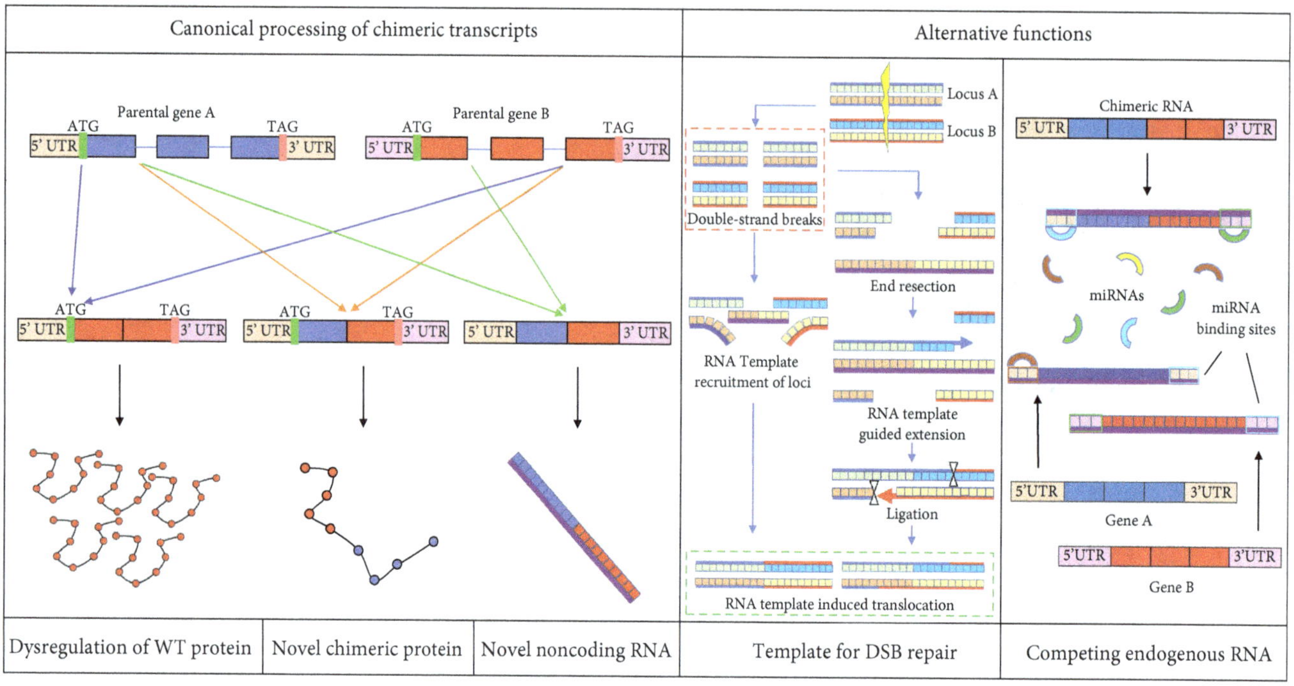

(a) (b) (c)

FIGURE 1: Implications of chimeric RNA in oncogenesis. (a) Canonical processing of chimeric transcripts. Colored rectangles represent exons, and connecting lines represent introns. Colored arrows indicate splicing configuration. Circles represent amino acids, and the nucleic acid with a purple backbone represents a mature mRNA transcript. Canonical processing includes dysregulation of a wild-type protein via splicing an ectopic UTR to a wild-type coding sequence, splicing of two in-frame coding sequences to produce a novel protein, and splicing into long noncoding RNA. (b) Chimeric RNA as a template for DSB repair. Two possible mechanisms are presented: chimeric RNA can serve as a template to recruit two distant genomic loci into proximity; chimeric RNA can serve as a homologous template for translocation of two distant genomic loci. (c) Chimeric RNA as ceRNA. Chimeric transcripts retain sequence homology with parental genes, thus potentially retaining miRNA binding sites to compete for local miRNAs.

signatures characteristic of different malignancies. These have been successfully used as diagnostic markers [13, 14] as well as therapeutic targets [15–17].

This is perhaps best exemplified by the *BCR-ABL1* fusion, which encodes a novel tyrosine kinase in chronic myelogenous leukemia [16]. The BCR-ABL1 fusion protein provides additional regulatory binding domains contained within BCR to the ABL1 tyrosine kinase, which increases the number of potential targets for the kinase [16]. The *BCR-ABL1* fusion has been used as a biomarker as well as a therapeutic target by the drug imatinib, which binds specifically to the kinase active site. As a result, patients diagnosed within the *BCR-ABL1* subtype have favorable prognoses [15, 16, 18].

Gene fusions can also induce oncogenesis without producing a novel protein. One such example combines the 5′ UTR of *TMPRSS2* to a member of the *ETS* transcription factor family (*TMPRSS2-ETS*). TMPRSS2 is a serine protease which is upregulated in response to androgen activation. The ETS family of transcription factors regulates a multitude of key cellular processes, and dysregulation can result in oncogenesis. ETS is overexpressed in 50% of all prostate cancers, of which 90% exhibit the *TMPRSS2-ETS* fusion. This fusion introduces an androgen-responsive regulatory element to ETS, which upregulates the ETS expression in response to androgen activation, leading to oncogenesis [14, 19, 20].

3. Intergenically Spliced Chimeric RNAs

Similar to fusion transcripts, chimeric RNAs generated by intergenic splicing can give rise to fusion proteins, which reflect the combined coding sequence of its parental genes (Figure 1(a)). Some of these transcripts are identical to those created by hallmark gene fusion events, which produce oncogenic proteins. Events which create these gene fusions at the DNA level result in constitutive overexpression of the chimeric RNA and therefore overexpression of the novel fusion protein. One prominent example is the *JAZF1-JJAZ1* gene fusion prevalent in endometrial stromal sarcoma. Both the chimeric RNA and protein are also present in normal endometrial stromal cells, and overexpression of the protein confers antiapoptotic activity, promoting cell survival [1, 21].

Intergenically spliced chimeric RNAs have also been shown to utilize the ETS family of transcription factors. Several such examples have been published including the *SLC45A3-ELK4* chimeras. Similar to *TMPRSS2*, *SLC45A3* (solute carrier family 45, member 3) is an androgen-responsive gene specifically expressed in the prostate. Rickman et al. described a chimera joining exon 1 of *SLC45A3* to exon 2 of *ELK4*. Notably, as *SLC45A3* exon 1 does not contain a coding sequence, the chimeric RNA adopts an androgen-responsive 5′ untranslated region while coding for wild-type ELK4 [22]. Maher et al. detected an isoform which joined *SLC45A3* exon 4 to *ELK4* exon 2 and also showed association with prostate cancer [23]. Further characterization of *SLC45A3-ELK4* chimeras showed that the transcript was created through *cis*-SAGe rather than *trans*-splicing [24], and most notably the exon 1/exon 2 form of the chimera functions as an androgen-responsive chimeric long noncoding RNA [25] (Figure 1(a)).

4. Chimeric RNA as Potential Templates for RNA-Guided DSB Repair and Rearrangement

An overlap between common loci for chromosomal translocation and parental genes involved in intergenic splicing may not be coincidental. As chimeric *trans*-splicing requires both parental transcripts to be present, it is likely that these events may be dependent upon the spatial proximity of the parental genes. It is well known that three-dimensional proximity of genomic regions increases the likelihood for translocation to occur between those regions through erroneous repair following double-strand breaks (DSB) [26–28]. Specific examples include *BCR-ABL1* and *MYC-IGH*, which are hallmarks of chronic myelogenous leukemia and Burkitt's lymphoma, respectively [28]. RNA templates or corresponding cDNA have been shown to mediate homologous recombination and DSB repair in the absence of a homologous chromosome [29–31]. Several authors have suggested that *trans*-spliced chimeric RNA or reverse-transcribed chimeric cDNA may serve as template for DNA rearrangement [3, 9, 32, 33], which would provide another mechanism for the induction of DNA-level gene fusion (Figure 1(b)). The occurrence of chimeric transcripts such as *JAZF1-JJAZ1* and *PAX3-FOXO1* (described hereafter), in both normal and neoplastic cells, supports this possibility.

5. Chimeric RNA as Potential Competing Endogenous RNA

In addition, similarity in sequence to parental genes presents chimeric RNAs as candidates to serve as competing endogenous RNAs (ceRNA), or micro RNA (miRNA) sponges, for both parental genes (Figure 1(c)). Recently, competing functions of transcribed noncoding regions of the genome have been described which are affected in certain subtypes of cancer [34]. Particular emphasis is placed on transcribed pseudogenes due to sequence homology, tissue-specific expression, and evolutionary conservation despite their lack of coding functionality [34–36]. Typically, ceRNAs are thought to compete with other transcripts of similar sequence by means of common miRNA binding sites. miRNA regulation has been implicated in many cancers, among other diseases [37, 38], and dysregulation of ceRNAs such as *HULC* or *PTENP1* can lead to oncogenesis [35, 39].

6. Chimeric and *Trans*-Spliced RNAs in Stem Cell Differentiation

Stem cell differentiation is generally considered a sequential process in which cells acquire new characteristics. These changes largely occur without alteration to the genome. Instead, iterative changes to the epigenome, primarily driven by the action of transcription factors (TF), coordinate cell fates [40–43]. Chromatin accessibility changes through the course of cell differentiation, induced by TF specific to cell type. These TF have been used to generate profiles indicative of cell stages through differentiation [40, 43]. TF regulation can affect cell differentiation [42, 44, 45] and can produce undifferentiated or dedifferentiated phenotypes characteristic of certain cancers [42, 45–47]. Further, the genome undergoes significant changes in higher-order chromatin organization through stages of differentiation [48, 49], which affect interaction frequencies between gene compartments as well as genes within these compartments.

Any of these changes have the potential to disrupt or introduce expression of chimeric RNAs. Thus, many chimeric transcripts show considerable tissue specificity [5, 50], several of which have been shown to be upregulated in cancer [4, 22–24, 51]. A subset of these are regulated through cell differentiation and can consist of TF parental genes [50]. One such example is a chimeric *PAX3-FOXO1* transcript which is formed through joining the DNA-binding domain of PAX3 to the transactivation domain of FOXO1 [52]. This chimeric RNA is identical in form to the *PAX3-FOXO1* hallmark gene fusion found in alveolar rhabdomyosarcoma (ARMS), a small blue round cell tumor with characteristic undifferentiation. The transcript is translated into a novel TF which regulates genes involved in myogenesis, myogenic signaling, and mesodermal development [53], and it has been shown to interfere with normal PAX3 and FOXO1 activity [54]. Chimeric *PAX3-FOXO1* is regulated through myogenesis, and its dysregulation interferes with proper differentiation [55].

Alternative intragenically *trans*-spliced RNAs (tsRNA) have also been shown to regulate embryonic stem cell differentiation. Through applying stringent criteria to predicted chimeric products, Wu et al. uncovered four noncollinear *trans*-spliced mRNAs which exhibited differential expression between *trans*-spliced and wild-type isoforms as well as differentiated and undifferentiated cell types. The tsRNAs also showed differing tissue specificity when compared to the wild-type transcripts and showed that the knockdown of one such long noncoding tsRNA impaired pluripotency maintenance through interaction with pluripotency-associated factors NANOG and SUZ12 [56].

7. Chimeric RNA Expression Profiling

Tissue and cell-stage specificity of chimeric RNAs and tsRNAs provides a strong basis for expression profiling. In fact, chimeric RNA profiling has been successfully used as a means to cluster cells from similar nonneoplastic tissue types [50] (Figure 2). Further, chimeric RNAs offer a unique opportunity to identify unknown cell of origin in undifferentiated tumor types. Exploring this possibility in ARMS, Xie et al. performed chimeric transcriptome profiling at four time points throughout myogenesis and found that the majority of chimeric RNAs were generated transiently and exclusively during differentiation. They were able to determine the chimeric RNA profile of RH30, an ARMS cell line, and found

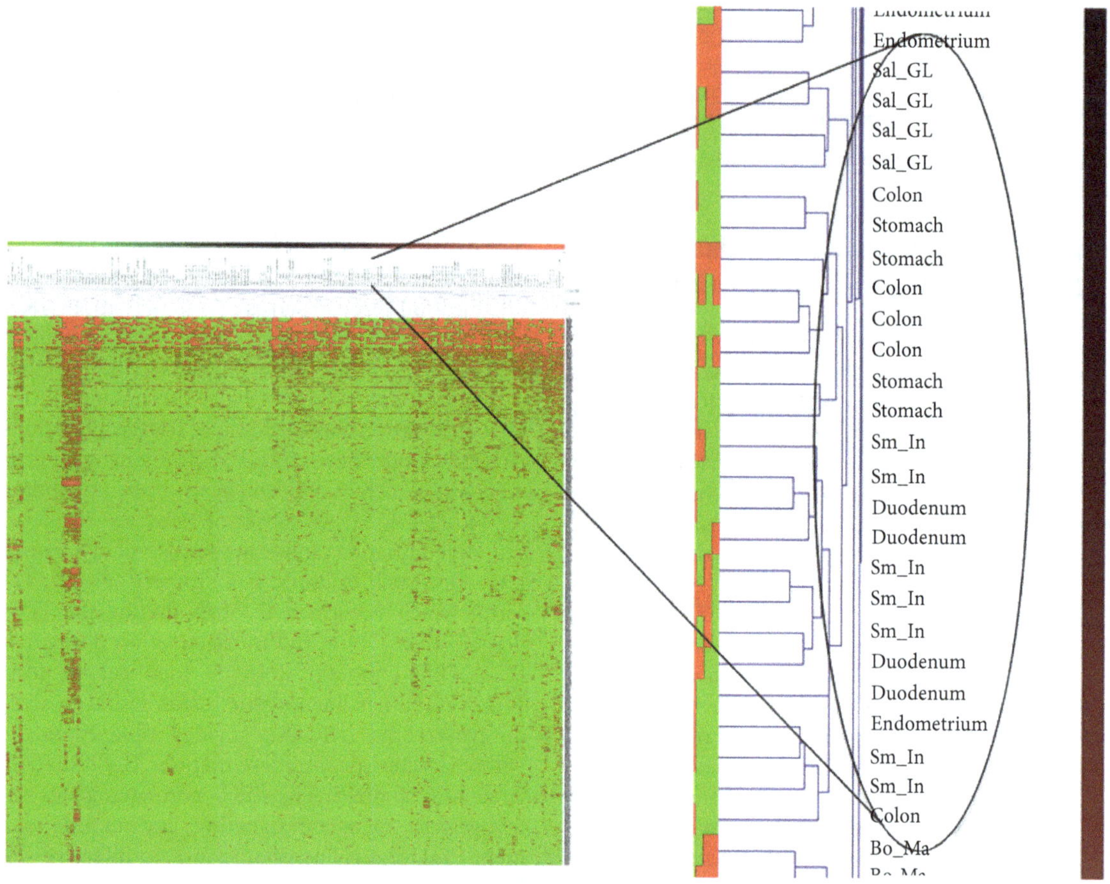

FIGURE 2: Unsupervised clustering of 27 nonneoplastic tissue samples from 171 RNA-Seq libraries by chimeric RNA expression group tissues with common developmental origin.

a set of 18 chimeric RNAs which appeared to be uniquely expressed by RH30 at one specific time point during myogenesis [50]. These findings are also in agreement with time-specific expression of myogenic expression of *PAX3-FOXO1* in an earlier study [2]. This methodology offers another valuable perspective to identifying cell of origin and may provide insight into other mysterious tumors.

8. Conclusion

Several exemplary cases of chimeric RNAs presented herein are shown to play roles in crucial cell processes; these are not likely isolated phenomena. Recurrent chimeric RNAs have been predicted and validated across various tissue types, and several have shown functional relevance in cell proliferation or motility [5, 24, 51]. The presence of chimeric RNAs in cancer and precancer lesions supports their potential as biomarkers and therapeutic targets. Chimeric transcripts may provide means for oncogenesis in cancers with notably low mutational burden such as acute myeloid leukemia [57, 58] or are perhaps veiled contributing factors to cancers with multiple oncogenic sources. Further, if proposed mechanisms for chimeric RNA-templated chromosomal translocation and activity as ceRNA are found to be true, controlled regulation of chimeric transcripts could play an important role in preventative cancer treatment.

Tissue and cell-stage specificity provides additional utility for the use of chimeric RNAs as diagnostic indicators. Increased accuracy in tissue profiling studies could improve specificity in treatments targeting particular cell types, and chimeric RNAs offer another avenue towards this end. The presence of chimeric RNAs which mirror hallmark cancerous fusions in precancer cells could also provide information on the cell of origin for mysterious tumors. Further, cell-stage specificity of chimeric RNA expression may give insight into particular pathologies for cancer progression.

In summary, while the mechanisms for chimeric RNA creation are not entirely clear, their importance and dynamic functionality continue to be proven. Chimeric RNA presents an underexplored library of biomarkers and regulatory pathways which could improve clinical treatment, provide insight into unknown oncogenic pathologies, and help to understand or classify mysterious differentiation states and tissues of origin.

Acknowledgments

We thank Drs. Mihaela Babiceanu and Zhongqiu Xie for

their assistance with chimeric RNA profiling. H.L. is currently supported by an American Cancer Society research scholar, a St. Baldrick's Foundation scholar, and NIH grant CA190713.

References

[1] H. Li, J. Wang, G. Mor, and J. Sklar, "A neoplastic gene fusion mimics trans-splicing of RNAs in normal human cells," *Science*, vol. 321, no. 5894, pp. 1357–1361, 2008.

[2] H. Yuan, F. Qin, M. Movassagh et al., "A chimeric RNA characteristic of rhabdomyosarcoma in normal myogenesis process," *Cancer Discovery*, vol. 3, no. 12, pp. 1394–1403, 2013.

[3] K. Jividen and H. Li, "Chimeric RNAs generated by intergenic splicing in normal and cancer cells," *Genes, Chromosomes and Cancer*, vol. 53, no. 12, pp. 963–971, 2014.

[4] F. Qin, Z. Song, M. Chang, Y. Song, H. Frierson, and H. Li, "Recurrent cis-SAGe chimeric RNA, *D2HGDH-GAL3ST2*, in prostate cancer," *Cancer Letters*, vol. 380, no. 1, pp. 39–46, 2016.

[5] M. Babiceanu, F. Qin, Z. Xie et al., "Recurrent chimeric fusion RNAs in non-cancer tissues and cells," *Nucleic Acids Research*, vol. 44, no. 6, pp. 2859–2872, 2016.

[6] K. Chwalenia, L. Facemire, and H. Li, "Chimeric RNAs in cancer and normal physiology," *Wiley Interdisciplinary Reviews: RNA*, vol. 8, no. 6, 2017.

[7] Y. Jia, Z. Xie, and H. Li, "Intergenically spliced chimeric RNAs in cancer," *Trends in Cancer*, vol. 2, no. 9, pp. 475–484, 2016.

[8] F. Qin, Z. Song, M. Babiceanu et al., "Discovery of CTCF-sensitive cis-spliced fusion RNAs between adjacent genes in human prostate cells," *PLoS Genetics*, vol. 11, no. 2, article e1005001, 2015.

[9] T. R. Gingeras, "Implications of chimaeric non-co-linear transcripts," *Nature*, vol. 461, no. 7261, pp. 206–211, 2009.

[10] X. Li, L. Zhao, H. Jiang, and W. Wang, "Short homologous sequences are strongly associated with the generation of chimeric RNAs in eukaryotes," *Journal of Molecular Evolution*, vol. 68, no. 1, pp. 56–65, 2009.

[11] R. Dorn, G. Reuter, and A. Loewendorf, "Transgene analysis proves mRNA trans-splicing at the complex *mod(mdg4)* locus in *Drosophila*," *Proceedings of the National Academy of Sciences of the United States of America*, vol. 98, no. 17, pp. 9724–9729, 2001.

[12] C. J. McManus, M. O. Duff, J. Eipper-Mains, and B. R. Graveley, "Global analysis of *trans*-splicing in *Drosophila*," *Proceedings of the National Academy of Sciences of the United States of America*, vol. 107, no. 29, pp. 12975–12979, 2010.

[13] E. Missiaglia, D. Williamson, J. Chisholm et al., "*PAX3/FOXO1* fusion gene status is the key prognostic molecular marker in rhabdomyosarcoma and significantly improves current risk stratification," *Journal of Clinical Oncology*, vol. 30, no. 14, pp. 1670–1677, 2012.

[14] S. A. Tomlins, D. R. Rhodes, S. Perner et al., "Recurrent fusion of *TMPRSS2* and ETS transcription factor genes in prostate cancer," *Science*, vol. 310, no. 5748, pp. 644–648, 2005.

[15] C. S. Huettner, P. Zhang, R. A. Van Etten, and D. G. Tenen, "Reversibility of acute B-cell leukaemia induced by *BCR-ABL1*," *Nature Genetics*, vol. 24, no. 1, pp. 57–60, 2000.

[16] R. Ren, "Mechanisms of BCR–ABL in the pathogenesis of chronic myelogenous leukaemia," *Nature Reviews Cancer*, vol. 5, no. 3, pp. 172–183, 2005.

[17] A. T. Shaw, B. Y. Yeap, B. J. Solomon et al., "Effect of crizotinib on overall survival in patients with advanced non-small-celllung cancer harbouring *ALK* gene rearrangement: a retrospective analysis," *The Lancet Oncology*, vol. 12, no. 11, pp. 1004-1012, 2011.

[18] O. Hantschel, U. Rix, and G. Superti-Furga, "Target spectrum of the BCR-ABL inhibitors imatinib, nilotinib and dasatinib," *Leukemia & Lymphoma*, vol. 49, no. 4, pp. 615–619, 2008.

[19] S. A. Tomlins, B. Laxman, S. Varambally et al., "Role of the *TMPRSS2-ERG* gene fusion in prostate cancer," *Neoplasia*, vol. 10, no. 2, pp. 177–188, 2008.

[20] F. Demichelis and M. A. Rubin, "*TMPRSS2-ETS* fusion prostate cancer: biological and clinical implications," *Journal of Clinical Pathology*, vol. 60, no. 11, pp. 1185-1186, 2007.

[21] H. Li, X. Ma, J. Wang, J. Koontz, M. Nucci, and J. Sklar, "Effects of rearrangement and allelic exclusion of *JJAZ1/SUZ12* on cell proliferation and survival," *Proceedings of the National Academy of Sciences of the United States of America*, vol. 104, no. 50, pp. 20001–20006, 2007.

[22] D. S. Rickman, D. Pflueger, B. Moss et al., "SLC45A3-ELK4 is a novel and frequent erythroblast transformation–specific fusion transcript in prostate cancer," *Cancer Research*, vol. 69, no. 7, pp. 2734–2738, 2009.

[23] C. A. Maher, C. Kumar-Sinha, X. Cao et al., "Transcriptome sequencing to detect gene fusions in cancer," *Nature*, vol. 458, no. 7234, pp. 97–101, 2009.

[24] Y. Zhang, M. Gong, H. Yuan, H. G. Park, H. F. Frierson, and H. Li, "Chimeric transcript generated by cis-splicing of adjacent genes regulates prostate cancer cell proliferation," *Cancer Discovery*, vol. 2, no. 7, pp. 598–607, 2012.

[25] F. Qin, Y. Zhang, J. Liu, and H. Li, "*SLC45A3-ELK4* functions as a long non-coding chimeric RNA," *Cancer Letters*, vol. 404, pp. 53–61, 2017.

[26] M. R. Branco and A. Pombo, "Intermingling of chromosome territories in interphase suggests role in translocations and transcription-dependent associations," *PLoS Biology*, vol. 4, no. 5, article e138, 2006.

[27] H. A. Foster, G. Estrada-Girona, M. Themis et al., "Relative proximity of chromosome territories influences chromosome exchange partners in radiation-induced chromosome rearrangements in primary human bronchial epithelial cells," *Mutation Research/Genetic Toxicology and Environmental Mutagenesis*, vol. 756, no. 1-2, pp. 66–77, 2013.

[28] J. M. Engreitz, V. Agarwala, and L. A. Mirny, "Three-dimensional genome architecture influences partner selection for chromosomal translocations in human disease," *PLoS One*, vol. 7, no. 9, article e44196, 2012.

[29] F. Storici, K. Bebenek, T. A. Kunkel, D. A. Gordenin, and M. A. Resnick, "RNA-templated DNA repair," *Nature*, vol. 447, no. 7142, pp. 338–341, 2007.

[30] H. Keskin, Y. Shen, F. Huang et al., "Transcript-RNA-templated DNA recombination and repair," *Nature*, vol. 515, no. 7527, pp. 436–439, 2014.

[31] H. Keskin, C. Meers, and F. Storici, "Transcript RNA supports precise repair of its own DNA gene," *RNA Biology*, vol. 13, no. 2, pp. 157–165, 2016.

[32] M. Nowacki, V. Vijayan, Y. Zhou, K. Schotanus, T. G. Doak, and L. F. Landweber, "RNA-mediated epigenetic programming of a genome-rearrangement pathway," *Nature*, vol. 451, no. 7175, pp. 153–158, 2008.

[33] W. Fang and L. F. Landweber, "RNA-mediated genome rearrangement: hypotheses and evidence," *BioEssays*, vol. 35, no. 2, pp. 84–87, 2013.

[34] L. Salmena, L. Poliseno, Y. Tay, L. Kats, and P. P. Pandolfi, "A *ceRNA* hypothesis: the Rosetta Stone of a hidden RNA language?," *Cell*, vol. 146, no. 3, pp. 353–358, 2011.

[35] L. Poliseno, L. Salmena, J. Zhang, B. Carver, W. J. Haveman, and P. P. Pandolfi, "A coding-independent function of gene and pseudogene mRNAs regulates tumour biology," *Nature*, vol. 465, no. 7301, pp. 1033–1038, 2010.

[36] R. C. Pink, K. Wicks, D. P. Caley, E. K. Punch, L. Jacobs, and D. R. Francisco Carter, "Pseudogenes: pseudo-functional or key regulators in health and disease?," *RNA*, vol. 17, no. 5, pp. 792–798, 2011.

[37] G. A. Calin, C. D. Dumitru, M. Shimizu et al., "Frequent deletions and down-regulation of micro- RNA genes *miR15* and *miR16* at 13q14 in chronic lymphocytic leukemia," *Proceedings of the National Academy of Sciences of the United States of America*, vol. 99, no. 24, pp. 15524–15529, 2002.

[38] M. Lu, Q. Zhang, M. Deng et al., "An analysis of human microRNA and disease associations," *PLoS One*, vol. 3, no. 10, article e3420, 2008.

[39] J. Wang, X. Liu, H. Wu et al., "CREB up-regulates long noncoding RNA, HULC expression through interaction with microRNA-372 in liver cancer," *Nucleic Acids Research*, vol. 38, no. 16, pp. 5366–5383, 2010.

[40] A. B. Stergachis, S. Neph, A. Reynolds et al., "Developmental fate and cellular maturity encoded in human regulatory DNA landscapes," *Cell*, vol. 154, no. 4, pp. 888-903, 2013.

[41] V. Azuara, P. Perry, S. Sauer et al., "Chromatin signatures of pluripotent cell lines," *Nature Cell Biology*, vol. 8, no. 5, pp. 532–538, 2006.

[42] A. M. Reimold, N. N. Iwakoshi, J. Manis et al., "Plasma cell differentiation requires the transcription factor XBP-1," *Nature*, vol. 412, no. 6844, pp. 300–307, 2001.

[43] L. Warren, D. Bryder, I. L. Weissman, and S. R. Quake, "Transcription factor profiling in individual hematopoietic progenitors by digital RT-PCR," *Proceedings of the National Academy of Sciences*, vol. 103, no. 47, pp. 17807–17812, 2006.

[44] S. Hori, T. Nomura, and S. Sakaguchi, "Control of regulatory T cell development by the transcription factor *Foxp3*," *Science*, vol. 299, no. 5609, pp. 1057–1061, 2003.

[45] H. Niwa, J. Miyazaki, and A. G. Smith, "Quantitative expression of Oct-3/4 defines differentiation, dedifferentiation or self-renewal of ES cells," *Nature Genetics*, vol. 24, no. 4, pp. 372–376, 2000.

[46] E. Batlle, E. Sancho, C. Francí et al., "The transcription factor Snail is a repressor of *E-cadherin* gene expression in epithelial tumour cells," *Nature Cell Biology*, vol. 2, no. 2, pp. 84–89, 2000.

[47] S. Cereghini, M. Yaniv, and R. Cortese, "Hepatocyte dedifferentiation and extinction is accompanied by a block in the synthesis of mRNA coding for the transcription factor HNF1/LFB1," *The EMBO Journal*, vol. 9, no. 7, pp. 2257–2263, 1990.

[48] J. R. Dixon, S. Selvaraj, F. Yue et al., "Topological domains in mammalian genomes identified by analysis of chromatin interactions," *Nature*, vol. 485, no. 7398, pp. 376–380, 2012.

[49] S. H. Kim, P. G. McQueen, M. K. Lichtman, E. M. Shevach, L. A. Parada, and T. Misteli, "Spatial genome organization during T-cell differentiation," *Cytogenetic and Genome Research*, vol. 105, no. 2–4, pp. 292–301, 2004.

[50] Z. Xie, M. Babiceanu, S. Kumar et al., "Fusion transcriptome profiling provides insights into alveolar rhabdomyosarcoma," *Proceedings of the National Academy of Sciences*, vol. 113, no. 46, pp. 13126–13131, 2016.

[51] K. E. Varley, J. Gertz, B. S. Roberts et al., "Recurrent read-through fusion transcripts in breast cancer," *Breast Cancer Research and Treatment*, vol. 146, no. 2, pp. 287–297, 2014.

[52] C. M. Linardic, "*PAX3–FOXO1* fusion gene in rhabdomyosarcoma," *Cancer Letters*, vol. 270, no. 1, pp. 10–18, 2008.

[53] J. Khan, R. Simon, M. Bittner et al., "Gene expression profiling of alveolar rhabdomyosarcoma with cDNA microarrays," *Cancer Research*, vol. 58, no. 22, pp. 5009–5013, 1998.

[54] M. Schmitt-Ney and G. Camussi, "The PAX3-FOXO1 fusion protein present in rhabdomyosarcoma interferes with normal FOXO activity and the TGF-β pathway," *PLoS One*, vol. 10, no. 3, article e0121474, 2015.

[55] F. Graf Finckenstein, V. Shahbazian, E. Davicioni, Y.-X. Ren, and M. J. Anderson, "PAX-FKHR function as pangenes by simultaneously inducing and inhibiting myogenesis," *Oncogene*, vol. 27, no. 14, pp. 2004–2014, 2008.

[56] C.-S. Wu, C. Y. Yu, C. Y. Chuang et al., "Integrative transcriptome sequencing identifies *trans*-splicing events with important roles in human embryonic stem cell pluripotency," *Genome Research*, vol. 24, no. 1, pp. 25–36, 2014.

[57] I. Martincorena and P. J. Campbell, "Somatic mutation in cancer and normal cells," *Science*, vol. 349, no. 6255, pp. 1483–1489, 2015.

[58] F. Rufflé, J. Audoux, A. Boureux et al., "New chimeric RNAs in acute myeloid leukemia," *F1000Research*, vol. 6, p. 1302, 2017.

5

Transfection of Peripheral Blood Monocytes with *SOX2* Enhances Multipotency, Proliferation, and Redifferentiation into Neohepatocytes and Insulin-Producing Cells

Ayman Hyder,[1] **Sabrina Ehnert**,[2] **Fred Fändrich**,[3] **and Hendrik Ungefroren**[4]

[1]*Faculty of Science, Damietta University, Damietta 34517, Egypt*
[2]*Siegfried Weller Institute for Trauma Research, Eberhard Karls University, Tübingen, Germany*
[3]*Institute for Applied Cell Therapy, University Hospital Schleswig-Holstein, Campus Kiel, Kiel, Germany*
[4]*First Department of Medicine, University Clinic Schleswig Holstein, Lübeck, Germany*

Correspondence should be addressed to Ayman Hyder; hyder@du.edu.eg

Guest Editor: Hyun Nam

Following a several-day incubation in medium containing IL-3 and M-CSF to generate a more plastic intermediate "reprogrammed multipotent cells of monocytic origin (RMCMO)," peripheral blood mononuclear cells (PBMCs) can be efficiently converted to hepatocyte-like cells (neohepatocytes) and insulin-producing cells. However, continuous efforts are devoted to enhancing the proliferative capacity of these multipotent cells while maintaining or further increasing their redifferentiation potential. In the present work, PBMCs were transfected with one pluripotency gene (*SOX2*) and the resulting RMCMO compared to standard RMCMO with respect to cell viability, proliferative activity, and redifferentiation potential. Ectopic *SOX2* expression increased the number of viable RMCMO, activated cell cycle genes, and enhanced proliferation as shown by quantitative RT-PCR and Ki67 immunofluorescent staining, respectively. Redifferentiation of RMCMO derived from *SOX2*-transfected PBMCs to neohepatocytes was more complete in comparison to control cells as revealed by higher urea and glucose secretion, increased activity of cytochrome P450 isoforms, and a phase II enzyme, while the same was true for insulin-producing cells as assessed by the expression of *INS*, *PDX1*, and *GLUT2* and glucose-stimulated insulin secretion. Our results indicate that *SOX2* transfection increases both multipotency and proliferation of RMCMO, eventually allowing production of neohepatocytes and insulin-producing cells of higher quality and quantity for transplantation purposes.

1. Introduction

Several studies have shown that hepatocyte-like cells can be generated from peripheral blood mononuclear cells (PBMCs) [1–4]. The procedure described by Ruhnke and colleagues initially involved a *de*differentiation step of the PBMCs in vitro to produce a cell type with stem cell-like characteristics termed "reprogrammed multipotent cells of monocytic origin" (RMCMO, formerly PCMO). This step was followed by *re*differentiation of RMCMO to either hepatocyte-like cells (neohepatocytes [3, 4]) or insulin-producing cells [3] with appropriate differentiation media.

The generation of neohepatocytes or insulin-producing cells may have impact on treatment of end-stage liver diseases or diabetes. Since transplantation of liver tissue or pancreatic islets is hampered by the shortage of donor tissues [5] and the lack of methodology to maintain primary hepatocytes and pancreatic β cells in a differentiated state in long-term in vitro culture [6], PBMCs may represent, after their tissue-specific *re*differentiation, a virtually unlimited source of cells for autologous transplantation. However, after the two-step reprogramming protocol of these cells, it was found that cell yields of neohepatocytes and insulin-producing cells were insufficient for transplantation purposes. A series of studies has been carried out with the goal of increasing the proliferative potential of these cells, including treatment with epidermal growth factor (EGF) during the redifferentiation step [6], or activin (s) or TGF-β during the *de*differentiation step [7]. However, these efforts resulted in only limited success.

One possibility to optimize neohepatocyte cell numbers is by increasing the plasticity of the RMCMO. Enhancing their stem cell features may induce their capacity for self-renewal until *re*differentiation is initiated. Application of the induced pluripotent stem cell (iPS) technology [8], in which embryonic stem cell-like cells have been generated from differentiated adult cells after introduction of four specific pluripotency genes, may enhance the plasticity of RMCMO leading to more efficient neohepatocyte redifferentiation. This technique has become safer and simpler by transferring the four genes by means of a plasmid vector rather than a virus [9, 10].

In the present study, the aim was to apply the iPS technology and generate iPS cells from PBMCs to increase proliferation and plasticity of the resulting RMCMO. However, transfecting the same plasmid used by Yu and colleagues [10] was unsuccessful due to a dramatic decrease in cell viability. Nevertheless, we were able to establish a transfection protocol with a plasmid encoding only *SOX2* that resulted in increased RMCMO proliferation and redifferentiation potential.

2. Materials and Methods

2.1. PBMC Isolation and Generation of RMCMO. PBMCs were isolated on day 0 from buffy coats of healthy donors by Histopaque density gradient centrifugation and further purified by adherence to T-75 culture flasks (Cell+, Sarstedt, Numbrecht, Germany) for 1–2 h in RPMI 1640 medium containing 10% human serum (Lonza, Cologne, Germany), 2 mmol/l glutamine, 100 U/ml penicillin, and 100 μg/ml streptomycin (Invitrogen, Darmstadt, Germany). Nonadherent cells were removed after 2 h, leaving the adherent PBMC fraction which consists of 60–70% CD14+ cells [3]. Subsequently, RMCMO were generated according to a previously published protocol [3] by culturing the adherent monocytes for 4 days in RPMI 1640 medium supplemented with 5 ng/ml M-CSF and 0.4 ng/ml IL-3 (both from R&D Systems, Wiesbaden, Germany), 90 μM 2-mercaptoethanol, and 10% human AB serum (Lonza, Verbier, Belgium).

2.2. SOX2 Cloning. Homo sapiens SRY- (sex determining region Y-) box 2 (*SOX2*, NM_003106.2) complete sequence was isolated from the plasmid pEP4 E02S EN2K provided by Addgene (Cambridge, MA, USA). The following primers were designed to amplify *SOX2* sequence: CTG*GAAT TC*ATGTACAACATGATGGAG, a forward primer with an *Eco*R1 restriction site and CAG*CTCGAG*TCACATGTGTG AGAGGG, a reverse primer with an *Xho*1 restriction site. The same restriction enzymes were used to cut the recipient plasmid pCAGGS [11]. PCR was performed using high-fidelity PCR mix, and both the product and vector were digested using FastDigest and the restriction enzymes *Eco*R1 and *Xho*1 (all from Fermentas/Thermo Fisher Scientific, Karlsruhe, Germany). Both the insert and vector were ligated using T4-Ligase Rapid kit (Fermentas). Ligation product was transformed overnight in DH5a *E. coli*, and the *SOX2* clones were then isolated using Fermentas jet plasmid miniprep. The identity of the product was verified by sequencing (MWG Biotech, Ebersberg, Germany).

2.3. Transfection. The plasmid pEP4 E02S EN2K was provided by Addgene and was originally deposited by Prof. James Thomson's lab [10]. It is used in the derivation of human iPS cells and expresses 4 pluripotency transcription factors: OCT3/4, SOX2, NANOG, and KLF4. The plasmid pCAGGS-sox2 was cloned as described. Lipofectamine 2000 (Invitrogen/Thermo Fisher Scientific, Germany) was used to transfect cultured PBMCs in 6-well plates on day 1 of culture according to manufacturers' instructions. Control cells were transfected with empty plasmids. Cell viability and counts were assessed two days later (on day 3) by Trypan blue staining, while parallel samples were subjected to RNA isolation and quantitative real-time RT-PCR (qPCR) to assess *SOX2* expression. Both control and *SOX2*-transfected cells were then cultured for another 4 days (days 3–7) in dedifferentiation medium to generate RMCMO as described before [6].

2.4. RNA Extraction and qPCR. RNA isolation was performed using the GeneJet purification kit (Fermentas). 1 μg of total RNA was reverse transcribed to cDNA using the high-capacity reverse transcription kit (Applied Biosystems/ Thermo Fisher Scientific, Germany). Gene expression was quantified by qPCR using SYBR Green (Applied Biosystems). Relative quantification was performed by $\Delta\Delta$Ct method. To normalize gene expression data, amplification of the housekeeping gene β-actin was used as an internal control. Primers used for PCR amplification were *ACTB* forward GATATCGCTGCGCTCGTC, reverse TCCATATCGTCCCA GTTGG; *SOX2* forward TGATGGAGACGGAGCTGAAG, reverse GCTTGCTGATCTCCGAGTTG; *NANOG* forward GATTTGTGGGCCTGAAGAAAACT, reverse AGGAGA GACAGTCTCCGTGTGAG; *ANAPC2* forward CCAGTA CAGGCGGTGATCTT, reverse GCTCTCGTCGTCACTGTC AA; *ABL-1* forward AACACCCTAACCTGGTGCAG, reverse CAAGTGGTTCTCCCCTACCA; *CDC2* forward GGGGTC AGCTCGTTACTCAA, reverse GATGCTAGGCTTCCTGG TTTC; *CDK4* forward CTGACCGGGAGATCAAGGTA, reverse AGCCAGCTTGACTGTTCCAC; *CDK6* forward TC CCAGGAGAAGAAGACTGG, reverse GGTCCTGGAAGT ATGGGTGA; *INS* forward GGGGAACGAGGCTTCTTC TA, reverse AGTTGCAGTAGTTCTCCAGC; *PDX1* forward AAGTCTACCAAAGCTCACGC, reverse GTTCAACATGA CAGCCAGCT; and *GLUT2* forward TTGGGCTGAGGAA GAGACTG, reverse AACCCCATCAAGAGAGCTCC.

2.5. Immunofluorescence. On day 7 of culture, adherent cells were fixed in 1% paraformaldehyde, incubated with anti-human CD14 antibody (BD Biosciences, Heidelberg, Germany) at room temperature for 2 h and Alexafluor 488-labeled secondary antibody (Invitrogen) for 1 h. After washing, cells were permeabilised using 0.5% Triton X-100 and incubated overnight with the anti-human Ki67 (BD Biosciences) at 4°C followed by Alexafluor 555-labeled secondary antibody (Invitrogen). Nuclei were stained with DAPI.

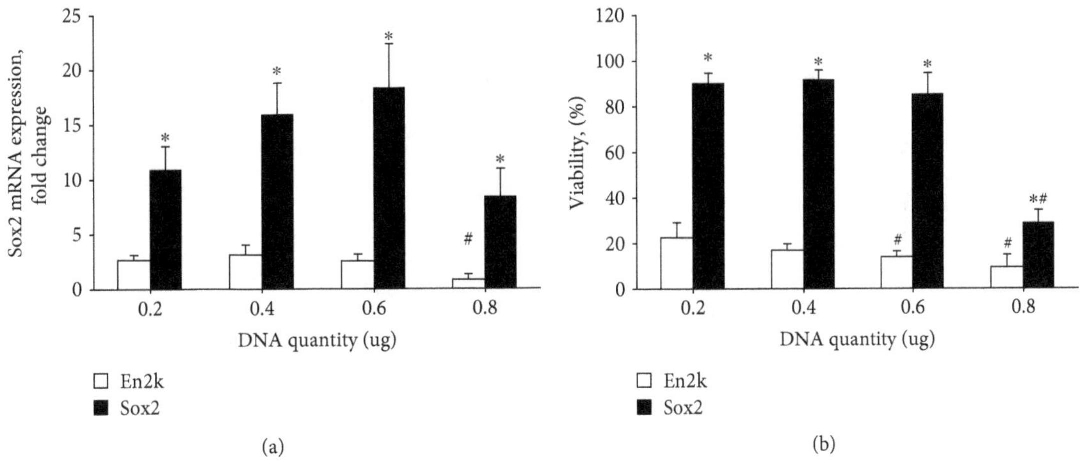

FIGURE 1: Transfection with *SOX2* plasmid increased *SOX2* mRNA expression and did not affect PBMC viability. PBMCs were transfected one day after plating with increasing concentrations of either the plasmid pEP4 E02S EN2K carrying the pluripotency genes *SOX2*, *KLF4*, *NANOG*, and *OCT3/4* (En2k) or pCAGGS plasmid carrying only *SOX2* (Sox2). The panels show *SOX2* mRNA expression as determined by qPCR (a) and the viability as determined by Trypan blue in the transfected cells by either plasmids (b) two days post transfection. Data are presented as mean ± SEM of $N = 3$. The symbol * denotes a significantly higher Sox2 group value than En2k value (t-test). The symbol # indicates a significant difference to the respective cells which received 0.2 μg DNA (Student's t-test after ANOVA $p < 0.05$).

Ki67-positive cells were counted and related to the cell count of CD14-positive PBMCs.

2.6. Redifferentiation of Transfected Cells to Neohepatocytes and Insulin-Producing Cells. Following completion of the dedifferentiation process of PBMCs on day 5 of culture, the resulting RMCMO were cultured for 2 weeks with either hepatocyte conditioning medium containing 3 ng/ml fibroblast growth factor-4 (FGF-4, R&D Systems, Wiesbaden, Germany) and 10% FBS for redifferentiation into neohepatocytes or islet cell-conditioning medium containing 10 ng/ml epidermal growth factor (EGF) and 20 ng/ml hepatocyte growth factor (HGF, both from Calbiochem, Darmstadt, Germany), 10 mmol/l nicotinamide (Sigma, Deisenhofen, Germany), and 5 mmol/l glucose for redifferentiation into insulin-producing cells [3]. The medium was changed every 3rd day. Redifferentiated cells were then subjected to analysis of hepatocyte or islet cell functions.

2.7. Functional Analyses of Neohepatocytes and Insulin-Producing Cells. The methodology for hepatocellular function was described in detail in our previous work [6]. For the measurement of insulin secretion, cells were washed twice with PBS and placed in 5% BSA blocking medium for 3 h, then incubated in secretion buffer containing different glucose concentrations for 2 h. The concentration of insulin in the medium was determined using ELISA kit (DRG diagnostics, Marburg, Germany) following the manufacturers' protocol. The method of rat islet isolation, culture, and rat insulin determination was described elsewhere [5]. Insulin-producing cells redifferentiated from RMCMO were also subjected to RNA extraction and conventional endpoint PCR to detect expression of *INS* (product size 202 bp), *PDX1* (product size 186 bp), and *GLUT2* (product size 192 bp) using the primers specified above.

2.8. Statistical Analysis. All samples were measured in duplicate. Values were expressed as mean ± SEM with $N = 3$ in all experiments. Statistical comparison between two groups was performed by Student's t-test. Statistical difference was considered significant if $p < 0.05$.

3. Results

3.1. Transfection with iPS Plasmid, but Not with a Plasmid Encoding SOX2 Alone, Decreased PBMC Viability. Initially, it was planned to generate iPS cells from PBMCs. To accomplish this, we transfected PBMCs with the plasmid pEP4 E02S EN2K encoding *OCT3/4*, *NANOG*, *SOX2*, and *KLF4*. It was observed that cultured PBMCs could not withstand the transfection process, with their viability decreasing dramatically with most plasmid concentrations (Figure 1(b)). Moreover, the transfection was not efficient enough, as revealed by qPCR, and largely failed to increase the expression of pluripotency genes exemplified by the expression of *Sox2* (Figure 1(a)). This brought us to the conclusion that the surviving cells were those that have not taken up the plasmid DNA. Therefore, it was thought to decrease the toxicity of the transfection by decreasing the plasmid size. However, similar results were obtained after transfecting PBMCs with a plasmid containing only 3 genes (*OCT3/4*, *NANOG*, and *KLF4*) (data not shown), indicating that reducing plasmid size was unable to reduce toxicity.

Next, we constructed pCAGGS-sox2, a plasmid containing only the *SOX2* cDNA. Following transfection of PBMCs with increasing amounts of this plasmid, no significant alterations in their viability were observed until an amount of 0.6 μg/well (Figure 1(b)). Meanwhile, the *SOX2* expression increased gradually and peaked at the same amount (Figure 1(a)), indicating a good efficiency of the *SOX2* transfection process.

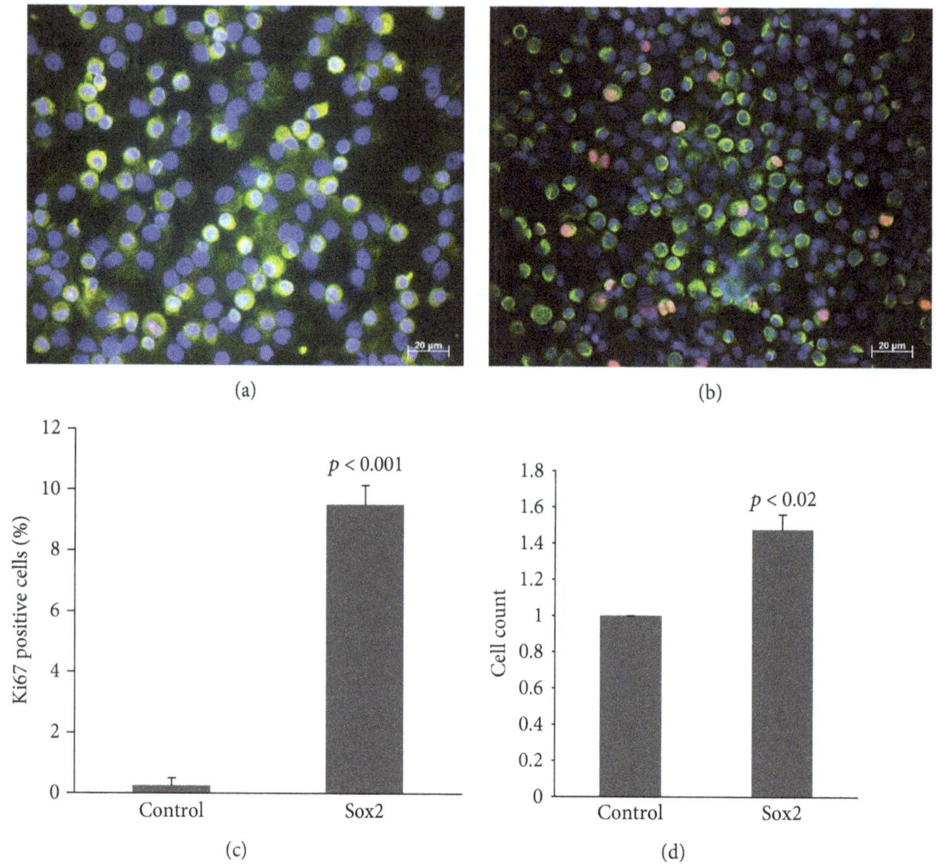

Figure 2: *SOX2* overexpression induces proliferation in RMCMO. Immunofluorescence of Ki67 expression (red) in normal RMCMO (a) or RMCMO generated after transfection of PBMCs with *SOX2* (b). Cells were also immunostained with anti-CD14 (green) as a monocyte-specific marker. Nuclei were stained with DAPI (blue). (c) Quantification of Ki67 in *SOX2*-overexpressing RMCMO. (d) RMCMO cell count (relative to control value set arbitrarily at 1) 4 days after *SOX2*-transfection. Control = empty vector-transfected RMCMO. Data ($N = 3$) are expressed as mean ± SEM. Statistical analysis was performed by unpaired Student's t-test.

3.2. SOX2 Overexpression Induces RMCMO Proliferation. Next, we examined the proliferative response of the PBMCs to *SOX2*-transfection. For this purpose, cells were stained by immunofluorescence for Ki67, a nuclear proliferation marker that is present only in mitotically active cells [12]. To assure the monocytic nature of the Ki67-positive cells, cultures were counterstained with anti-CD14, a cell surface marker of monocytes. The results showed no signs of proliferation in control RMCMOs (Figures 2(a) and 2(c)), while 8.5 ± 1% of *SOX2*-transfected RMCMO were positive for Ki67 (Figures 2(b) and 2(c)). Four days post transfection, cell counts were compared in both groups. It was found that cell numbers of *SOX2*-transfected cells significantly increased by 47.5 ± 9% over the control group (Figure 2(d)). Taken together, the data clearly show that *SOX2* can induce mitotic activity in RMCMO.

3.3. Ectopic SOX2 Expression Is Associated with Transcriptional Upregulation of Genes Involved in Cell Cycle Regulation and Pluripotency. The Ki67 data suggest that the increase in cell numbers in *SOX2*-overexpressing cells was the result of increased mitotic activity. Since mitotic activity involves transcriptional changes in key cell cycle regulators, we examined by qPCR analysis whether *SOX2*-induced proliferation was associated with the upregulation of genes that have regulatory roles in different stages of the cell cycle. As seen in Figure 3(a), *SOX2* overexpression significantly upregulated the mRNA expression of the ANAPC2, ABL-1, CDC2, CDK4, and CDK6 genes. These transcriptional effects on cell cycle genes are in agreement with the promitotic role of SOX2 and are likely mediated by its transcription factor function.

To reveal whether ectopic expression of *SOX2* in PBMCs impacts transcriptional regulation of other pluripotency-determining genes, we measured expression of *NANOG* and *OCT3/4* in the resulting RMCMO by qPCR. Interestingly, in *SOX2*-transfected cells, both *NANOG* and *OCT3/4* mRNA were significantly upregulated compared to control-transfectants (Figures 3(b) and 3(c)). This shows that *SOX2* does not only increase mitotic activity but also induces expression of other essential pluripotency-associated factors and, thereby, might enhance the plasticity/redifferentiation potential of RMCMO.

3.4. SOX2 Enhances Hepatocyte-Specific Functions of Neohepatocytes. The observation of *SOX2*-mediated upregulation of *OCT3/4* and *NANOG* suggested the possibility that *SOX2* can establish a regulatory network with other

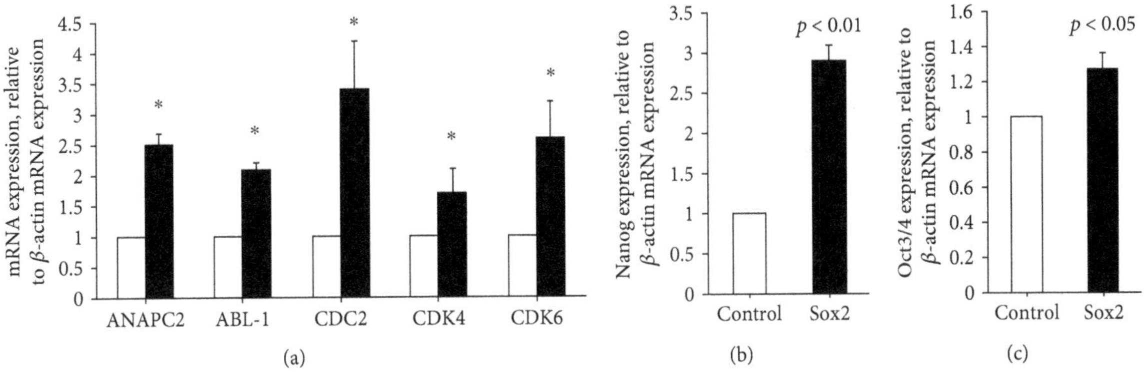

FIGURE 3: *SOX2* overexpression upregulates cell cycle and pluripotency gene expression in RMCMO. qPCR-based measurement of gene expression of five cell cycle regulatory genes (a) and the pluripotency genes, *NANOG* (b) and *OCT3/4* (c), in RMCMO derived from *SOX2*- (black columns) and control-transfected (white columns) PBMCs. Data for the gene of interest (mean ± SEM, $N = 3$, duplicates) were normalized to the gene expression level of β-actin. Statistical analysis between *SOX2*-transfected and empty vector-transfected cells was performed by unpaired Student's t-test.

pluripotency factors that ultimately result in an increase in RMCMO plasticity. Hence, it was tested whether the overexpression of *SOX2* in PBMCs would change the functional parameters of RMCMO-derived neohepatocytes. After the 4-day culture period necessary for PBMC *de*differentiation to RMCMO, control and *SOX2*-transfected cells were allowed to redifferentiate into neohepatocytes for 2 weeks. At the end of this period, cells were analysed for hepatic cell-specific functions (Figures 4(a)–4(c)). Neohepatocytes exhibited phase I enzyme activities. The activity of three different cytochrome P450 isoforms (1A1/2, 2D6, and 3A4) was investigated. All cells showed activity of the 3 enzymes. For all enzymes, the activity was significantly higher in neohepatocytes obtained after *SOX2* transfection than in control standard neohepatocytes. Both neohepatocytes and control cells secreted urea, and the addition of ammonium chloride (NH_4Cl) significantly increased urea formation in all preparations. However, urea secretion was higher in neohepatocytes obtained from *SOX2*-overexpressing RMCMO (Figure 4(d)). As well, all neohepatocytes including the controls were shown to secrete glucose. To measure the ability of the cells to perform gluconeogenesis, the sodium pyruvate-containing incubation buffer was supplemented with lactate. Stimulation with pyruvate/lactate induced higher glucose secretion compared to that from cultures with pyruvate only (Figure 4(e)). As for urea formation, the gluconeogenesis was significantly higher in neohepatocytes obtained from *SOX2*-transfected RMCMO. These data show that *SOX2* transfection impacts the functional state of the redifferentiated "end product," the neohepatocyte, most likely because of a RMCMO of higher plasticity.

3.5. SOX2 Enhances the Differentiated Phenotype of Insulin-Producing Cells. The *SOX2*-transfected RMCMO were also allowed to redifferentiate to insulin-producing cells. The islet cell-like differentiation was confirmed by the expression of the β cell-specific genes *INS*, *PDX1*, and *GLUT2*, and downregulation of *NANOG* as tested by standard endpoint PCR (Figure 5(a)). Moreover, *SOX2*-transfected cells exhibited concentration-dependent glucose-stimulated insulin secretion (Figure 5(b)), albeit the secretion level was low as compared to that of intact islets (Figure 5(c)). In addition, insulin-producing cells derived from *SOX2*-expressing RMCMO from individual donors responded quite differently to glucose stimulation (Figure 5(d)). The insulin response (stimulatory index) was calculated by dividing the secretion level at 22.2 mmol/l glucose by the basal value at 2.8 mmol/l. Some donor cells did not respond or showed only a weak response, while others displayed a high stimulatory index (Figure 5(d)).

4. Discussion

PBMCs were shown to be able to acquire stem cell-like features, and the resulting RMCMO have some advantageous features over other types of stem cells. These include ease of isolation from peripheral blood, absence of risk of oncogenicity because RMCMO lack telomerase expression [13], and their autologous transplantation without the need for immunosuppressive drugs. Yet, they also share with embryonic stem cells the expression of some major pluripotency genes such as *OCT3/4*, *NANOG* [12], *c-MYC* [14], and *KLF4*, the latter of which exhibits high constitutive expression in monocytes [13, 15]. However, the use of PBMCs as a cellular source for regenerative purposes in the clinical setting also has some disadvantages, i.e., a comparatively low number in peripheral blood and a limited proliferation potential in vitro [7]. To be considered as a cellular source for transplantation, it is therefore mandatory to increase cell yields by expanding them in vitro. Thus, it was the main goal of the present work to enhance the proliferation potential of PBMCs/RMCMO during culture and—at the same time—improve their redifferentiation potential towards hepatocyte-like and insulin-producing cells. We, therefore, initially attempted to induce pluripotency in plastic-adherent PBMCs by iPS technology, a technique that has opened up possibilities for diverse clinical applications. The iPS cells are able to self-renew and differentiate similarly to embryonic stem cells. They are generated by reprogramming of any kind of somatic cell of any

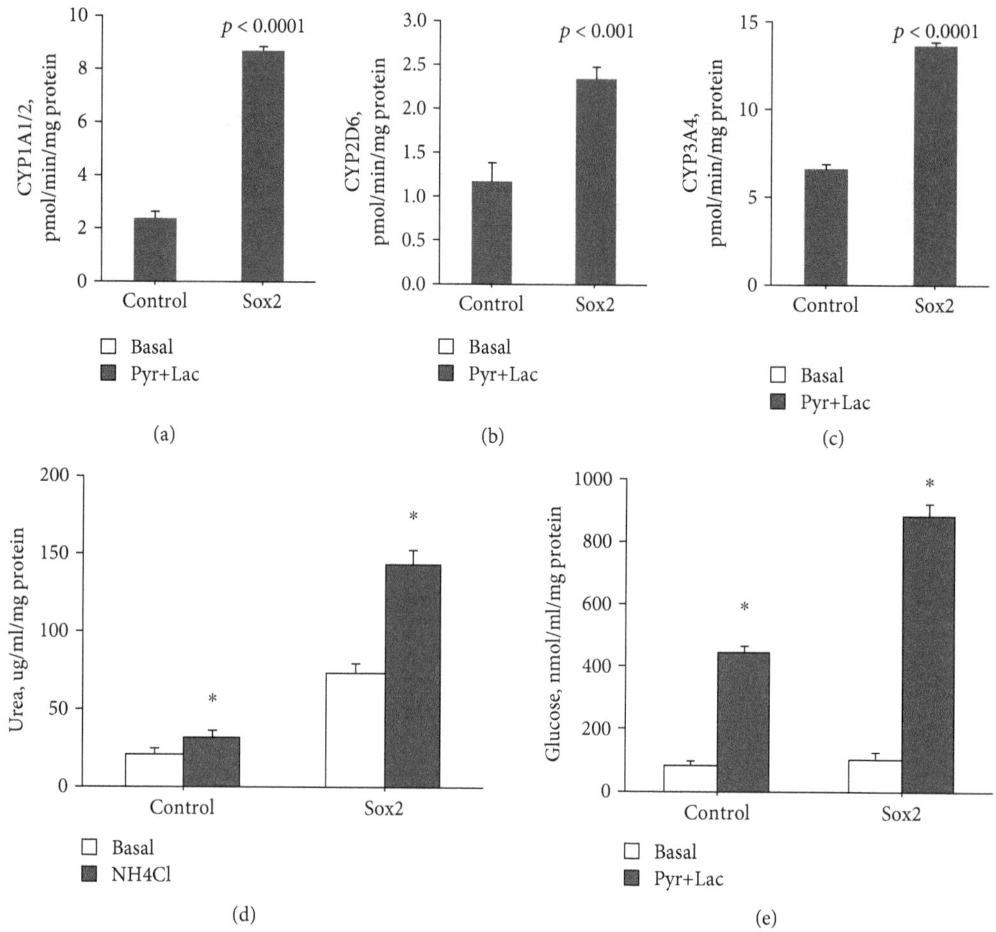

Figure 4: *SOX2*-overexpression improves hepatic cell function in RMCMO-derived neohepatocytes. RMCMO derived from *SOX2*-transfected PBMCs were cultured in hepatocyte conditioning medium for 2 weeks before subjecting them to analysis of cytochrome P450 (CYP) isoforms 1A1/2, 2D6, and 3A4, urea metabolism, and glucose metabolism. Activities and secretion levels were normalized to protein content (mg) of each sample. Data are presented as mean ± SEM of $N = 3$. Statistical analysis between *SOX2*-transfected and nontransfected control cells was performed by unpaired Student's t-test. Pyr, pyruvate; Lac, lactate.

person and therefore represent an ultimate source of personal cells. The iPS cells were initially produced using retroviral vectors encoding four transcription factors that are found at high levels in embryonic stem cells, OCT3/4, NANOG, SOX2, and KLF4. However, retroviral vectors leave a footprint in the resulting iPS cells, which could cause oncogene activation. Since this is a serious drawback for clinical applications [16], virus-free methods—like plasmid vector-mediated transfer—were developed to reduce the oncogenic risk [10]. In our hands, however, PBMCs did not tolerate the transfection procedure with the pEP4 E02S EN2K plasmid or the same vector carrying only three of the four genes. This could be attributed to either the large size of both plasmids containing the complete coding sequences of the four and three pluripotency genes, respectively, or alternatively, to the presence of a sequence that is poisonous to PBMCs. Fortunately, however, PBMCs were easily transfectable with another (smaller) plasmid containing only the *SOX2* cDNA.

Pluripotency is associated with self-renewal/proliferation. Moreover, *SOX2* has been shown to prevent exiting of the cell cycle [17, 18] which is in line with the enhanced proliferative activity in SOX2-transfected RMCMO. The proliferative activity of RMCMO derived from *SOX2*-transfected PBMCs was verified by an increase in cell counts and by nuclear Ki67 staining. The present data also showed upregulation at the mRNA level of cell cycle regulatory genes *ANAPC2*, *ABL-1*, *CDC2*, *CDK4*, and *CDK6* in RMCMO overexpressing *SOX2*. ANAPC2 controls the regulation of the G1/S and G2/M transitions, ABL-1 regulates the S-phase and DNA replication, CDC2 takes part in M-phase regulation, and CDK4 and CDK6 participate in the G1/S transition [19]. Inhibition of ANAPC2 and CDC2 has been reported to induce cell cycle arrest at G2/M [20]. Activation of the cell cycle and mitosis led to induction of proliferation as assessed by Ki67 immunofluorescence and the increases in total cell counts.

Ideally, modifications to the procedure of RMCMO generation from PBMCs should enhance not only proliferation but also the multipotent state/plasticity of these cells in a way that the resulting neohepatocytes become more hepatocyte like. Interestingly, ectopic *SOX2* expression further enhanced both *NANOG* and *OCT3/4* mRNA expression over that seen in standard RMCMO [13]. Given the already high constitutive expression of *KLF4* in monocytes [15], it is likely

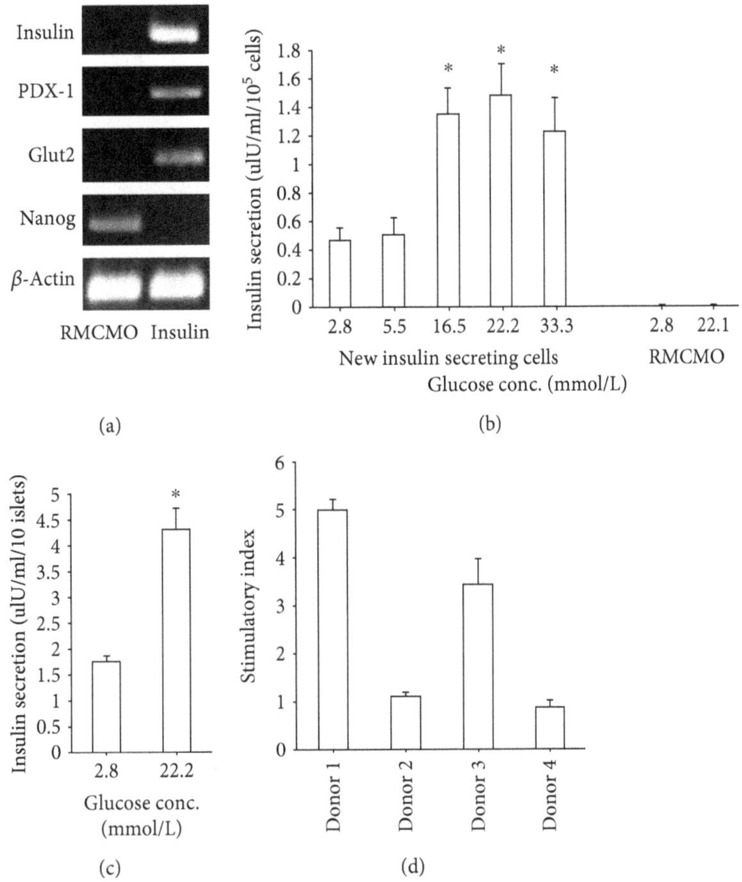

FIGURE 5: RMCMO generated from *SOX2*-transfected PBMCs are efficiently redifferentiated into insulin-producing cells. (a) Standard RMCMO or RMCMO generated from *SOX2* transfection of PBMCs (insulin) were cultured in islet cell-conditioning medium for 2 weeks and subsequently subjected to analysis of β cell-specific gene expression. (b) Insulin-producing cells obtained after redifferentiation of *SOX2*-transfected RMCMO (new insulin-secreting cells) or standard RMCMO were cultured with increasing glucose concentrations to determine their ability to secrete insulin. Insulin secretion was quantified from 1×10^5 cells. (c) Glucose-stimulated insulin secretion in intact islets for comparison. Insulin secretion was quantified from 10 islets. (d) Insulin secretion response of insulin-producing cells obtained after redifferentiation of *SOX2*-transfected RMCMO from four different donors to glucose stimulation. The stimulatory index was calculated as glucose-stimulated secretion/basal secretion. Data are presented as mean ± SEM of $N = 3$. Statistical analysis between basal and stimulated secretions was performed by unpaired Student's t-test.

that the elevated protein expression of all four iPS factors in the *SOX2*-transfectants accounted for an increase in multipotency/plasticity. This, in turn, may have caused the neohepatocytes derived from *SOX2*-transfectants to more closely resemble primary hepatocytes with respect to CYP activity, urea production, and glucose metabolism.

5. Conclusions

Although PBMCs were refractory to transfection with an iPS plasmid, they can successfully be transfected with a plasmid carrying one pluripotency gene (*SOX2*). Ectopic *SOX2*-expression resulted in the enhancement of both RMCMO proliferation and redifferentiation into hepatocyte-like and insulin-producing cells.

Acknowledgments

This work was supported in part by a grant from the "Bundesministerium für Bildung und Forschung" (01 GN 0985). We are grateful to H. Hinz for excellent technical assistance.

References

[1] M. Kuwana, Y. Okazaki, H. Kodama et al., "Human circulating CD14$^+$ monocytes as a source of progenitors that exhibit mesenchymal cell differentiation," *Journal of Leukocyte Biology*, vol. 74, no. 5, pp. 833–845, 2003.

[2] Y. Zhao, D. Glesne, and E. Huberman, "A human peripheral blood monocyte-derived subset acts as pluripotent stem cells," *Proceedings of the National Academy of Sciences of the United States of America*, vol. 100, no. 5, pp. 2426–2431, 2003.

[3] M. Ruhnke, H. Ungefroren, A. Nussler et al., "Differentiation of in vitro–modified human peripheral blood monocytes into hepatocyte-like and pancreatic islet-like cells," *Gastroenterology*, vol. 128, no. 7, pp. 1774–1786, 2005.

[4] M. Ruhnke, A. K. Nussler, H. Ungefroren et al., "Human

monocyte-derived neohepatocytes: a promising alternative to primary human hepatocytes for autologous cell therapy," *Transplantation*, vol. 79, no. 9, pp. 1097–1103, 2005.

[5] A. Hyder, C. Laue, and J. Schrezenmeir, "Metabolic aspects of neonatal rat islet hypoxia tolerance," *Transplant International*, vol. 23, no. 1, pp. 80–89, 2010.

[6] A. Hyder, S. Ehnert, H. Hinz, A. K. Nüssler, F. Fändrich, and H. Ungefroren, "EGF and HB-EGF enhance the proliferation of programmable cells of monocytic origin (PCMO) through activation of MEK/ERK signaling and improve differentiation of PCMO-derived hepatocyte-like cells," *Cell Communication and Signaling: CCS*, vol. 10, no. 1, pp. 23–32, 2012.

[7] H. Ungefroren, A. Hyder, H. Hinz et al., "Pluripotency gene expression and growth control in cultures of peripheral blood monocytes during their conversion into programmable cells of monocytic origin (PCMO): evidence for a regulatory role of autocrine activin and TGF-β," *PLoS One*, vol. 10, no. 2, article e0118097, 2015.

[8] K. Takahashi and S. Yamanaka, "Induction of pluripotent stem cells from mouse embryonic and adult fibroblast cultures by defined factors," *Cell*, vol. 126, no. 4, pp. 663–676, 2006.

[9] K. Okita, M. Nakagawa, H. Hyenjong, T. Ichisaka, and S. Yamanaka, "Generation of mouse induced pluripotent stem cells without viral vectors," *Science*, vol. 322, no. 5903, pp. 949–953, 2008.

[10] J. Yu, K. Hu, K. Smuga-Otto et al., "Human induced pluripotent stem cells free of vector and transgene sequences," *Science*, vol. 324, no. 5928, pp. 797–801, 2009.

[11] M. Zenhom, A. Hyder, I. Kraus-Stojanowic, A. Auinger, T. Roeder, and J. Schrezenmeir, "PPARγ-dependent peptidoglycan recognition protein 3 (PGlyRP3) expression regulates proinflammatory cytokines by microbial and dietary fatty acids," *Immunobiology*, vol. 216, no. 6, pp. 715–724, 2011.

[12] T. Scholzen and J. Gerdes, "The Ki-67 protein: from the known and the unknown," *Journal of Cellular Physiology*, vol. 182, no. 3, pp. 311–322, 2000.

[13] H. Ungefroren, S. Groth, A. Hyder et al., "The generation of programmable cells of monocytic origin involves partial repression of monocyte/macrophage markers and reactivation of pluripotency genes," *Stem Cells and Development*, vol. 19, no. 11, pp. 1769–1780, 2010.

[14] J. Lee, K. Mehta, M. B. Blick, J. U. Gutterman, and G. Lopez-Berestein, "Expression of c-fos, c-myb, and c-myc in human monocytes: correlation with monocytic differentiation," *Blood*, vol. 69, no. 5, pp. 1542–1545, 1987.

[15] M. W. Feinberg, A. K. Wara, Z. Cao et al., "The Kruppel-like factor KLF4 is a critical regulator of monocyte differentiation," *The EMBO Journal*, vol. 26, no. 18, pp. 4138–4148, 2007.

[16] J. A. Desmarais, C. Unger, I. Damjanov, M. Meuth, and P. Andrews, "Apoptosis and failure of checkpoint kinase 1 activation in human induced pluripotent stem cells under replication stress," *Stem Cell Research & Therapy*, vol. 7, no. 1, p. 17, 2016.

[17] M. Bylund, E. Andersson, B. G. Novitch, and J. Muhr, "Vertebrate neurogenesis is counteracted by Sox 1-3 activity," *Nature Neuroscience*, vol. 6, no. 11, pp. 1162–1168, 2003.

[18] V. Graham, J. Khudyakov, P. Ellis, and L. Pevny, "SOX2 functions to maintain neural progenitor identity," *Neuron*, vol. 39, no. 5, pp. 749–765, 2003.

[19] J. M. Enserink and R. D. Kolodner, "An overview of Cdk1-controlled targets and processes," *Cell Division*, vol. 5, no. 1, p. 11, 2010.

[20] D. W. Heilman, M. R. Green, and J. G. Teodoro, "The anaphase promoting complex: a critical target for viral proteins and anticancer drugs," *Cell Cycle*, vol. 4, no. 4, pp. 560–563, 2005.

6

Efficient Promotion of Autophagy and Angiogenesis using Mesenchymal Stem Cell Therapy Enhanced by the Low-Energy Shock Waves in the Treatment of Erectile Dysfunction

Guan Qun Zhu,[1] Seung Hwan Jeon,[1] Woong Jin Bae,[1,2] Sae Woong Choi,[1] Hyun Cheol Jeong,[1] Kang Sup Kim,[1] Su Jin Kim,[3] Hyuk Jin Cho,[1] U. Syn Ha,[1] Sung Hoo Hong,[1] Ji Youl Lee,[1] Eun Bi Kwon,[4] and Sae Woong Kim[1,2]

[1]*Department of Urology, College of Medicine, The Catholic University of Korea, Seoul, Republic of Korea*
[2]*Catholic Integrative Medicine Research Institute, College of Medicine, The Catholic University of Korea, Seoul, Republic of Korea*
[3]*Department of Urology, Wonju College of Medicine, Yonsei University, Wonju, Republic of Korea*
[4]*KEMIMEDI, Seoul, Republic of Korea*

Correspondence should be addressed to Sae Woong Kim; ksw1227@catholic.ac.kr

Academic Editor: Valeria Sorrenti

Background. Mesenchymal stem cell therapy (MSCT) and defocused low-energy shock wave therapy (ESWT) has been shown to ameliorate erectile dysfunction (ED). However, the interactions and effects of action between MSCT and ESWT remain poorly understood. In this study, we investigated the mechanisms of combination therapy with MSCT and ESWT in a rat model of diabetic ED. *Materials and Methods.* Eight-week-old male Sprague-Dawley rats were randomly divided into 2 parts. Diabetic rats induced by streptozotocin (65 mg/kg) were randomly divided into 4 groups: (1) DM control group, (2) DM + ESWT group, (3) DM + MSCT group, and (4) DM + ESWT + MSCT group. The sham group was a normal control group (without streptozotocin). MSCT and (or) ESWT were, respectively, administered to each group according to the proposal for 8 weeks. Immediately after recording of intracavernous pressure (ICP), the penis was then harvested for histologic analysis, ELISA, and Western blotting. *Results.* The ratio of ICP/MAP was significantly higher in the DM + ESWT + MSCT group than in ESWT or MSCT treated group ($P < 0.05$). Also, the treatment stimulated angiogenesis and vasodilatation in the corpus cavernosum ($P < 0.05$). ESWT increased the quantity of MSCs in the corpus cavernosum and also induced MSCs to express more VEGF in vitro and vivo ($P < 0.05$) which activated the PI3K/AKT/mTOR and NO/cGMP signaling pathways in the corpus cavernosum. The combination approach stimulated autophagy and decreased apoptosis in the corpus cavernosum. NGF and BDNF expressions were higher in the DM + ESWT + MSCT group than in the DM control group ($P < 0.01$). Furthermore, the treatment promoted the MSC recruitment by inducing penile tissues to express more PECAM and SDF-1. *Conclusions.* Combination of LI-ESWT and MSCT can get a better result than a single treatment by expressing more VEGF which can take part in autophagy by triggering the PI3K/AKT/mTOR signaling pathway. This cooperative therapy would provide a new research direction in ED treatment for the future.

1. Introduction

Diabetic patients suffer from a higher incidence of erectile dysfunction (ED), which is less responsive to drugs than nondiabetic individuals, and this diabetes mellitus (DM) erectile dysfunction (DMED) seriously influences the quality of life of diabetic patients [1–3]. Now, phosphodiesterase 5 inhibitor (PDE5I) represents the first-line treatment for ED, but there are still poor therapeutic effects for some DMED patients [4–6]. So it is extremely urgent to find a new and therapeutic approach to treat the drug-useless DMED patients.

As a relatively novel approach in regeneration medicine, defocused low-energy shock wave therapy (DL-ESWT) has shown great potential and promising evidences, especially for the treatment of various disorders such as tissue trauma and defects [7–11]. At present, ESWT has been applied to clinical therapy for ED, and many studies have shown that ESWT can achieve satisfactory therapeutic effects [12–14]. The main mechanism of ESWT is considered that can stimulate angiogenesis and restore blood flow to the disorder area, through promoting regeneration and repair [15]. Hayashi et al. [7] reported that the expressions of various proangiogenic factors, such as vascular endothelial growth factor (VEGF) and endothelial nitric oxide synthase (eNOS), could be upregulated by DL-ESWT in diabetic mice. Another reason for ED therapy using DL-ESWT is that it can enhance the recruitment of endothelial progenitor cells by upregulating stromal cell-derived factor-1 (SDF-1) in wound tissues [16]. Li et al. [17] found that DL-ESWT could promote the recruitment of endogenous progenitor cells and activation of Schwann cells, coinciding with angiogenesis, tissue, and nerve generation in a rat model of pelvic neurovascular injuries.

Now, some researchers [18–20] suggest that as a new approach, mesenchymal stem cell (MSC) therapy can be a good remedial method for ED. Gokce et al. [21] consider that the reason and mechanism of ED stem cell therapy are that stem cells can stimulate endothelial cell proliferation and inhibit endothelial cell apoptosis by a paracrine mechanism. But MSCs' survival rate is still a problem through intracavernous injection. Liu et al. [22] consider that in the DMED rat model hyperglycemia can induce cell apoptosis, but oxidative stress also can increase MSC autophagy by cell self-defense, and augmentation of autophagy can reduce apoptosis, prolong MSC survival, and improve MSC-based therapeutic efficacy for DMED. Also, some studies [23, 24] prove that not all MSCs, through intracavernous injection, will be apoptotic, dead immediately, or flowing away by migrating into the circulatory system. So we believe that mesenchymal stem cell therapy (MSCT) will be a potential and promising ED treatment.

Since both ESWT and MSCT can be an approach for ED treatment by paracrine growth factors to promote cellular proliferation, we have reasons to believe that combination of both for ED treatment will get a better result. In this report, we proved that combination of LI-EWST and MSCT might be a better way to improve ED by promoting angiogenesis, regeneration, and autophagy. Our study also proved that ESWT can drive homing of MSCs. Also, this cooperative therapy combining stem cells with machine provides a theoretic and experimental basis for clinic treatment.

2. Materials and Methods

2.1. Cell Cultures. MSCs come from the surplus stock of frozen cells at a cell bank (SL BIGEN, Seongnam, Korea). Cells were cultured in a special medium (mesenchymal stem cell proliferation media; SL BIGEN) and maintained at 37°C with 5% CO_2 in a humidified atmosphere. Two days later, nonadherent cells were removed and fresh culture medium was added. The culture medium was changed every 2 days. Cells were passaged when they reached approximately 90% confluence. The ESWT on cultured MSCs was performed by an extracorporeal shock wave machine (Urontech, Hwaseong, Korea). The shock wave probe was kept in contact with the culture flask containing adherent MSCs by means of a water-filled cushion covered with common ultrasound gel. The cells were subjected to 200 impulses of ESWT at an energy flux density of 0.09 mJ/mm^2 with a frequency of 120/min as described previously [25]. ESWT was performed after cell attachment. Every generation only accepted ESWT one time.

2.2. Effect of ESWT on Activating MSCs In Vitro. We quantified the VEGF in the cell culture supernatants by species-specific VEGF immunoassay ELISA kits (R&D Systems Europe, Abingdon, United Kingdom) according to the manufacturer's instructions. After ESWT, MSCs (each well seeded the same quantity of MSCs and from the first passage to the fifth passage of MSCs was seeded in a discrete 6 cm culture dish) were cultured for 12 h in a constant-temperature incubator, and then 1 mL of medium was collected and stored at −80°C until used. Absorbance was read at a wavelength of 450 nm in a microplate reader (Synergy H1 M, Biotek, USA). At least 3 separate dishes of cells were assayed for each clone.

2.3. Experimental Animal and Study Design. Eight-week-old male Sprague-Dawley rats weighing 270–300 g (Orient Bio Co., Seongnam, Korea) were used in this study. All animal experiments in this study were approved by the Institutional Animal Care and Use Committee of the Catholic University of Korea. DM was induced by an intraperitoneal injection of streptozotocin (STZ, Sigma-Aldrich chemical company, USA) at a dose of 65 mg/kg body weight (prepared STZ in 50 mM citrated buffer pH 4.5) as described previously [26], and the sham rats were injected in an equal vehicle (0.1 mol/L citrate-phosphate buffer, pH 4.5). After 72 h, DM was confirmed by blood glucose levels above 300 mg/dL to determine by the Accu-Chek Active blood glucose monitor (Hoffmann-La Roche Ltd., Basel, Switzerland), and blood samples were obtained from tail veins (the percentage of diabetic animals after STZ injection was about 70%). Unhealthy rats showing ruffled hair, poor appearance, vocalization, and lack of appetite were not included in our experiment. After 12 weeks, evaluation of erectile function was performed for these rats and rats with normal erectile function were excluded. In brief, streptozotocin-induced rats were put into a rearing cage with an adult female rat. If seminal stain was not found in the cage in 1 week, the experimental rat was included in the next process. If seminal stain was found, the rat was excluded. The included rats were randomly divided into 4 groups ($N = 10$ per group): (1) DM control group, (2) DM + ESWT group, (3) DM + MSCT group, and (4) DM + ESWT + MSCT group, and the sham group ($N = 10$, without STZ) was the normal control group.

2.4. MSC Injection and ESWT. All experimental rats (including DM control, DM + ESWT, DM + MSCT, and DM + ESWT + MSCT groups) underwent bilateral intracavernous injection. Briefly, animals in experimental groups were anesthetized by inhalational 2.0% isoflurane, and then each rat was placed in the back position with its lower abdomen shaved and the penis was drawn out of the prepuce. Before MSC injection, we labeled the MSCs with a fluorescent dye (CellTracker™ CM-DiI; Molecular Probes, Eugene, OR) to track the location of MSCs according to the manufacturer's protocol. Rats in DM + ESWT and DM + ESWT + MSCT groups received bilateral intracavernous injection of 200 μL PBS solution containing 1×10^6 MSCs (P3) as described previously [23, 27], and the DM control and DM + ESWT groups received bilateral intracavernous injection of just 200 μL PBS. MSCT was repeated 1 time per week, for a total duration of 4 weeks.

After MSC injection, rats in the DM + ESWT and DM + ESWT + MSCT groups were treated with shock waves. Under anesthesia, the penis was drawn out of the prepuce in a supine position. Ultrasonic gel was applied to the penis, and then the shock wave applicator (Urontech, Hwaseong, Korea) was placed on the penis. Each penis was subjected to 300 impulses of ESWT at an energy flux density of 0.1 mJ/mm^2 with a frequency of 120/min which is based on other studies [17, 28]. ESWT was repeated 3 times per week with one day's break, for a total duration of 4 weeks.

2.5. Erectile Function Evaluation. Under anesthesia, the carotid artery and cavernous nerve were exposed via midline laparotomy. The corpus cavernosum of the penis was cannulated with a 25-gauge butterfly needle filled with heparin (250 U/mL) via insertion at the crura. The cannula was connected to a pressure transducer (Grass model S48 K; Astro-Med Inc., West Warwick, RI) for continuous assessment and recording of intracavernous pressure (ICP). BD Intramedic PE-50 tubing (BD, Franklin Lakes, NJ) was inserted into the carotid artery for the measurement of MAP. Both ICP and mean arterial blood pressure (MAP) were recorded continuously as previously described [23, 29, 30]. The stimulus parameters were 1.5 mA, 20 Hz, pulse width 0.2 ms, and duration 50 s. The maximal ICP during nerve electrostimulation was calculated from an isometric force transducer and recorded on a computer with a PowerLab commercial data acquisition system (AD Instruments, Dunedin, New Zealand). The ratio of ICP to MAP was used to evaluate the level of erectile function. The penis was then harvested for histologic analysis, ELISA, and Western blotting.

2.6. Histology and Immunofluorescence Staining. Animals were sacrificed by intraperitoneal injection with sodium pentobarbital (50 mg/kg), followed by bilateral thoracotomy. Penile midshaft tissues were freshly harvested and fixed [23], and immunofluorescence staining was performed as previously described [31]. The corpus cavernosum paraffin sections were immunostained with VEGF (diluted 1 : 200 Santa Cruz Biotechnologies, Santa Cruz, US), neuronal nitric oxide synthase (nNOS, diluted 1 : 200 Santa Cruz Biotechnologies, Santa Cruz, CA), brain-derived neurotrophic factor (BDNF, diluted 1 : 200; Abcam, Cambridge, UK), nerve growth factor (NGF, diluted 1 : 200; Abcam, Cambridge, UK), stromal cell-derived factor-1 (SDF-1 diluted 1 : 200; Abcam, Cambridge, UK), and neuron-specific β-III tubulin (diluted 1 : 200; Abcam, Cambridge, UK) and mounted with 4,6-diamidino-2-phenylindole (DAPI; Vector Laboratories Inc., Burlingame, CA) to stain the nuclei. The collagen and vascular smooth muscle was evaluated after tissue staining with the Masson trichrome technique using the method previously described [32]. Digital images were obtained using a Zeiss LSM 510 Meta confocal microscope (Zeiss, Oberkochen, Germany), and the mean intensity was calculated using ZEN 2009 (Zeiss).

2.7. Analysis of Apoptosis and Autophagy In Vivo. We assessed the apoptosis in vivo using Western blotting to test the poly-ADP-ribose polymerase (PARP) as previously described [33]. We also analyzed the autophagy in penile tissue by Western blotting to detect light chain 3 (LC3) [34]. The antibodies of PARP and LC3 were listed in Western blot analysis.

2.8. Effect of Combination between ESWT and MSCT In Vivo. 60 mg of penile tissue from both normal control and experimental animals was immersed with 350 mL of 0.1 M HCL, and silica beads were added (BioSec Enviro Inc., Guelph, Canada). The treated sample was homogenized in 2 mL lysate buffer (Precellys 24; Bertin Technologies, Montigny-le-Bretonneux, France) and centrifuged at 14,000 ×g for 10 minutes at 4°C, and then its supernatant was extracted. The protein concentration in each sample was determined by bicinchoninic acid (BCA) assay according to the manufacturer's instructions. The cGMP (cyclic guanosine monophosphate) direct immunoassay kit (K372, BioVision, San Francisco, US) was used for detection of cavernous cGMP levels according to the manufacturer's protocol.

2.9. Western Blot Analysis. Corpus cavernosum tissue was homogenized using ice-cold RIPA buffer (Cell Signaling Technology, Danvers, US) containing ethylenediaminetetraacetic acid-free protease inhibitor cocktail and phosphatase inhibitor cocktail (Roche Diagnostics GmbH). The homogenized sample was then centrifuged at 12,000 ×g for 10 minutes at 4°C and its supernatant extracted. This supernatant was electrophoresed on NuPAGE 4%–12% bis-Tris gel (Invitrogen, Carlsbad, CA) and then transferred onto a nitrocellulose membrane. After the transfer, the membrane was blocked with 5% skim milk at room temperature for 1 hour and then incubated with the primary antibodies including endothelial nitric oxide synthase (eNOS diluted 1 : 500 Santa Cruz Biotechnologies, Santa Cruz, CA), phosphorylated endothelial nitric oxide synthase (p-eNOS diluted 1 : 500 Santa Cruz Biotechnologies, Santa Cruz, CA), AKT (diluted 1 : 500; Cell Signaling Technology, Danvers, US), p-AKT (diluted 1 : 500; Cell Signaling Technology, Danvers, US), PARP (diluted 1 : 500; Abcam, Cambridge, UK), LC3 (diluted 1 : 500; Abcam, Cambridge, UK), platelet endothelial cell adhesion molecule (PECAM, diluted 1 : 500; Abcam, Cambridge, UK), and β-actin (diluted 1 : 1000; Abcam, Cambridge, UK). After this, the membrane was incubated with a secondary antibody conjugated to horseradish peroxidase for 1 hour at room temperature. The enhanced chemiluminescence method (Amersham, Arlington Heights, IL) was used for protein detection. The resulting images were analyzed using ImageJ (National Institutes of Health, Bethesda, MD, US) to determine the integrated density for each protein band.

2.10. Image and Statistical Analysis. The images were quantified by ImageJ and Image-Pro Plus (Media Cybernetics, Silver Spring, MD, USA). The results were analyzed using SPSS 20.0 software (SPSS Inc., Chicago, IL, USA). The measurement data are presented as mean ± standard deviation (SD), and the multigroup comparisons were made with (ANOVA) followed by the Tukey-Kramer test for post hoc comparisons. Data expressed as proportions were assessed with a chi square test. Values of $P < 0.05$ were considered to indicate a statistically significant difference.

3. Results

3.1. ESWT + MSCT Can Improve ED Significantly. ICP results are shown in Figure 1. As we can see from Figure 1(a), the ICP result of the DM + ESWT + MSCT group is apparently higher than the result of the DM control group. In quantitative results (Figure 1(b)), the sham group is 0.73 ± 0.08. The experimental groups including DM control, DM + ESWT, DM + MSCT, and DM + ESWT + MSCT groups are, in order, 0.21 ± 0.08, 0.43 ± 0.07, 0.41 ± 0.11, and 0.59 ± 0.09. Both ESWT and MSCT can improve ED; their quantitative results are higher than in the DM control group ($P < 0.05$). The ratio of ICP/MAP was significantly higher in the DM + ESWT + MSCT group than in the DM + ESWT and DM + MSCT groups ($P < 0.05$). The quantitative result of the DM + ESWT + MSCT group is very close to the result of the sham group. So we can hold the opinion that ED treatment is more effective by DM + ESWT + MSCT than by a single way (ESWT or MSCT).

3.2. ESWT + MSCT Stimulates Angiogenesis and Vasodilatation in DMED Rats' Corpus Cavernosum. The result of Masson staining (Figure 2(a)) shows that the vascular smooth muscle of the DM + ESWT + MSCT group is obviously more, in comparison with vascular smooth muscle of the DM group. These results show that both EWST and MSCT can stimulate angiogenesis, compared with the DE group ($P < 0.05$). The result was significantly higher in the DM + ESWT + MSCT group than in the DM + ESWT or DM + MSCT groups ($P < 0.05$), which proved that DM + ESWT + MSCT could stimulate angiogenesis and vasodilatation, significantly. It is also emphasized that angiogenesis and vasodilatation (Figure 2(a)) in the DM + ESWT + MSCT group is approximated to the sham group. One of the primary reasons for DM is vascular damage caused by oxidative stress response and hyperglycemia [35, 36]. Insufficient blood supply results from vascular damage leading to ED. So increasing the angiogenesis and recovering vascular function are key to restoring erectile function. Now, PDE5I is the first-line treatment for ED, but there are still poor therapeutic effects for some DMED patients especially with damaged vascular endothelium [4–6]. As we can see from our results (Figure 2), ESWT + MSCT can obviously increase the blood supply in the corpus cavernosum. So we believe that after ESWT + MSCT, the erectile function of DMED patients will be improved significantly.

3.3. ESWT Increases the Quantity of MSCs in the Corpus Cavernosum. After MSC intracavernous injection, we made a MSCT successively. In our results (Figure 3), we found that ESWT can increase the quantity of MSCs in the corpus cavernosum obviously. So we made a quantitative analysis of staining results. As we can see from the quantitative results (Figure 4(c)), we found after MSC intracavernous injection that the quantity of MSCs with MSCT was higher than the quantity of MSCs without EWST ($P < 0.05$). This result tells us that ESWT can increase MSCs.

3.4. ESWT Can Induce MSCs to Express More VEGF In Vitro and In Vivo. We found after ESWT that MSCs could express more VEGF (Figure 4(a)) than without ESWT in vitro ($P < 0.05$). In order to research the effect of ESWT on the MSCs in vivo, we injected MSCs into the corpus cavernosum of DMED rats and then carried out ESWT. From the results (Figures 3(a) and 3(D)), we found that VEGF expression in the DN + DMED + ESWT group was higher than others ($P < 0.05$). So we consider that after ESWT, the MSCs can express more VEGF in vivo. From Figures 3(D) and 3(d), we found that penile tissues of DMED rats scarcely expressed VEGF. This phenomenon leads to endothelial proliferation slowly and angiogenesis barely. But in the DM + ESWT or DM + MSCT groups, there was still some VEGF in the corpus cavernosum. This is one reason why ESWT and MSCT can improve DMED.

3.5. VEGF Activates the PI3K/AKT/mTOR and NO/cGMP Signaling Pathway in the Corpus Cavernosum. Some researchers [37, 38] believe that VEGF can activate the PI3K/AKT/mTOR pathway, so we detected the expression quantity of AKT and p-AKT. The results (Figures 5(a) and 5(b)) show that with ESWT + MSCT, the expression quantity of p-AKT/AKT is apparently higher than others ($P < 0.05$). Combining with the result (Figure 3(D)), we consider after ESWT + MSCT that plentiful VEGF triggers the PI3K/AKT/mTOR pathway in the DMED corpus cavernosum. Some researchers [39] consider that NO mediates vasodilatation by increasing soluble guanylate cyclase (sGC) in the smooth muscle of vessels. According to the NO/cGMP pathway [40], we detected the quantity of eNOS/p-eNOS, nNOS, and cGMP expression. The results (Figures 4(b), 5, and 6) indicate that with ESWT + MSCT, the quantity of p-eNOS/eNOS and cGMP is apparently higher than others ($P < 0.05$). Combining with the result (Figure 3(D)), we believe that, after ESWT + MSCT, much of VEGF activates the NO/cGMP pathway. As in the above, we believe that ESWT + MSCT can increase the expression of VEGF, and plenty of VEGF can trigger the PI3K/AKT/mTOR and NO/cGMP pathways.

3.6. ESWT + MSCT Can Stimulate Autophagy and Decrease Apoptosis in the Corpus Cavernosum. Some researchers [20, 41, 42] believe that activating the PI3K/AKT/mTOR pathway can induce autophagy by reducing mechanistic

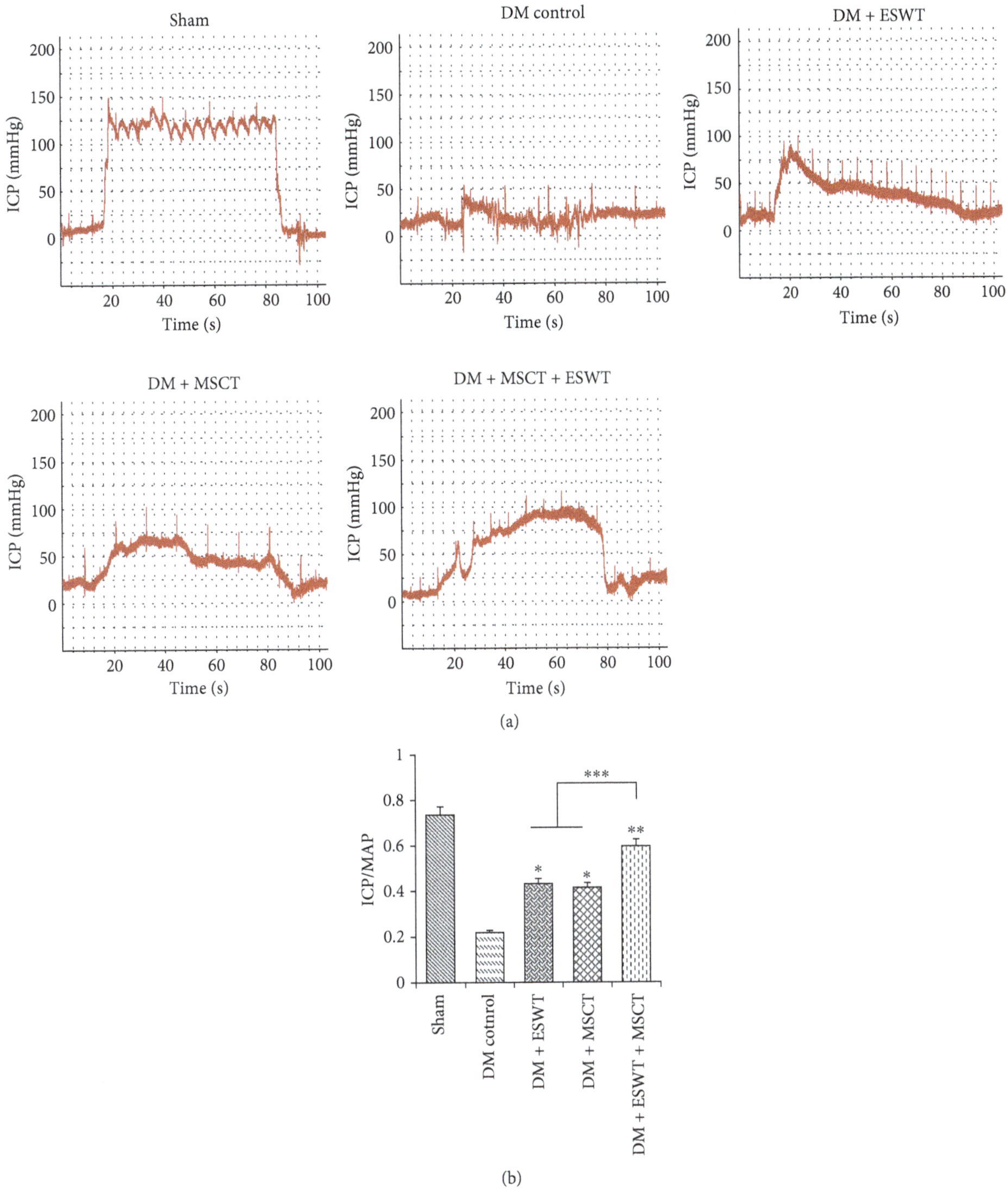

FIGURE 1: Erectile function of each group. (a) Representative images of intracavernous pressure (ICP) in response to electrical stimulation of the cavernosal nerve. (b) Results of ratio ICP to mean MAP of each group. Each bar shows the mean values (standard deviation). $^{*}p < 0.05$ compared with DMED rats. $^{**}p < 0.01$ compared with DMED rats. $^{***}p < 0.05$ compared with DM + ESWT and DM + MSCT groups.

target of rapamycin complex (mTORC) 1 kinase activity and Rheb levels. As a type of self-defense, autophagy can offset losses caused by apoptosis [22]. We found (Figure 4(c)) that after ESWT, the quantity of MSCs increased significantly ($P < 0.05$). So we made a hypothesis that ESWT induced MSCs to express more VEGF, and then VEGF triggered the PI3K/AKT/mTOR pathway for increasing autophagy. The results of autophagy and apoptosis assay (Figure 7) show that ESWT can activate autophagy of the penile tissues and decrease apoptosis effectively. Also, we found that NGF (Figures 3(a) and 3(A)) and BDNF (Figures 3(c) and 3(C)) expression was higher in the DM + ESWT + MSCT group than in the DM group ($P < 0.01$), which has been considered to defend apoptosis [43, 44]. These results proved our hypothesis that ESWT could stimulate autophagy and decrease apoptosis in the corpus cavernosum.

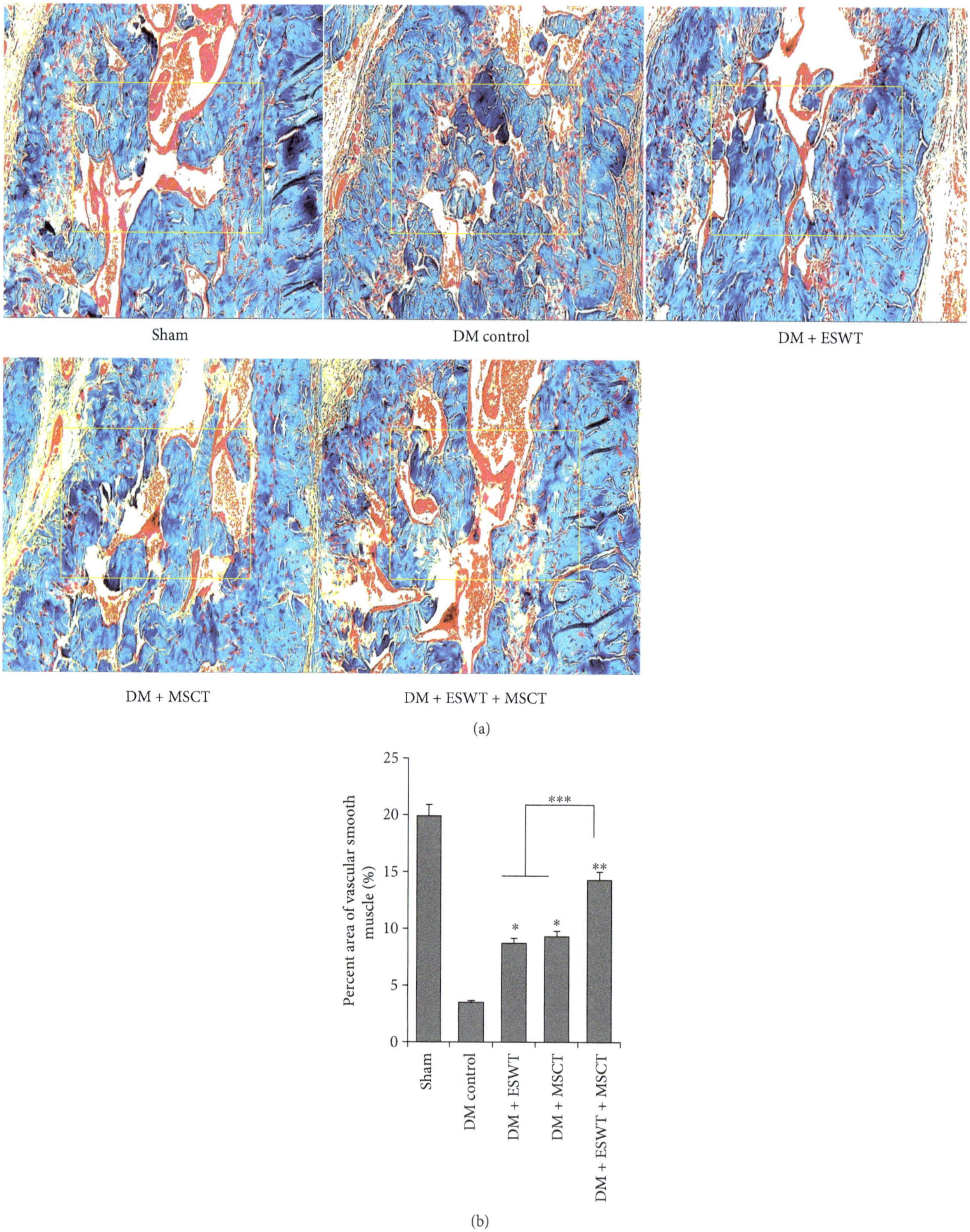

FIGURE 2: Masson staining of corpus cavernosum (a) Representative images of Masson trichrome stain for each group. Red is vascular smooth muscle, and blue is collagen. Original magnification: ×200. (b) Percentage area of endothelial cell smooth muscle cells for each group. Each bar shows the mean values (standard deviation). $^{*}P < 0.05$ compared with the DM control group. $^{**}P < 0.01$ compared with the DM control group. $^{***}P < 0.05$ compared with the DM + ESWT and DM + MSCT groups.

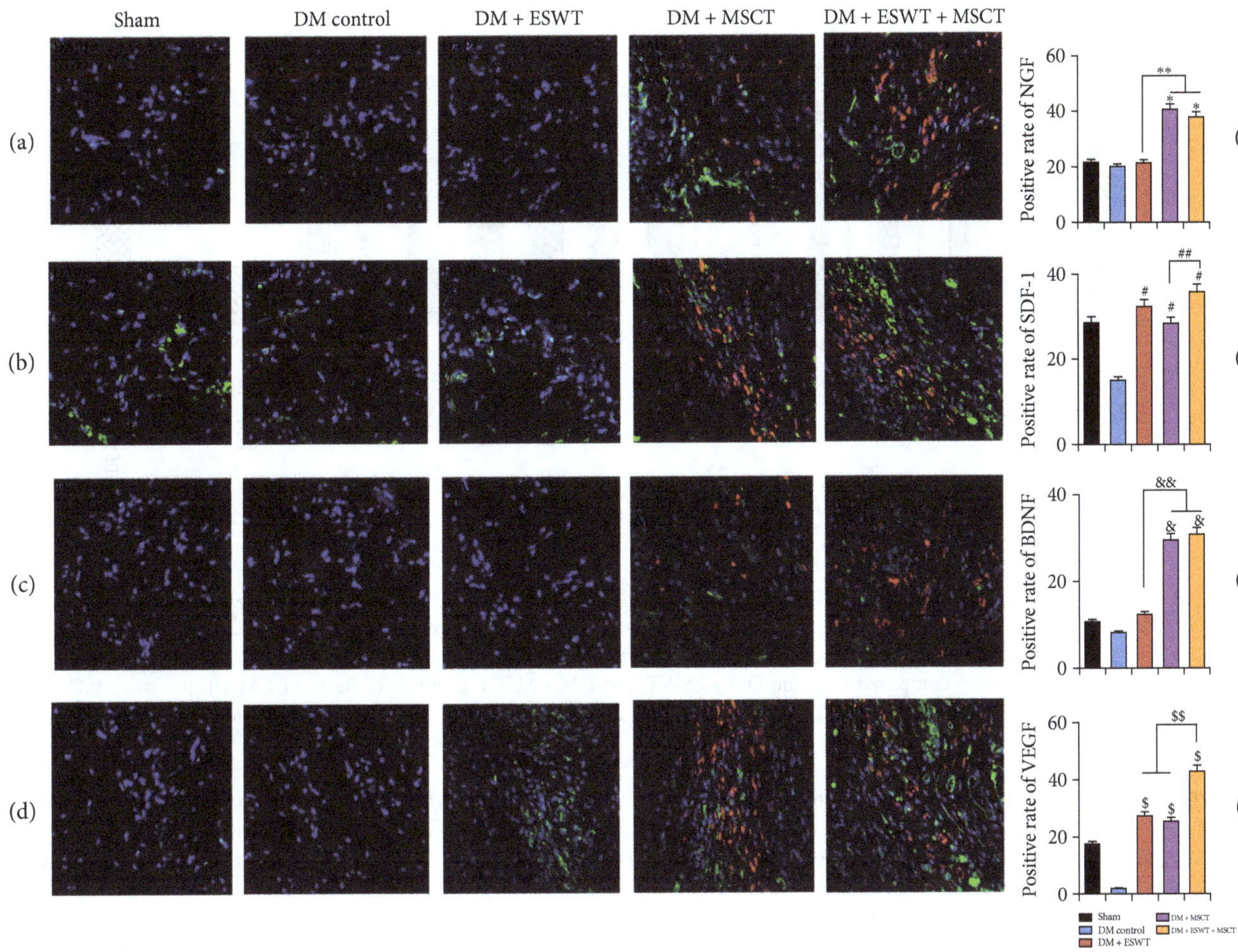

FIGURE 3: ESWT + MSCT promoted proliferation and migration in vivo. (a) Representative images of NGF stain for each group. Original magnification: ×200. (B) Positive rate of NGF for each group. Each bar shows the mean values (standard deviation). $^{*}P < 0.01$ compared with the DM control group, $^{**}P < 0.01$. (b) Representative images of SDF-1 stain for each group. Original magnification: ×200. (B) Positive rate of SDF-1 for each group. Each bar shows the mean values (standard deviation). $^{\#}P < 0.01$ compared with the DM control group, $^{\#\#}P < 0.05$. (b) Representative images of BDNF stain for each group. Original magnification: ×200. (B) Positive rate of BDNF for each group. Each bar shows the mean values (standard deviation). $^{\&}P < 0.01$ compared with the DM control group, $^{\&\&}P < 0.01$. (b) Representative images of VEGF stain for each group. Original magnification: ×200. (b) Positive rate of VEGF for each group. Each bar shows the mean values (standard deviation). $^{\$}P < 0.01$ compared with the DM control group, $^{\$\$}P < 0.05$.

3.7. ESWT Can Promote MSC Recruitment by Inducing Penile Tissues to Express More SDF-1 and PECAM. Finally, in order to explore other reasons why ESWT can increase MSCs, we detected SDF-1 and PECAM. Fandel et al. [23] believe that SDF-1 can attract intracavernously injected stem cells. PECAM is a chemokine like SDF-1 and can direct cell trafficking. Our results (Figures 3(b) and 3(B) and 5) indicate that after ESWT, there are lots of SDF-1 and PECAM expression in the corpus cavernosum ($P < 0.05$). So combining with the Figure 4(c), we hold the opinion that ESWT can drive recruitment of MSCs.

4. Discussion

DL-ESWT and MSCT have been studied as a treatment of ED for several years [45–47]. Some findings [48, 49] have been used clinically as a novel ED therapy, but translation of MSCT studies to clinic remains slow, and the molecular mechanisms of the effect of LI-ESWT remain confusing [50]. So we want to provide more theoretic and experimental bases for clinical treatment. In our study, we found that DL-ESWT could stimulate MSCs to express more VEGF in vitro and vivo. We also found that ESWT + MSCT could be a better ED therapy than by a single way. We also verified that VEGF took part in the PI3K/AKT/mTOR signaling pathway to induce autophagy and activated the NO/cGMP signaling pathway to induce vasodilatation and angiogenesis in vivo. Meanwhile, our study verified that ESWT can increase the quantity of MSCs in the corpus cavernosum.

There are many reasons for DMED, but the primary reason is vascular damage caused by oxidative stress response

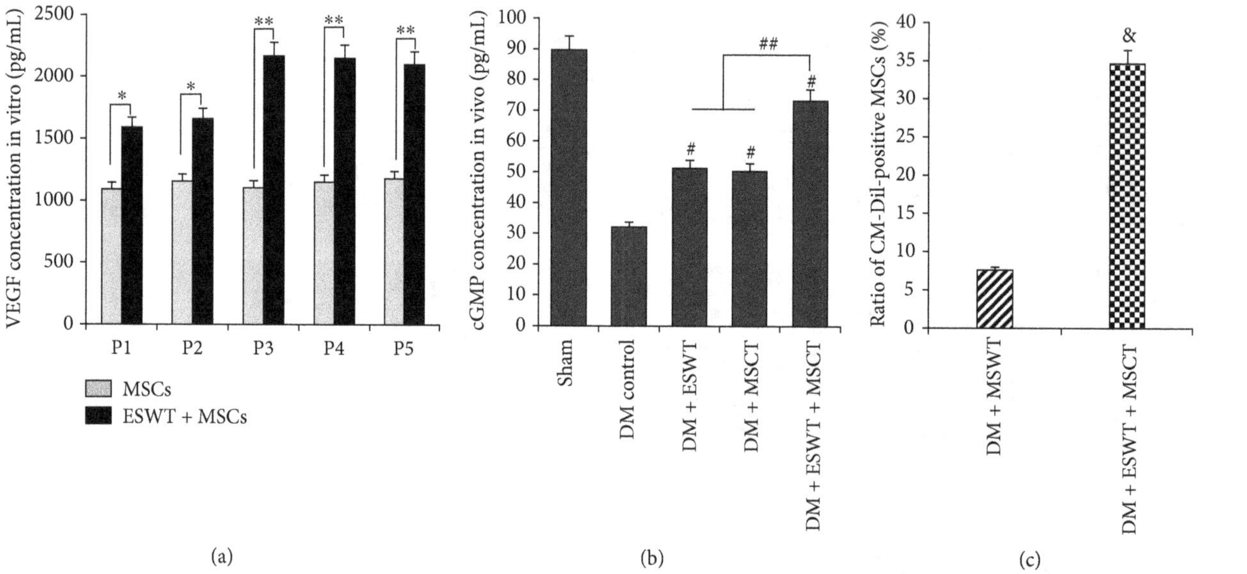

FIGURE 4: (a) VEGF concentration in vitro from P1 to P5 after ESWT or not, by ELISA. $^{*}P < 0.05$, with untreated MSCs; treated MSCs secreted higher levels of VEGF. $^{**}P < 0.01$, with untreated MSCs; treated MSCs secreted higher levels of VEGF. (b) cGMP concentration of each group in vivo, by ELISA. $^{\#}P < 0.05$, with untreated MSCs; treated MSCs secreted higher levels of cGMP. $^{\#}P < 0.05$ compared with the DM control group. $^{\#\#}P < 0.05$ compared with the DM + ESWT and DM + MSCT groups. (c) Ratio of CM-Dil-positive MSCs in the corpus cavernosum. $^{\&}P < 0.01$; in the DM + ESWT + MSCT group, the quantity of MSCs is higher than in the DM + MSCT group.

and hyperglycemia [35, 36]. On the one hand, vascular damage can cause penis insufficient blood supply leading to erectile disorder. On the other hand, oxidative stress response can cause neurocyte damage and endothelial apoptosis, which can reduce eNOS and nNOS in the corpus cavernosum, and these can decrease NO and then lead to DMED [51, 52]. Tepekoylu et al. [53] proved that ESWT could induce angiogenesis and lead to mobilization of endogenous endothelial cells. Prieto et al. [54] show that MSCT can stimulate angiogenesis in vascular homeostasis, and our study also shows similar consequences. What is more, our results indicate that ESWT + MSCT can improve erectile function more effectively than by a single way. Accordingly, these results confirm our hypothesis that combination of both ESWT and MSCT for ED treatment will get a better result than by a single way. In our results, we find that in vitro and vivo MSCs after ESWT can express more VEGF. So we believe that the VEGF content in the penile tissues is the key to recovering erectile function.

In some studies [23, 24], the quantity of MSCs after injection will decrease rapidly and only a few MSCs can reach the target area. They believed that most of MSCs would flow away via migration into the circulatory system. But in this experiment, we verified that ESWT could increase the quantity of MSCs in the corpus cavernosum. Also, these MSCs can be beneficial for ED treatment. Fandel et al. [23] considered that nerve injury upregulated SDF-1 expression in the ganglion and thereby attracted intracavernously injected stem cells. They injected MSCs into penile tissues and detected the labeled MSCs in the major pelvic ganglia. In our study, similarly we injected MSCs to the penile tissues, and after ESWT we found a high expression of SDF-1 and PECAM, which can drive MSCs to stay in the corpus cavernosum. We also found after ESWT the quantity of MSCs increased in the corpus cavernosum. So it is proved that ESWT could drive recruitment of MSCs. This is why ESWT can keep the MSCs in the corpus cavernosum adequately.

Some researchers [55, 56] consider that NO can trigger cavernous smooth muscle cell relaxation, which can allow blood to enter into the sinusoids during sexual arousal. They indicated that it was a crucial reason why increasing NO could improve ED. But according to the latest study, Yoshida et al. [57] consider that the level of NO in the corpus cavernosum can induce vasodilatation and stimulate angiogenesis, which is another important reason that NO could improve ED. On the basis of the NO/cGMP pathway [40, 58], we believe that more nNOS and cGMP can improve ED, efficiently. Komori et al. [59] consider that VEGF can stimulate angiogenesis by activating the NO/cGMP signaling pathway. We find that after ESWT and MSCT, VEGF expression is higher than without ESWT or MSCT. So we believe that after ESWT and MSCT the NO/cGMP signaling pathway should be activated in the corpus cavernosum. Wu et al. [60] conclude that VEGF plays an important role in NO/cGMP signaling pathway activation in the process of promoting angiogenesis. Similarly, our results demonstrated that as nNOS and cGMP in the penile tissues increase, the level of NO in the penile tissues could augment, which can relax vessels and stimulate angiogenesis, and then improve erectile function. To sum up the above arguments, we can conclude that ESWT + MSCT can be a great ED treatment because of better regeneration and repair compared with a single ESWT or MSCT.

Some researchers [22, 61] consider that there is an important relationship between apoptosis and autophagy,

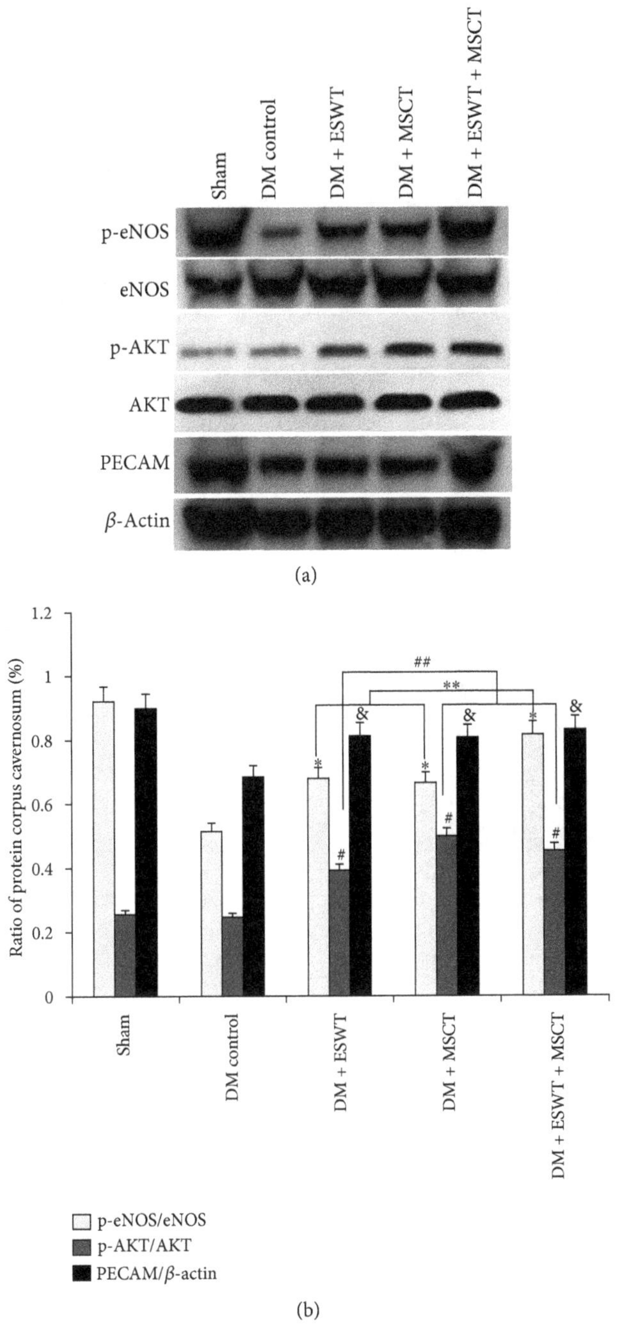

FIGURE 5: ESWT increases proteins of proliferation, autophagy, and migration. (a) All groups were compared for p-eNOS, eNOS, p-AKT, AKT, and PECAM in the corpus cavernosum using Western blotting. (b) Quantity analysis of Western blotting, including p-eNOS/eNOS, p-AKT/AKT, and PECAM/β-actin. $^{*}P < 0.05$ compared with values from the DM control group. $^{**}P < 0.05$ compared with the DM + ESWT and DM + MSCT groups. $^{\#}P < 0.05$ compared with the DM control group. $^{\#\#}P < 0.05$ compared with the DM + MSCT and DM + ESWT + MSCT groups. $^{\&}P < 0.05$ compared with the DM control group.

which means the increased autophagy can decrease apoptosis. In DMED rats' corpus cavernosum, oxidative stress response induces apoptosis [22]. The apoptosis aggravates corpus cavernosum ischemia and then weaken erectile function [62]. Autophagy [63, 64] is a self-protection that cells can get nutriment needed to sustain survival, and autophagy is an important self-regulation system of cells to inhibit apoptosis. Our results show that in the DM + ESWT + MSCT group, the number of apoptosis in the corpus cavernosum is lower than in other groups, which is close to the normal group. So we consider that ESWT + MSCT can increase autophagy to defend apoptosis in the DMED rats' corpus cavernosum. Wei et al. [37] consider that VEGF can activate the PI3K/AKT/mTOR signaling pathway and then stimulate autophagy. In our results, we found that in the DM + ESWT + MSCT group p-akt/akt expression was higher than in others. So we consider that VEGF plays an important role in the PI3K/AKT/mTOR signaling pathway in the process of improving erectile function. In brief, we believe that after being treated by DL-ESWT and MSCT, the corpus cavernosum can express a lot of VEGF, and these VEGF can bind to VEGF receptors in the corpus cavernosum. On the one hand, VEGF can stimulate the PI3K/AKT/mTOR signaling pathway, induce autophagy, and then improve erectile function. On the other hand, VEGF can trigger the NO/cGMP signaling pathway, activate vasodilatation and angiogenesis, and then improve ED. We tested the VEGF expression in each group, and the results show that the expression in the DM + ESWT + MSCT group is higher than in other groups. This result also proves that combination of LI-ESWT and MSCT can express more VEGF than a single treatment. VEGF can reach the cell surface and bind to VEGF receptors via the paracrine, which regulates autophagy and apoptosis by activating the PI3K/AKT/mTOR and NO/cGMP signaling pathway. These also explained why LI-ESWT and MSCT could induce vasodilatation and angiogenesis to improve ED. In the next experiment, we want to test the further relationship between VEGF and these two pathways. We will block the VEGF receptors on the cell surface, which cannot make VEGF and VEGF receptors combined. These experiments will find out if VEGF can trigger the PI3K/AKT/mTOR and NO/cGMP pathways exactly. Berrak et al. [65] inhibited the PI3K/AKT/mTOR pathway to test the relationship between autophagy and apoptosis in the prostate cancer cells, and some researchers [66] inhibited the NO pathway to detect the proliferation ability of endothelial cells. So next we will, respectively, inhibit the PI3K/AKT/mTOR and NO/cGMP pathways and find out these two pathways' influences on ED. If these results coincide with our results in this report, we will conclude that a combination of LI-ESWT and MSCT can be a great potential and promising way to improve ED by activating the PI3K/AKT/mTOR pathway which can increase autophagy and decrease apoptosis and the NO/cGMP pathway which can induce vasodilatation and angiogenesis.

Our experiment does have some places for improvement. Firstly, the rats in our experiment are 8 weeks old, so we do not know if LI-ESWT and MCST have the same effect on older DMED rats. Secondly, the number of MSCs in the corpus cavernosum by intracavernous injection is hard to control in each DMED rat, so it is difficult to avoid errors. At last, about the pathway, we just made an animal

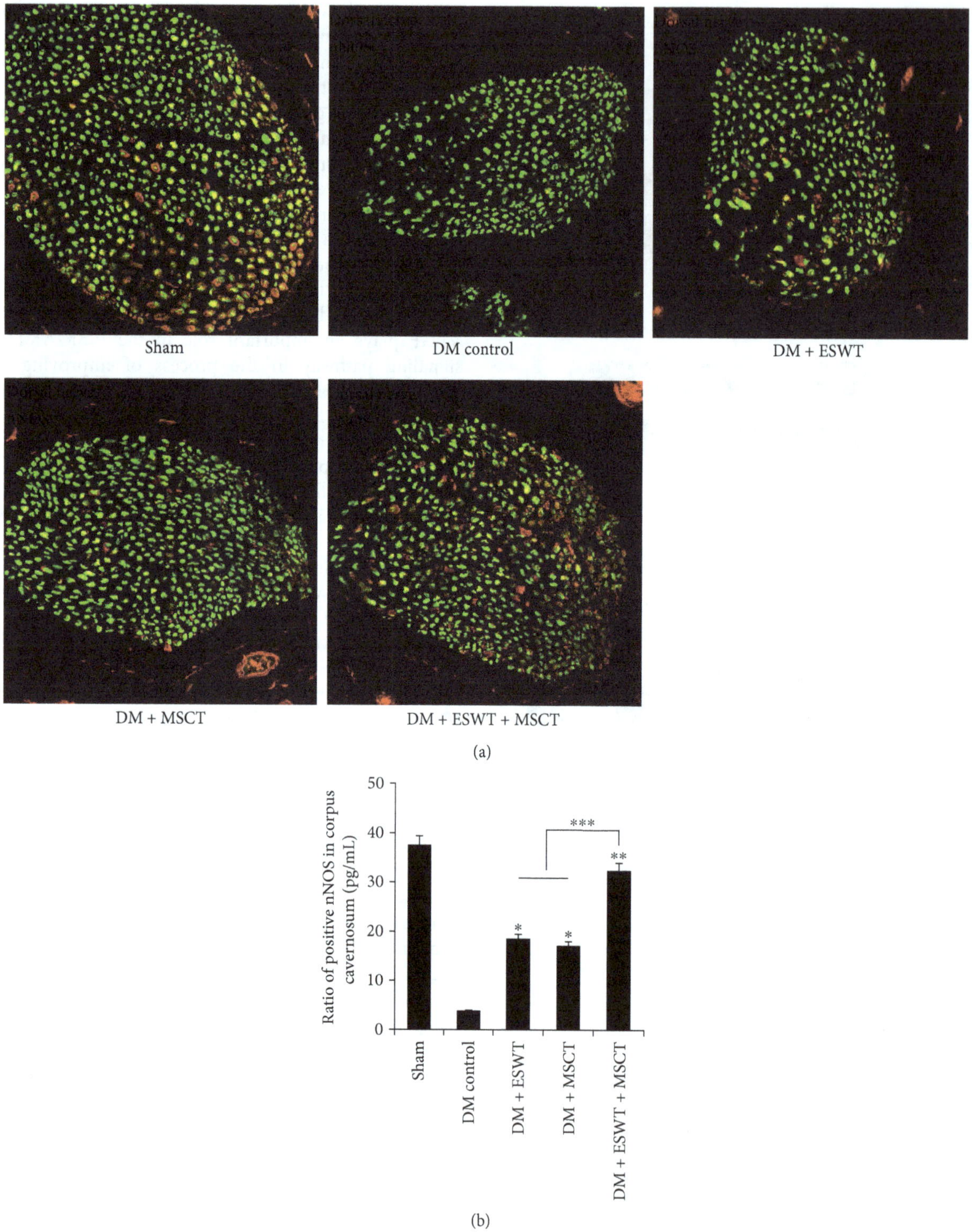

FIGURE 6: ESWT + MSCT induce nNOS expression in the corpus cavernosum. (a) Representative images of nNOS staining in the corpus cavernosum. (b) Ratio of positive nNOS of each group. Each bar shows the mean values (standard deviation). Original magnification: ×400. $^{*}P < 0.05$ compared with the DM control group. $^{**}P < 0.01$ compared with the DM control group. $^{***}P < 0.05$ compared with the DM + ESWT and DM + MSCT groups.

experiment, but no cell experiment. So in the next step, we will inhibit the PI3K/AKT/mTOR and NO/cGMP pathways and control the related gene expression to verify our animal experiment.

5. Conclusion

Our experiment has proved that combination of LI-ESWT and MSCT can get a better result than by a single way as a

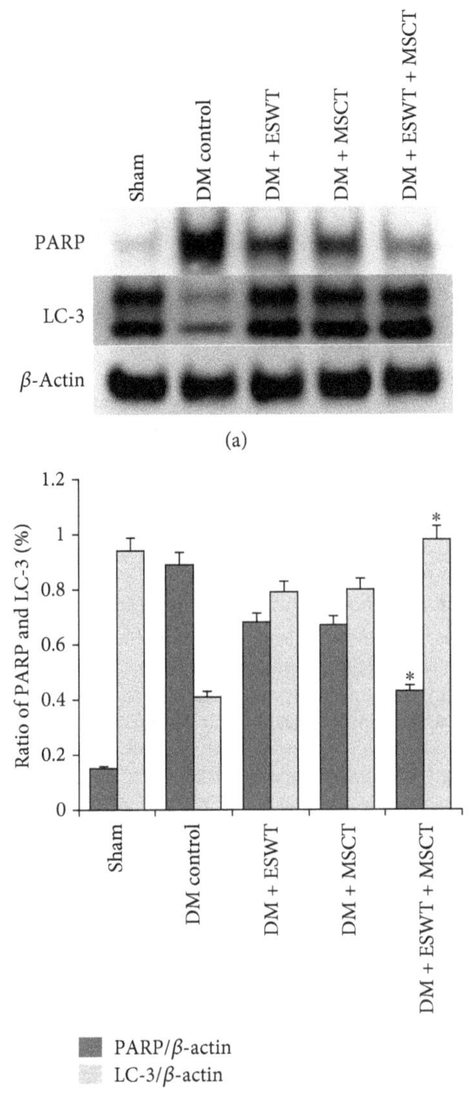

FIGURE 7: ESWT can activate autophagy and decrease apoptosis in vivo. (a) All groups were compared for PARP and LC-3 in vivo by Western blotting. (b) Quantity analysis of Western blotting, including PARP/β-actin and LC-3/β-actin. $^*P < 0.01$ compared with values from the DM control group.

novel ED treatment. This is because combination of LI-ESWT and MSCT can express more VEGF than a single treatment, which can take part in autophagy by triggering the PI3K/AKT/mTOR signaling pathway. LI-ESWT and MSCT can induce vasodilatation and angiogenesis by activating the NO/cGMP signaling pathway. Our study has proved that ESWT can drive homing of MSCs in the corpus cavernosum. Our study provides a theoretic and experimental basis for clinical treatment. This cooperative therapy combined with stem cells and machine also provides a new research direction in ED treatment for the future.

Abbreviations

BCA: Bicinchoninic acid
BDNF: Brain-derived neurotrophic factor
cGMP: Cyclic guanosine monophosphate
DAPI: 4,6-Diamidino-2-phenylindole
DL-ESWT: Defocused low-energy shock wave therapy
DMED: Diabetes mellitus erectile dysfunction
ED: Erectile dysfunction
eNOS: Endothelial nitric oxide synthase
ICP: Intracavernous pressure
NGF: Nerve growth factor
NO: Nitric oxide
PDE5I: Phosphodiesterase 5 inhibitor
SDF-1: Stromal cell-derived factor-1
LC3: Light chain 3
MAP: Mean arterial blood pressure
MSCs: Mesenchymal stem cells
MSCT: Mesenchymal stem cell therapy
mTORC: Mechanistic target of rapamycin complex
nNOS: Neuronal nitric oxide synthase
PARP: Poly-ADP-ribose polymerase
PECAM: Platelet endothelial cell adhesion molecule
sGC: Soluble guanylate cyclase
STZ: Streptozotocin
VEGF: Vascular endothelial growth factor.

Authors' Contributions

Guan Qun Zhu, first author, was responsible for the conception, design data analysis and interpretation, and manuscript writing. Seung Hwan Jeon was responsible for the collection and assembly of data and data analysis. Woong Jin Bae was responsible for the conception and design, assembly of data, data analysis and interpretation, and revision of the manuscript. Sae Woong Choi, Hyun Cheol Jeong, Kang Sup Kim, and Su Jin Kim were responsible for the collection and assembly of data. Hyuk Jin Cho, U. Syn Ha, Sung Hoo Hong, and Eun Bi Kwon were responsible for the provision of study material and animal models. Ji Youl Lee was responsible for the conception and design, data analysis, and interpretation. Sae Woong Kim, corresponding author, was responsible for the conception and design, financial support, drafting and revision of the manuscript, and final approval of the manuscript. All authors read and approved the final manuscript.

Acknowledgments

This research was supported by a grant of the Korean Health Technology R&D Project through the Korea Health Industry Development Institute (KHIDI), funded by the Ministry of Health and Welfare, Republic of Korea (Grant HI17C1944).

References

[1] D. F. Penson, D. M. Latini, D. P. Lubeck, K. L. Wallace, J. M. Henning, and T. F. Lue, "Do impotent men with diabetes have more severe erectile dysfunction and worse quality of life than the general population of impotent patients? Results from the Exploratory Comprehensive Evaluation of Erectile Dysfunction (ExCEED) database," *Diabetes Care*, vol. 26, no. 4, pp. 1093–1099, 2003.

[2] G. De Berardis, M. Franciosi, M. Belfiglio et al., "Erectile dysfunction and quality of life in type 2 diabetic patients: a serious problem too often overlooked," *Diabetes Care*, vol. 25, no. 2, pp. 284–291, 2002.

[3] V. S. Thorve, A. D. Kshirsagar, N. S. Vyawahare, V. S. Joshi, K. G. Ingale, and R. J. Mohite, "Diabetes-induced erectile dysfunction: epidemiology, pathophysiology and management," *Journal of Diabetes and its Complications*, vol. 25, no. 2, pp. 129–136, 2011.

[4] V. Phé and M. Rouprêt, "Erectile dysfunction and diabetes: a review of the current evidence-based medicine and a synthesis of the main available therapies," *Diabetes & Metabolism*, vol. 38, no. 1, pp. 1–13, 2012.

[5] L. S. Malavige and J. C. Levy, "Erectile dysfunction in diabetes mellitus," *The Journal of Sexual Medicine*, vol. 6, no. 5, pp. 1232–1247, 2009.

[6] M. S. Rendell, J. Rajfer, P. A. Wicker, M. D. Smith, and for the Sildenafil Diabetes Study Group, "Sildenafil for treatment of erectile dysfunction in men with diabetes: a randomized controlled trial," *JAMA*, vol. 281, no. 5, pp. 421–426, 1999.

[7] D. Hayashi, K. Kawakami, K. Ito et al., "Low-energy extracorporeal shock wave therapy enhances skin wound healing in diabetic mice: a critical role of endothelial nitric oxide synthase," *Wound Repair and Regeneration*, vol. 20, no. 6, pp. 887–895, 2012.

[8] C. B. Foldager, C. Kearney, and M. Spector, "Clinical application of extracorporeal shock wave therapy in orthopedics: focused versus unfocused shock waves," *Ultrasound in Medicine and Biology*, vol. 38, no. 10, pp. 1673–1680, 2012.

[9] A. Aqil, M. R. Siddiqui, M. Solan, D. J. Redfern, V. Gulati, and J. P. Cobb, "Extracorporeal shock wave therapy is effective in treating chronic plantar fasciitis: a meta-analysis of RCTs," *Clinical Orthopaedics and Related Research*, vol. 471, no. 11, pp. 3645–3652, 2013.

[10] T. Cayton, A. E. Harwood, G. E. Smith, J. P. Totty, D. Carradice, and I. C. Chetter, "Extracorporeal shockwave therapy for the treatment of lower limb intermittent claudication: study protocol for a randomised controlled trial (the SHOCKWAVE 1 trial)," *Trials*, vol. 18, no. 1, p. 104, 2017.

[11] A. Zissler, P. Steinbacher, R. Zimmermann et al., "Extracorporeal shock wave therapy accelerates regeneration after acute skeletal muscle injury," *The American Journal of Sports Medicine*, vol. 45, no. 3, pp. 676–684, 2017.

[12] I. Gruenwald, B. Appel, and Y. Vardi, "Low-intensity extracorporeal shock wave therapy—a novel effective treatment for erectile dysfunction in severe ED patients who respond poorly to PDE5 inhibitor therapy," *The Journal of Sexual Medicine*, vol. 9, no. 1, pp. 259–264, 2012.

[13] R. I. Clavijo, T. P. Kohn, J. R. Kohn, and R. Ramasamy, "Effects of low-intensity extracorporeal shockwave therapy on erectile dysfunction: a systematic review and meta-analysis," *The Journal of Sexual Medicine*, vol. 14, no. 1, pp. 27–35, 2017.

[14] Z. Lu, G. Lin, A. Reed-Maldonado, C. Wang, Y. C. Lee, and T. F. Lue, "Low-intensity extracorporeal shock wave treatment improves erectile function: a systematic review and meta-analysis," *European Urology*, vol. 71, no. 2, pp. 223–233, 2017.

[15] B. Wang, H. Ning, A. B. Reed-Maldonado et al., "Low-intensity extracorporeal shock wave therapy enhances brain-derived neurotrophic factor expression through PERK/ATF4 signaling pathway," *International Journal of Molecular Sciences*, vol. 18, no. 2, p. 433, 2017.

[16] A. Aicher, C. Heeschen, K. Sasaki, C. Urbich, A. M. Zeiher, and S. Dimmeler, "Low-energy shock wave for enhancing recruitment of endothelial progenitor cells: a new modality to increase efficacy of cell therapy in chronic hind limb ischemia," *Circulation*, vol. 114, no. 25, pp. 2823–2830, 2006.

[17] H. Li, M. P. Matheu, F. Sun et al., "Low-energy shock wave therapy ameliorates erectile dysfunction in a pelvic neurovascular injuries rat model," *The Journal of Sexual Medicine*, vol. 13, no. 1, pp. 22–32, 2016.

[18] N. Mangır and L. Türkeri, "Stem cell therapies in post-prostatectomy erectile dysfunction: a critical review," *The Canadian Journal of Urology*, vol. 24, no. 1, pp. 8609–8619, 2017.

[19] R. Yiou, M. Mahrouf-Yorgov, C. Trébeau et al., "Delivery of human mesenchymal adipose-derived stem cells restores multiple urological dysfunctions in a rat model mimicking radical prostatectomy damages through tissue-specific paracrine mechanisms," *Stem Cells*, vol. 34, no. 2, pp. 392–404, 2016.

[20] A. Takayanagi, M. Sasaki, Y. Kataoka-Sasaki et al., "Intravenous preload of mesenchymal stem cells rescues erectile function in a rat model of cavernous nerve injury," *The Journal of Sexual Medicine*, vol. 12, no. 8, pp. 1713–1721, 2015.

[21] A. Gokce, Z. Y. Abd Elmageed, G. F. Lasker et al., "Intratunical injection of genetically modified adipose tissue-derived stem cells with human interferon α-2b for treatment of erectile dysfunction in a rat model of tunica albugineal fibrosis," *The Journal of Sexual Medicine*, vol. 12, no. 7, pp. 1533–1544, 2015.

[22] G. Y. Liu, X. X. Jiang, X. Zhu et al., "ROS activates JNK-mediated autophagy to counteract apoptosis in mouse mesenchymal stem cells *in vitro*," *Acta Pharmacologica Sinica*, vol. 36, no. 12, pp. 1473–1479, 2015.

[23] T. M. Fandel, M. Albersen, G. Lin et al., "Recruitment of intracavernously injected adipose-derived stem cells to the major pelvic ganglion improves erectile function in a rat model of cavernous nerve injury," *European Urology*, vol. 61, no. 1, pp. 201–210, 2012.

[24] F. Zhou, Y. Hui, Y. Xu et al., "Effects of adipose-derived stem cells plus insulin on erectile function in streptozotocin-induced diabetic rats," *International Urology and Nephrology*, vol. 48, no. 5, pp. 657–669, 2016.

[25] C. M. Schuh, P. Heher, A. M. Weihs et al., "*In vitro* extracorporeal shock wave treatment enhances stemness and preserves multipotency of rat and human adipose-derived stem cells," *Cytotherapy*, vol. 16, no. 12, pp. 1666–1678, 2014.

[26] Z. H. Wang, Y. Y. Shang, S. Zhang et al., "Silence of TRIB3 suppresses atherosclerosis and stabilizes plaques in diabetic Apo $E^{-/-}$/LDL receptor$^{-/-}$ mice," *Diabetes*, vol. 61, no. 2, pp. 463–473, 2012.

[27] X. Wang, C. Liu, Y. Xu et al., "Combination of mesenchymal stem cell injection with icariin for the treatment of diabetes-associated erectile dysfunction," *PLoS One*, vol. 12, no. 3, article e0174145, 2017.

[28] J. Liu, F. Zhou, G. Y. Li et al., "Evaluation of the effect of different doses of low energy shock wave therapy on the erectile function of streptozotocin (STZ)-induced diabetic rats," *International Journal of Molecular Sciences*, vol. 14, no. 5, pp. 10661–10673, 2013.

[29] X. Qiu, T. M. Fandel, L. Ferretti et al., "Both immediate and delayed intracavernous injection of autologous adipose-

derived stromal vascular fraction enhances recovery of erectile function in a rat model of cavernous nerve injury," *European Urology*, vol. 62, pp. 720–727, 2012.

[30] M. Albersen, T. M. Fandel, H. Zhang et al., "Pentoxifylline promotes recovery of erectile function in a rat model of postprostatectomy erectile dysfunction," *European Urology*, vol. 59, no. 2, pp. 286–296, 2011.

[31] A. J. Bella, G. Lin, M. M. Garcia et al., "Upregulation of penile brain-derived neurotrophic factor (BDNF) and activation of the JAK/STAT signalling pathway in the major pelvic ganglion of the rat after cavernous nerve transection," *European Urology*, vol. 52, no. 2, pp. 574–581, 2007.

[32] P. Linharattanaruksa, S. Srisuwatanasagul, S. Ponglowhapan, M. Khalid, and K. Chatdarong, "Collagen and glycosaminoglycan profiles in the canine cervix during different stages of the estrous cycle and in open- and closed-cervix pyometra," *The Journal of Veterinary Medical Science*, vol. 76, no. 2, pp. 197–203, 2014.

[33] R. V. Talanian, C. Quinlan, S. Trautz et al., "Substrate specificities of caspase family proteases," *The Journal of Biological Chemistry*, vol. 272, no. 15, pp. 9677–9682, 1997.

[34] K. R. Drake, M. Kang, and A. K. Kenworthy, "Nucleocytoplasmic distribution and dynamics of the autophagosome marker EGFP-LC3," *PLoS One*, vol. 5, no. 3, article e9806, 2010.

[35] G. N. Yin, S. H. Park, K. M. Song et al., "Establishment of in vitro model of erectile dysfunction for the study of high-glucose-induced angiopathy and neuropathy," *Andrology*, vol. 5, no. 2, pp. 327–335, 2017.

[36] M. H. Kwon, J. K. Ryu, W. J. Kim et al., "Effect of intracavernous administration of angiopoietin-4 on erectile function in the streptozotocin-induced diabetic mouse," *The Journal of Sexual Medicine*, vol. 10, no. 12, pp. 2912–2927, 2013.

[37] J. Wei, H. Jiang, H. Gao, and G. Wang, "Blocking mammalian target of rapamycin (mTOR) attenuates HIF-1α pathways engaged-vascular endothelial growth factor (VEGF) in diabetic retinopathy," *Cellular Physiology and Biochemistry*, vol. 40, no. 6, pp. 1570–1577, 2016.

[38] H. V. Rodrigues, D. Ke, J. Lim et al., "Phase I combination of pazopanib and everolimus in PIK3CA mutation positive/PTEN loss patients with advanced solid tumors refractory to standard therapy," *Investigational New Drugs*, vol. 33, no. 3, pp. 700–709, 2015.

[39] X. Liu, M. A. El-Mahdy, J. Boslett et al., "Cytoglobin regulates blood pressure and vascular tone through nitric oxide metabolism in the vascular wall," *Nature Communications*, vol. 8, article 14807, 2017.

[40] S. Moncada, R. M. Palmer, and E. A. Higgs, "Nitric oxide: physiology, pathophysiology, and pharmacology," *Pharmacological Reviews*, vol. 43, no. 2, pp. 109–142, 1991.

[41] M. Nakaoka, E. Iwai-Kanai, M. Katamura, Y. Okawa, Y. Mita, and S. Matoba, "An alpha-adrenergic agonist protects hearts by inducing Akt1-mediated autophagy," *Biochemical and Biophysical Research Communications*, vol. 456, no. 1, pp. 250–256, 2015.

[42] G. Wan, W. Xie, Z. Liu et al., "Hypoxia-induced *MIR155* is a potent autophagy inducer by targeting multiple players in the MTOR pathway," *Autophagy*, vol. 10, no. 1, pp. 70–79, 2014.

[43] S. A. Mok, K. Lund, and R. B. Campenot, "A retrograde apoptotic signal originating in NGF-deprived distal axons of rat sympathetic neurons in compartmented cultures," *Cell Res*, vol. 19, no. 5, pp. 546–560, 2009.

[44] K. Kawamura, N. Kawamura, Y. Kumazawa, J. Kumagai, T. Fujimoto, and T. Tanaka, "Brain-derived neurotrophic factor/tyrosine kinase B signaling regulates human trophoblast growth in an in vivo animal model of ectopic pregnancy," *Endocrinology*, vol. 152, no. 3, pp. 1090–1100, 2011.

[45] Y. Vardi, B. Appel, A. Kilchevsky, and I. Gruenwald, "Does low intensity extracorporeal shock wave therapy have a physiological effect on erectile function? Short-term results of a randomized, double-blind, sham controlled study," *The Journal of Urology*, vol. 187, no. 5, pp. 1769–1775, 2012.

[46] A. B. Olsen, M. Persiani, S. Boie, M. Hanna, and L. Lund, "Can low-intensity extracorporeal shockwave therapy improve erectile dysfunction? A prospective, randomized, double-blind, placebo-controlled study," *Scandinavian Journal of Urology*, vol. 49, no. 4, pp. 329–333, 2015.

[47] S. Chitale, M. Morsey, L. Swift, and K. Sethia, "Limited shock wave therapy vs sham treatment in men with Peyronie's disease: results of a prospective randomized controlled double-blind trial," *BJU International*, vol. 106, no. 9, pp. 1352–1356, 2010.

[48] V. S. Srini, R. K. Reddy, T. Shultz, and B. Denes, "Low intensity extracorporeal shockwave therapy for erectile dysfunction: a study in an Indian population," *The Canadian Journal of Urology*, vol. 22, no. 1, pp. 7614–7622, 2015.

[49] C. H. Yee, E. S. Chan, S. S. Hou, and C. F. Ng, "Extracorporeal shockwave therapy in the treatment of erectile dysfunction: a prospective, randomized, double-blinded, placebo controlled study," *International Journal of Urology*, vol. 21, no. 10, pp. 1041–1045, 2014.

[50] M. Fode, L. Lowenstein, and Y. Reisman, "Low-intensity extracorporeal shockwave therapy in sexual medicine: a questionnaire-based assessment of knowledge, clinical practice patterns, and attitudes in sexual medicine practitioners," *Sexual Medicine*, vol. 5, no. 2, pp. e94–e98, 2017.

[51] W. D. Dunsmuir and S. A. Holmes, "The aetiology and management of erectile, ejaculatory, and fertility problems in men with diabetes mellitus," *Diabetic Medicine*, vol. 13, no. 8, pp. 700–708, 1996.

[52] A. L. Burnett, C. J. Lowenstein, D. S. Bredt, T. S. Chang, and S. H. Snyder, "Nitric oxide: a physiologic mediator of penile erection," *Science*, vol. 257, no. 5068, pp. 401–403, 1992.

[53] C. Tepekoylu, F. S. Wang, R. Kozaryn et al., "Shock wave treatment induces angiogenesis and mobilizes endogenous CD31/CD34-positive endothelial cells in a hindlimb ischemia model: implications for angiogenesis and vasculogenesis," *The Journal of Thoracic and Cardiovascular Surgery*, vol. 146, no. 4, pp. 971–978, 2013.

[54] C. P. Prieto, M. C. Ortiz, A. Villanueva et al., "Netrin-1 acts as a non-canonical angiogenic factor produced by human Wharton's jelly mesenchymal stem cells (WJ-MSC)," *Stem Cell Research & Therapy*, vol. 8, no. 1, p. 43, 2017.

[55] T. F. Lue, "Erectile dysfunction," *The New England Journal Medicine*, vol. 342, no. 24, pp. 1802–1813, 2000.

[56] C. S. Lin, G. Lin, and T. F. Lue, "Original research—basic science: cyclic nucleotide signaling in cavernous smooth muscle," *The Journal of Sexual Medicine*, vol. 2, pp. 478–491, 2005.

[57] S. Yoshida, K. Aihara, Y. Ikeda et al., "Androgen receptor promotes sex-independent angiogenesis in response to ischemia and is required for activation of vascular endothelial growth factor receptor signaling," *Circulation*, vol. 128, no. 1, pp. 60–71, 2013.

[58] C. G. McMahon, C. N. McMahon, L. J. Leow, and C. G. Winestock, "Efficacy of type-5 phosphodiesterase inhibitors in the drug treatment of premature ejaculation: a systematic review," *BJU International*, vol. 98, no. 2, pp. 259–272, 2006.

[59] K. Komori, A. Tsujimura, T. Takao et al., "Nitric oxide synthesis leads to vascular endothelial growth factor synthesis via the NO/cyclic guanosine 3′,5′-monophosphate (cGMP) pathway in human corpus cavernosal smooth muscle cells," *The Journal of Sexual Medicine*, vol. 5, no. 7, pp. 1623–1635, 2008.

[60] M. H. Wu, S. Y. Yuan, and H. J. Granger, "The protein kinase MEK1/2 mediate vascular endothelial growth factor- and histamine-induced hyperpermeability in porcine coronary venules," *The Journal of Physiology*, vol. 563, no. 1, pp. 95–104, 2005.

[61] R. Kang, H. J. Zeh, M. T. Lotze, and D. Tang, "The beclin 1 network regulates autophagy and apoptosis," *Cell Death & Differentiation*, vol. 18, no. 4, pp. 571–580, 2011.

[62] F. N. Salloum, R. A. Ockaili, M. Wittkamp, V. R. Marwaha, and R. C. Kukreja, "Vardenafil: a novel type 5 phosphodiesterase inhibitor reduces myocardial infarct size following ischemia/reperfusion injury via opening of mitochondrial K_{ATP} channels in rabbits," *Journal of Molecular and Cellular Cardiology*, vol. 40, no. 3, pp. 405–411, 2006.

[63] M. R. Warr, M. Binnewies, J. Flach et al., "FOXO3A directs a protective autophagy program in haematopoietic stem cells," *Nature*, vol. 494, no. 7437, pp. 323–327, 2013.

[64] B. Fang, M. Qin, Y. Li et al., "Electroacupuncture preconditioning and postconditioning inhibit apoptosis and neuroinflammation induced by spinal cord ischemia reperfusion injury through enhancing autophagy in rats," *Neuroscience Letters*, vol. 642, pp. 136–141, 2017.

[65] O. Berrak, E. D. Arisan, P. Obakan-Yerlikaya, A. Coker-Gürkan, and N. Palavan-Unsal, "mTOR is a fine tuning molecule in CDK inhibitors-induced distinct cell death mechanisms via PI3K/AKT/mTOR signaling axis in prostate cancer cells," *Apoptosis*, vol. 21, no. 10, pp. 1158–1178, 2016.

[66] H. N. Kung, C. L. Chien, G. Y. Chau, M. J. Don, K. S. Lu, and Y. P. Chau, "Involvement of NO/cGMP signaling in the apoptotic and anti-angiogenic effects of beta-lapachone on endothelial cells in vitro," *Journal of Cellular Physiology*, vol. 211, no. 2, pp. 522–532, 2007.

7

Altered Expression of Hematopoiesis Regulatory Molecules in Lipopolysaccharide-Induced Bone Marrow Mesenchymal Stem Cells of Patients with Aplastic Anemia

Chandra Prakash Chaturvedi, Naresh Kumar Tripathy, Ekta Minocha, Akhilesh Sharma, Khaliqur Rahman, and Soniya Nityanand

Stem Cell Research Facility, Department of Hematology, Sanjay Gandhi Postgraduate Institute of Medical Sciences (SGPGIMS), Raebareli Road, Lucknow 226014, India

Correspondence should be addressed to Soniya Nityanand; soniya_nityanand@yahoo.co.in

Academic Editor: Hector Mayani

We have investigated the expression of RNA transcripts of hematopoiesis regulatory molecules, viz., macrophage inflammatory protein (MIP)-1α, tumor necrosis factor (TNF)-α, granulocyte colony-stimulating factor (G-CSF), stromal cell-derived factor (SDF)-1α, stem cell factor (SCF), and transforming growth factor (TGF)-β in lipopolysaccharide-induced bone marrow mesenchymal stem cells (BM-MSCs) and levels of their soluble forms in the culture supernatants of BM-MSCs and BM plasma of patients with acquired aplastic anemia (AA) ($n = 29$) and controls ($n = 29$). The BM-MSCs of AA patients as compared to controls had markedly lower expression of MIP-1α transcripts ($p < 0.001$), higher expression of TNF-α ($p < 0.001$), G-CSF ($p < 0.001$), and SDF-1α ($p < 0.01$) transcripts, and no difference in the expression of SCF and TGF-β transcripts. The culture supernatants of BM-MSCs and BM plasma of AA patients in comparison to controls also had lower levels of MIP-1α ($p < 0.01$ and $p < 0.001$, respectively) and higher levels of TNF-α ($p < 0.05$ for both) and G-CSF ($p < 0.05$ and $p < 0.001$, respectively) but with no difference in the levels of SDF-1α and SCF. The levels of TGF-β were although similar in culture supernatants of BM-MSCs of both the groups, but they were significantly lower in BM plasma of the patients than controls ($p < 0.001$). Our data shows that BM-MSCs of AA patients have altered expression of hematopoiesis regulatory molecules suggesting that they may have a role in the pathogenesis of the disease.

1. Introduction

Acquired aplastic anemia (AA) is a state of bone marrow failure characterized by peripheral pancytopenia and a hypoplastic bone marrow (BM) where the normal hematopoietic cells are replaced by fat cells. The majority of the cases of AA are idiopathic where the cause is not known and most studies have focused on intrinsic hematopoietic stem cell defect or immune-mediated destruction of hematopoietic stem cells (HSCs) in the pathogenesis of AA, but a precise pathogenic mechanism of the disease remains unclear till now [1, 2].

BM mesenchymal stem cells (BM-MSCs) and their differentiated cells constitute the hematopoietic niche in the BM and have a vital role in maintaining long-term hematopoiesis [2].We and other groups have reported an increased adipogenic and/or decreased osteogenic differentiation potential of BM-MSCs in AA patients [3–5]. An increase in the adipogenesis and a decrease in the osteogenesis in the BM negatively affect hematopoiesis [6, 7], and hence, these alterations in the differentiation potential of BM-MSCs of AA patients may contribute to the deficient hematopoiesis in AA. In addition, using crossover coculture experiments, it has also been demonstrated that BM-MSCs of AA patients have deficient hematopoiesis-supportive activity [8, 9]. Since BM-MSCs interact with HSCs mainly by secreting paracrine molecules including cytokines, chemokines, and growth factors to maintain hematopoietic homeostasis [2, 10], hence our hypothesis is that an altered expression of hematopoietic regulatory molecules may be involved in mediating these functional abnormalities of BM-MSCs in AA.

Therefore, the aim of the present study was to study the expression of hematopoietic regulatory molecules including macrophage inflammatory protein (MIP)-1α, tumor necrosis factor (TNF)-α, granulocyte colony-stimulating factor (G-CSF), stromal cell-derived factor (SDF)-1α, stem cell factor (SCF), and transforming growth factor (TGF)-β by BM-MSCs of AA patients.

2. Materials and Methods

2.1. Subjects. Twenty-nine AA patients (12 females, 17 males) with a mean age of 32.86 ± 16.43 years (range 12–64 years) and the same number of age- and sex-matched controls were recruited in the study. Diagnosis and grading of severity of AA was done as per published criteria [11]. Controls included 10 healthy donors and 19 patients with immune thrombocytopenic purpura who had undergone a diagnostic BM testing but had normal marrow. After informed consent, 5 ml of BM from the posterior superior iliac crest of each subject was aspirated into heparinized tube for isolation and culture of BM-MSC.

2.2. Isolation, Culture, and Immunophenotypic Characterization of BM-MSCs. The BM-MSCs were isolated, cultured, and characterized as described earlier [3]. Briefly, mononuclear cells obtained from the BM aspirates by density gradient centrifugation were cultured in 25 cm^2 flasks (BD Biosciences, USA) at 37°C in 5% CO_2 using 5 ml of complete culture media consisting of α-MEM, 1% GlutaMAX, 16.5% fetal bovine serum, 100 U/ml penicillin, and 100 μg/ml streptomycin (all from Gibco and Thermo Fisher Scientific, USA). After 48 hours, nonadherent cells were removed and medium was replaced. When culture reached 70–80% confluency, adherent cells were harvested using 0.05% trypsin (Gibco) and replated for further expansion. The cells of the 3rd passage were used in all the experiments.

For immunophenotypic characterization, the BM-MSCs were stained by incubating the cells for 30 minutes with the following preconjugated antibodies: CD73 (PE), CD90 (PE), CD105 (PE), CD166 (PE), CD34 (FITC), CD45 (FITC), HLA-DR (FITC), and CD13 (PE) (all from Serotec, (http://www.abdserotec.com)). Cells stained with isotype-matched antibodies served as controls. After washing, the cells were acquired on a BD FACS-Canto flow cytometer (BD Biosciences, San Jose, CA, USA) and the data analysis was done using the FACS express software.

2.3. Differentiation of BM-MSCs into Adipocytic and Osteocytic Lineages. Differentiation of BM-MSCs into adipocytic and osteocytic cells was carried out using the adipogenesis and osteogenesis kits, respectively (both from Gibco, Gaithersburg, MD, USA) as per the manufacturer's instructions and already reported by us [3]. For adipogenic and osteogenic differentiation, the cells were fixed and stained with oil red O stain after 18 days, and with alizarin red stain after 21 days of incubation in the differentiation medium, respectively.

Table 1: List of primer sequences used for RT-qPCR.

SDF-1 (CXCL12)	
Forward	5′-ATGAACGCCAAGGTCGTGGTC-3′
Reverse	5′-GGTCTGTTGTGCTTACTTGTTT-3′
SCF (c-kit ligand)	
Forward	5′-ACT GAC TCT GGA ATC TTT CTC AGG-3′
Reverse	5′-GAT GTT TTG CCA AGT CAT TGT TGG-3′
G-CSF	
Forward	5′-TCTGAGTTTCATTCTCCTGCCTG-3′
Reverse	5′-ATTTACCTATCTACCTCCCAGTCCAG-3′
TNF-α	
Forward	5′CCCAGGGACCTCTCTCTAATCA-3′
Reverse	5′AGCTGCCCCTCAGCTTGAG-3′
TGF-β1	
Forward	5′-AGTGGACATCAACGGGTTCAG-3′
Reverse	5′-CATGAGAAGCAGGAAAGGCC-3′
MIP-1α (CCL3)	
Forward	5′-TGCCTGCTGCTTCTCCTACA-3′
Reverse	T5′-TGGACCCAGGTCTCTTTGGA-3′
GAPDH	
Forward	5′-CCCCTTCATTGACCTCAACTAC-3′
Reverse	5′GATGACAAGCTTCCCGTTCTC-3′

2.4. RNA Extraction and Quantitative Real-Time PCR (qRT-PCR). BM-MSCs obtained from the 3rd passage semi-confluent cultures were cultured for further 24 hours in plain alpha MEM medium (Gibco) supplemented with 500 ng/ml lipopolysaccharide (LPS; Sigma-Aldrich, St. Louis, Missouri, USA) and trypsinized after 24 hours and total RNA was extracted using TRIzol reagent (Invitrogen, Waltham, Massachusetts, USA). The cDNA synthesis and quantitative real-time PCR were performed as previously established in the lab [3]. The fold expression change was calculated using $2^{-\Delta\Delta Ct}$ method. The oligonucleotides used as primers (from MWG Biotech Pvt. Limited, Bangalore, India) for RT-qPCR are given in Table 1.

2.5. Quantization of Hematopoietic Regulatory Cytokines in BM-MSC Culture Supernatants and BM Plasma. To prepare culture supernatant, the 3rd passage BM-MSCs were cultured for 24 hours in 2.5 ml of plain alpha MEM medium (Gibco) containing 500 ng/ml of LPS. The culture supernatant of these cultures was harvested and centrifuged at 1000g for 10 minutes to remove any cellular debris. The BM plasma was collected by centrifuging the marrow aspirate at 1000g for 10 minutes. The culture supernatant and BM plasma were stored at −20°C until use. Quantitative estimation of G-CSF, SCF, SDF-1, MIP-1α, TNF-α, and TGF-β in the culture

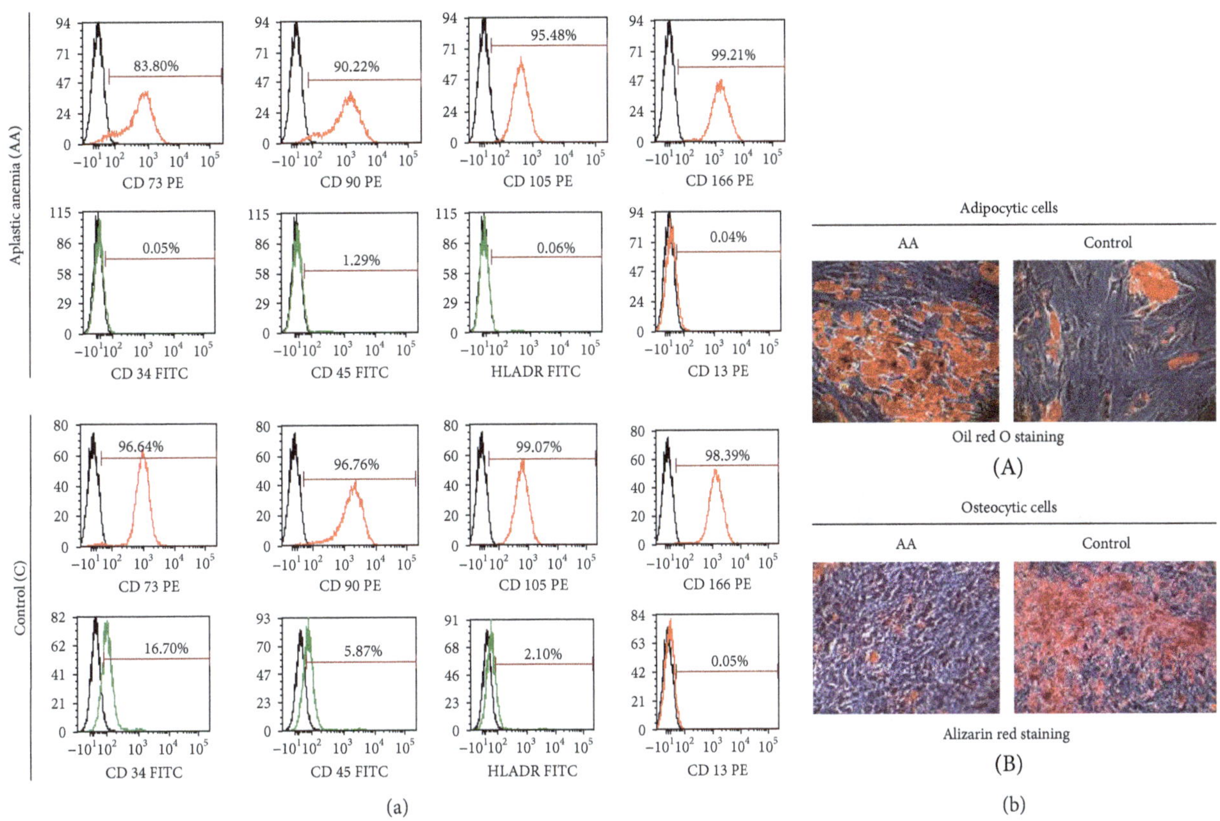

FIGURE 1: Immunophenotypic and differentiation characterization of BM-MSCs of aplastic anemia (AA) patients. (a) Representative flow cytometric histograms showing immunophenotype of BM-MSCs of AA patients and controls. (b) (A) Oil red O staining of adipocytes differentiated from BM-MSCs of AA patients and controls. (b) (B) Alizarin red staining of osteocytes differentiated from BM-MSCs of AA patients and controls.

supernatants and concomitantly in the BM plasma of each subject was performed by ELISA kits (R&D Systems, Minneapolis, MN, USA), as per manufacturer's instructions.

2.6. Statistical Analysis. The results were calculated as mean ± SE. The statistical significance was determined by Student's t-test using the GraphPad Prism Software Version 5 (GraphPad, San Diego, CA, USA). The p values < 0.05 were considered to be statistically significant.

3. Results

3.1. Morphology and Immunophenotypic Characterization. The BM-MSCs of AA patients showed fibroblast-like spindle-shaped morphology similar to BM-MSCs of controls. The flow cytometric analysis of their phenotypic markers showed that BM-MSCs of AA patients as well as of controls expressed comparable levels of MSC markers CD73, CD89, CD105, and CD166 and lacked the expression of CD13, CD34, CD45, and HLA-DR (Figure 1(a)).

3.2. Adipogenic and Osteogenic Differentiation of BM-MSCs. The oil red O staining of the adipocytes differentiated from AA BM-MSCs showed higher density and larger size of lipid droplets suggesting a higher adipogenic potential of AA BM-MSCs as compared to control BM-MSCs (Figure 1(b)). However, BM-MSCs of the AA patients showed a lesser osteogenic potential as compared to the control MSCs as reveled by alizarin red staining (Figure 1(b)).

3.3. Expression of Hematopoiesis Regulatory Genes in BM-MSCs. The BM-MSC of AA patients ($n = 29$) in comparison to controls ($n = 29$) showed no difference in the constitutive expression of transcripts of MIP-1α, TNF-α, TGF-β1, G-CSF, SDF-1α, and SCF. However, following LPS stimulation, the transcript levels of MIP-1α were dramatically lower (fold decrease: 7.1; $p < 0.001$) while those of TNF-α (fold increase: 7.0; $p < 0.001$), G-CSF (fold increase: 2.38; $p < 0.001$), and SDF-1α (fold increase: 1.36; $p < 0.01$) were significantly higher with no difference in the levels of the SCF and TGF-β1 transcripts, between patients and controls (Figure 2(a)).

3.4. Secretion of Hematopoiesis Regulatory Molecules by AA BM-MSCs. The culture supernatants of BM-MSCs of AA patients ($n = 29$) compared to controls ($n = 29$) showed no difference in the levels of MIP-1α, TNF-α, TGF-β1, G-CSF, SDF-1α, and SCF levels. However, following LPS stimulation, the culture supernatants of BM-MSCs of the patients compared to controls also had significantly lower levels of MIP-1α (216.7 ± 58.72 vs 670.1 ± 72.85; $p < 0.01$) and higher levels of TNF-α (172.32 ± 32.05 vs 44.76 ± 10.89 $p < 0.05$), and G-CSF (306.8 ± 56.90 vs 123.2 ± 17.68; $p < 0.05$) with no difference in the levels of SCF (24.32 ± 3.09 vs $31.98 \pm$

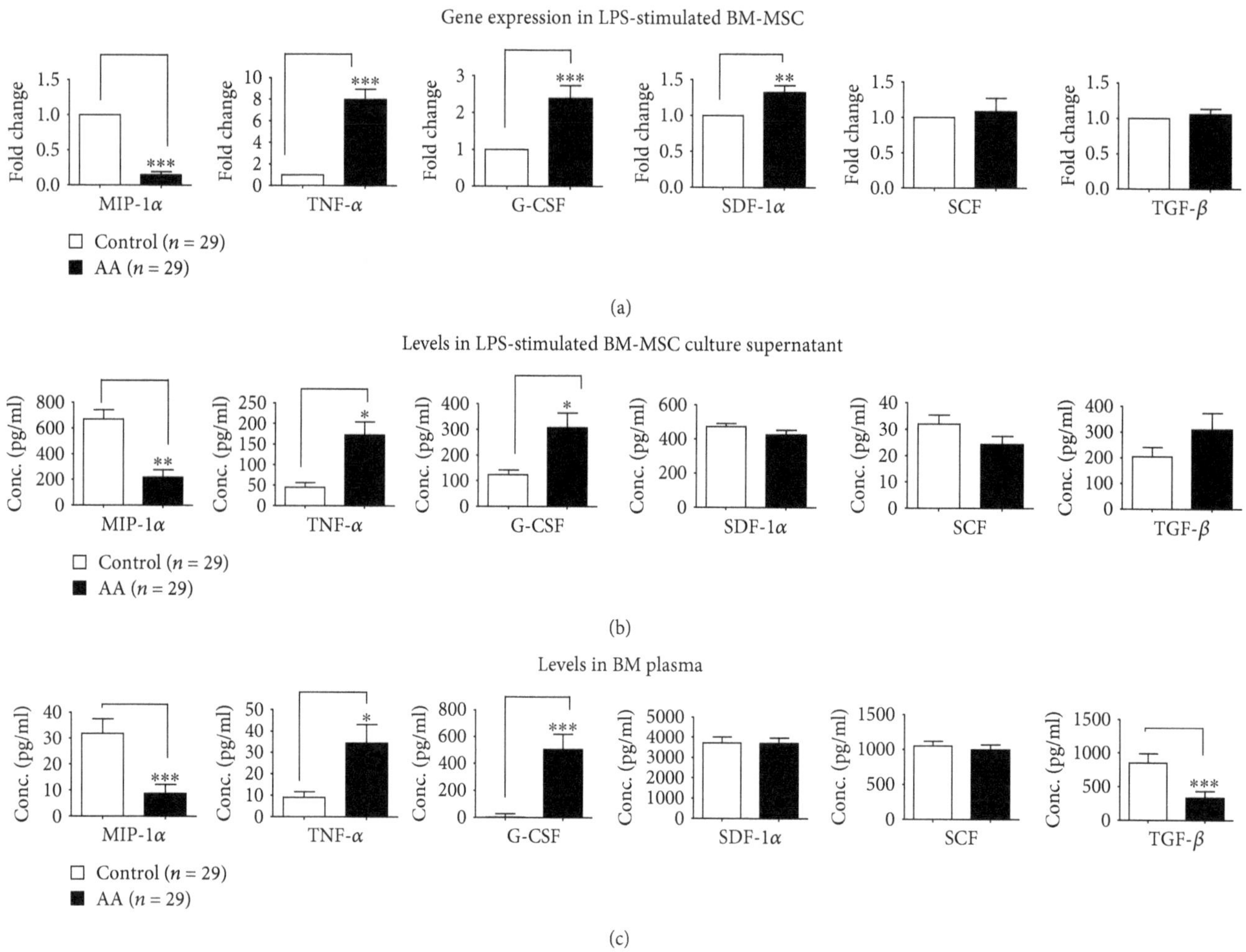

FIGURE 2: Expression of the hematopoietic regulatory molecules: MIP-1α, TNF-α, G-CSF, SDF-1α, SCF, and TGF-β1. (a) Relative fold changes in mRNA expression of hematopoietic regulatory cytokine genes in AA BM-MSCs as compared to control BM-MSCs by qRT-PCR after LPS stimulation. (b) Levels of the hematopoietic regulatory molecules in culture supernatants of LPS-stimulated AA and control BM-MSCs as detected by ELISA. (c) Levels of the hematopoietic regulatory molecules in the BM plasma of AA patients and controls as detected by ELISA. Values represent mean ± SE. $^{***}p < 0.001$, $^{**}p < 0.01$, and $^{*}p < 0.05$ between AA patients and controls.

3.45; $p > 0.05$) and TGF-β1 (310.0 ± 63.68 vs 204.70 ± 36.37; $p > 0.05$)(Figure 2(b)).

3.5. Levels of Hematopoiesis Regulatory Molecules in BM Plasma. The BM plasma of AA patients ($n = 29$) in comparison to that of controls ($n = 29$) also showed significantly lower levels of MIP-1α (8.70 ± 3.51 vs 31.91 ± 5.58; $p < 0.001$) and higher levels of TNF-α (34.26 ± 8.87 vs 9.07 ± 2.47; $p < 0.05$), and G-CSF (505.32 ± 112.80 vs 3.48 ± 5.99; $p < 0.001$), with no difference in the levels of SCF (996.20 ± 67.68 vs 1050 ± 64.70; $p > 0.05$) and SDF-1α (3695.0 ± 268.4 vs 3706.0 ± 296.0; $p > 0.05$). However, the levels of TGF-β1 were significantly lower in BM plasma of patients than controls (335.2 ± 97.07 vs 850.7 ± 139; $p < 0.001$) (Figure 2(c)).

4. Discussion

We observed that BM-MSCs of AA patients although have a morphology and phenotype similar to controls but have a higher adipogenic and lower osteogenic differentiation potential, which is consistent with previous reports of our and other groups [3–5]. To study the role of BM-MSC derived hematopoiesis regulatory molecules in AA, we initially evaluated the expression of MIP-1α, TNF-α, G-CSF, SDF-1α, SCF, and TGF-β1 transcripts in BM-MSCs of AA patients and controls as well as levels of soluble forms of these hematopoiesis regulatory molecules in the culture supernatants of BM-MSCs of both the groups under constitutive conditions but observed no significant difference between the two groups either in the expression of the transcripts of these molecules or in their soluble protein levels in the cell culture supernatants. Therefore, we measured these hematopoiesis regulatory cytokines following stimulation of BM-MSCs with LPS, which is a potent stimulant of these cells and induces their activation via binding to their Toll-like receptors [12, 13]. The LPS-stimulated BM-MSCs of AA patients as compared to controls exhibited markedly lower expression of MIP-1α and higher expression of TNF-α, G-CSF, and SDF-1α transcripts as well as lower MIP-1α

and higher TNF-α and G-CSF levels in the culture supernatants with no difference in the levels of SDF-1α, SCF, and TGF-β1. The BM plasma of AA patients also had alterations in the levels of these hematopoiesis regulatory molecules corroborating with the alterations in the levels in the culture supernatants, except for TGF-β1 where the levels were reduced in the BM plasma though the levels were comparable in the culture supernatants of patients and controls. Although a few sporadic reports are available in literature on these hematopoiesis regulatory molecules in bone marrow mononuclear cells of AA patients, but to the best of our knowledge, this is the first study on transcripts of these molecules in BM-MSCs and their protein levels in the culture supernatant of BM-MSCs as well as in BM plasma of AA patients.

There is no previous report on MIP-1α transcripts or proteins in BM-MSCs of patients with AA. However, a single report on long-term marrow cultures of AA patients has shown elevated levels of MIP-1α in the baseline culture supernatants of 14 of 20 AA patients, and following IL-1α stimulation of the cultures, the levels further increased in 7 patients but markedly decreased in remaining 7 patients as observed by us in the present study [14]. MIP-1α is reported to suppress proliferation of primitive HSCs probably to maintain their quiescence while promoting proliferation of mature HSCs highlighting its bidirectional role in hematopoiesis [15]. In addition, MIP-1α is also important in mediating interaction between MSCs and HSCs or immune cells of the BM to modulate their functional properties [16]. Hence, our observation on the almost absent expression of MIP-1α in BM-MSCs and the corresponding decrease in its levels in BM plasma of AA patients is likely to impair the cell-cell interaction of HSCs with MSCs and in turn the hematopoiesis supporting functions of BM-MSCs.

TNF-α is reported to cause bone marrow aplasia in AA by inducing apoptotic cell death of HSCs through Fas-Fas ligand and/or TNF-related apoptosis-inducing ligand pathways [17]. Increased levels of TNF-α have been reported in AA, and T-cells present in marrow of the patients are considered to be the main source of TNF-α [18, 19]. Our demonstration of higher expression of TNF-α at transcript as well as protein levels in BM-MSCs of patients with AA is the first report showing that BM-MSCs are also an important source of TNF-α in BM of AA patients. Our previous study showing increased levels of TNF-α in BM plasma but no expression in marrow T-cells also supports our current observation [20].

The BM-MSCs of AA patients had higher expression of G-CSF transcripts with corresponding higher levels in culture supernatants. It is an important member of the hematopoietic cytokine family secreted by stromal and other cell types. Similar to our observation, elevated levels of G-CSF transcripts have been reported in BM stromal cells and their culture supernatants [21, 22]. On the one hand, increased expression of G-CSF is considered to represent a compensatory supraphysiological response of BM-MSCs to boost reduced hematopoiesis in AA. On the other hand, an inverse correlation of higher G-CSF levels with numbers of myeloid cells has been reported in AA patients. However, after BM transplantation or immunosuppressive therapy, the G-CSF levels have been shown to return to normal levels in AA patients, which together suggest an antimyelopoietic effect of G-CSF in AA [23, 24]. The expression of SDF-1α transcripts in BM-MSCs of patients with AA although was statistically higher as compared to controls, but the levels in the culture supernatant were similar to controls. The levels of SCF, which is solely produced by marrow stromal cells, were comparable to controls at both the gene and protein levels. Data of previous studies on SDF-1α and SCF in marrow stromal cells corroborates with our observation [25, 26].

In order to ascertain the alterations in these hematopoiesis regulatory molecules *in vivo* in the marrow microenvironment as well, we analyzed their levels in BM plasma of patients with AA. It was observed that similar to their levels in culture supernatant of BM-MSCs, the BM plasma of AA patients as compared to controls had lower levels of MIP-1α and higher levels of TNF-α and G-CSF with no difference in the levels of SCF and SDF-1α. The alterations in the BM plasma levels of these cytokines also corroborated with the levels of the mRNA transcripts in LPS-stimulated BM-MSCs of AA patients, but since there is widespread adipogenesis in the marrow of AA patients, hence BM adipocytes and other cell-like macrophages/T-cells may also have an important contribution to the alterations of these cytokines in BM plasma of AA patients. The levels of TGF-β1 were significantly lower in BM plasma of the patients than controls, unlike the comparable expression in the culture supernatants of BM-MSCs implying a deficient production of this cytokine by other marrow cell-like T-cells and/or macrophages. Similar to our observation, lower levels of TGF-β1 have been reported previously in long-term marrow cultures of AA patients [27]. Since one of the main functions of TGF-β1 is to mediate expansion of regulatory T-cells, the reduced level of this cytokine may be responsible for the decreased numbers of Tregs reported in the marrow of AA patients [5]. Future studies exploring the role of MIP-1α, TNF-α, and G-CSF in hematopoietic and immunomodulatory functions of BM-MSCs of AA would be important for better understanding the pathophysiology of the disease.

5. Conclusion

Our data shows that BM-MSCs of AA patients have markedly lower expression of MIP-1α and higher expression of TNF-α and G-CSF transcripts with corresponding alteration of their levels in the culture supernatant as well as in BM plasma, collectively highlighting an abnormality of BM-MSCs in AA.

Authors' Contributions

SN, NKT, and CPC contributed to the research design, analysis, and interpretation of the data. NKT and CPC wrote the paper and SN revised the paper. CPC, NKT, EM, and AS carried out the laboratory work. SN, CPC, and KR provided the reagents and tools for the research work. KR contributed to the laboratory work-up of the AA patients. Chandra Prakash Chaturvedi and Naresh Kumar Tripathy contributed equally to this work.

Acknowledgments

This work was supported by an Intramural Grant (PGI/DIR/RC/304/2014) of SGPGIMS, Lucknow, sanctioned to SN and Ramalingaswami Re-entry Fellowship Grant of Department of Biotechnology, Government of India (BT/RLF/Re-Entry/45/2012) sanctioned to CPC.

References

[1] P. C. Boddu and T. M. Kadia, "Updates on the pathophysiology and treatment of aplastic anemia: a comprehensive review," *Expert Review of Hematology*, vol. 10, no. 5, pp. 433–448, 2017.

[2] Y. Zeng and E. Katsanis, "The complex pathophysiology of acquired aplastic anaemia," *Clinical & Experimental Immunology*, vol. 180, no. 3, pp. 361–370, 2015.

[3] N. K. Tripathy, S. P. Singh, and S. Nityanand, "Enhanced adipogenicity of bone marrow mesenchymal stem cells in aplastic anemia," *Stem Cells International*, vol. 2014, Article ID 276862, 6 pages, 2014.

[4] Y. Xu, Y. Takahashi, Y. Wang et al., "Downregulation of GATA-2 and overexpression of adipogenic gene-PPARγ in mesenchymal stem cells from patients with aplastic anemia," *Experimental Hematology*, vol. 37, no. 12, pp. 1393–1399, 2009.

[5] J. Li, S. Lu, S. Yang et al., "Impaired immunomodulatory ability of bone marrow mesenchymal stem cells on $CD4^+$ T cells in aplastic anemia," *Results in Immunology*, vol. 2, pp. 142–147, 2012.

[6] R. Sugimura and L. Li, "Shifting in balance between osteogenesis and adipogenesis substantially influences hematopoiesis," *Journal of Molecular Cell Biology*, vol. 2, no. 2, pp. 61-62, 2010.

[7] O. Naveiras, V. Nardi, P. L. Wenzel, P. V. Hauschka, F. Fahey, and G. Q. Daley, "Bone-marrow adipocytes as negative regulators of the haematopoietic microenvironment," *Nature*, vol. 460, no. 7252, pp. 259–263, 2009.

[8] H. S. Juneja and F. H. Gardner, "Functionally abnormal marrow stromal cells in aplastic anemia," *Experimental Hematology*, vol. 13, no. 3, pp. 194–199, 1985.

[9] E. Hamzic, K. Whiting, E. Gordon Smith, and R. Pettengell, "Characterization of bone marrow mesenchymal stromal cells in aplastic anaemia," *British Journal of Haematology*, vol. 169, no. 6, pp. 804–813, 2015.

[10] B. A. Anthony and D. C. Link, "Regulation of hematopoietic stem cells by bone marrow stromal cells," *Trends in Immunology*, vol. 35, no. 1, pp. 32–37, 2014.

[11] S. B. Killick, N. Bown, J. Cavenagh et al., "Guidelines for the diagnosis and management of adult aplastic anaemia," *British Journal of Haematology*, vol. 172, no. 2, pp. 187–207, 2016.

[12] X. He, H. Wang, T. Jin, Y. Xu, L. Mei, and J. Yang, "TLR4 activation promotes bone marrow MSC proliferation and osteogenic differentiation via Wnt3a and Wnt5a signaling," *PLoS One*, vol. 11, no. 3, article e0149876, 2016.

[13] X. Wang, Y. Zhu, B. Xu, J. Wang, and X. Liu, "Identification of TLR2 and TLR4-induced microRNAs in human mesenchymal stem cells and their possible roles in regulating TLR signals," *Molecular Medicine Reports*, vol. 13, no. 6, pp. 4969–4980, 2016.

[14] L. A. Holmberg, K. Seidel, W. Leisenring, and B. Torok-Storb, "Aplastic anemia: analysis of stromal cell function in long-term marrow cultures," *Blood*, vol. 84, no. 11, pp. 3685–3690, 1994.

[15] H. Mayani, M. T. Little, W. Dragowska, G. Thornbury, and P. M. Lansdorp, "Differential effects of the hematopoietic inhibitors MIP-1 alpha, TGF-beta, and TNF-alpha on cytokine-induced proliferation of subpopulations of CD34+ cells purified from cord blood and fetal liver," *Experimental Hematology*, vol. 23, no. 5, pp. 422–427, 1995.

[16] Y. Suehiro, K. Muta, T. Umemura, Y. Abe, J. Nishimura, and H. Nawata, "Macrophage inflammatory protein 1α enhances in a different manner adhesion of hematopoietic progenitor cells from bone marrow, cord blood, and mobilized peripheral blood," *Experimental Hematology*, vol. 27, no. 11, pp. 1637–1645, 1999.

[17] Y. Chen, Z. Zou, Z. Wu et al., "TNF-α-induced programmed cell death in the pathogenesis of acquired aplastic anemia," *Expert Review of Hematology*, vol. 8, no. 4, pp. 515–526, 2015.

[18] J. C. Schultz and N. T. Shahidi, "Detection of tumor necrosis factor-α in bone marrow plasma and peripheral blood plasma from patients with aplastic anemia," *American Journal of Hematology*, vol. 45, no. 1, pp. 32–38, 1994.

[19] T. Hara, K. Ando, H. Tsurumi, and H. Moriwaki, "Excessive production of tumor necrosis factor-alpha by bone marrow T lymphocytes is essential in causing bone marrow failure in patients with aplastic anemia," *European Journal of Haematology*, vol. 73, no. 1, pp. 10–16, 2004.

[20] S. Dubey, P. Shukla, and S. Nityanand, "Expression of interferon-gamma and tumor necrosis factor-alpha in bone marrow T cells and their levels in bone marrow plasma in patients with aplastic anemia," *Annals of Hematology*, vol. 84, no. 9, pp. 572–577, 2005.

[21] G. Martínez-Jaramillo, E. Flores-Figueroa, E. Gómez-Morales, E. Sánchez-Valle, and H. Mayani, "Tumor necrosis factor-alpha levels in long-term marrow cultures from patients with aplastic anemia: modulation by granulocyte-macrophage colony-stimulating factor," *American Journal of Hematology*, vol. 68, no. 3, pp. 144–148, 2001.

[22] F. M. Gibson, J. Scopes, S. Daly, S. Ball, and E. C. Gordon-Smith, "Haemopoietic growth factor production by normal and aplastic anaemia stroma in long-term bone marrow culture," *British Journal of Haematology*, vol. 91, no. 3, pp. 551–561, 1995.

[23] Y. Hirayama, Y. Kohgo, T. Matsunaga, S. Ohi, S. Sakamaki, and Y. Niitsu, "Cytokine mRNA expression of bone marrow stromal cells from patients with aplastic anaemia and myelodysplastic syndrome," *British Journal of Haematology*, vol. 85, no. 4, pp. 676–683, 1993.

[24] K. Shinohara, E. Oeda, J. Nomiyama et al., "The levels of granulocyte colony-stimulating factor in the plasma of the bone marrow aspirate in various hematological disorders," *Stem Cells*, vol. 13, no. 4, pp. 421–427, 1995.

[25] M. Park, C. J. Park, S. Jang et al., "Reduced expression of osteonectin and increased natural killer cells may contribute to the pathophysiology of aplastic anemia," *Applied Immunohistochemistry & Molecular Morphology*, vol. 23, no. 2, pp. 139–145, 2015.

[26] S. Kojima, T. Matsuyama, and Y. Kodera, "Plasma levels and production of soluble stem cell factor by marrow stromal cells in patients with aplastic anaemia," *British Journal of Haematology*, vol. 99, no. 2, pp. 440–446, 1997.

[27] S. Rizzo, S. B. Killick, S. Patel et al., "Reduced TGF-β1 in patients with aplastic anaemia *in vivo* and *in vitro*," *British Journal of Haematology*, vol. 107, no. 4, pp. 797–803, 1999.

8

Osteogenic Potential of Human Umbilical Cord Mesenchymal Stem Cells on Coralline Hydroxyapatite/Calcium Carbonate Microparticles

A. G. E. Day,[1] W. R. Francis,[1] K. Fu,[2] I. L. Pieper,[1] O. Guy,[3] and Z. Xia[1]

[1]*Institute of Life Science, Swansea University Medical School, Swansea SA2 8PP, UK*
[2]*Department of Orthopaedic Surgery, The First Affiliated Hospital of Hainan Medical College, Hainan, China*
[3]*College of Engineering, Swansea University, Swansea SA2 8PP, UK*

Correspondence should be addressed to K. Fu; fudh168@hotmail.com and Z. Xia; z.xia@swansea.ac.uk

Academic Editor: Zhi-Yong Zhang

Coralline hydroxyapatite/calcium carbonate (CHACC) is a biodegradable and osteoconductive bone graft material with promising clinical performance. CHACC has been shown to support proliferation and osteogenic differentiation of human bone marrow mesenchymal stem cells (MSCs) *in vitro* and demonstrated to work as a functional scaffold for bone formation *in vivo*. Umbilical cord matrix is a more accessible and abundant tissue source of MSCs, but its osteogenic capacity in comparison to human bone marrow when cultured on CHACC has not yet been demonstrated. In this study, we assessed the osteogenic differentiation capacity of human MSCs, isolated from bone marrow and umbilical cord matrix and characterised by flow cytometry, when cultured on 200–300 μm CHACC granules. The 3D cultures were characterised by brightfield and scanning electron microscopy (SEM). Osteogenic potential was assessed by immunocytochemistry and qPCR for key markers of bone differentiation (alkaline phosphatase, runx2, type I collagen, and osteocalcin). By day 1, the MSCs had enveloped the surface of the CHACC granules to form organoids, and by day 7, cells had proliferated to bridge nearby organoids. Extracellular matrix deposition and osteogenic differentiation were demonstrated by MSCs from both tissue sources at day 21. However, MSCs from bone marrow demonstrated superior osteogenic differentiation capability compared to those from umbilical cord matrix. In conclusion, it is possible to culture and induce osteogenic differentiation of umbilical cord matrix MSCs on CHACC. Further research is required to optimise the osteogenicity of umbilical cord matrix MSCs to release their full potential as a readily available, accessible, and abundant tissue source for bone tissue engineering.

1. Introduction

Of the diverse range of scaffolds available for use in maxillofacial surgery and dentistry, autografts have been reported to be the "gold standard" with respect to bone grafting procedures [1]. However, harvesting of autografts, usually from the iliac crest, requires surgical intervention, which is associated with additional risks of blood loss, infection, and morbidity, and supply is limited [2, 3]. Other types of grafts include allografts and xenografts, but these can cause an immunological reaction and be rejected by the recipient [3]; so, it is vital to identify suitable alternative materials.

Synthetic biomaterials, such as hydroxyapatite, tricalcium phosphate ceramics and cements, and bioglass, are alternative sources for bone graft substitutes. However, these synthetic biomaterials do not mimic the architecture, porosity, and organic components of the natural bone and are not optimal in regard to biodegradation and host tissue integration or practical to implant or inject. Naturally occurring coral exoskeleton has a porous architecture that is similar to the human trabecular bone [4]. Since its main composition is calcium carbonate, a hydrothermal technique was developed to completely convert the calcium carbonate to be coralline hydroxyapatite (CHA) ceramics for clinical application [5–8].

We have previously reported a coralline hydroxyapatite/calcium carbonate (CHACC) material which shows promising clinical performance when implanted in sizes ranging from 10–100 × 10 × 10 mm^3 [9, 10]. This material not only has properties such as porosity, surface structure, and osteoconductivity of coralline hydroxyapatite (CHA) as previously investigated [5–7] but also improves host tissue integration and can be completely biodegraded during bone remodelling [9]. Herein, we are focusing on smaller-sized CHACC, 200–300 μm particles, with the potential to be injected facilitating administration for maxillofacial and dentistry applications.

To increase the functionality of bone biomaterials by hopefully contributing towards remodelling and host integration, stem cells are commonly added [11]. *In vitro* cellular 3D structures [12] created from stem cells resembling living tissue are known as organoids and have been developed as models for translational medicine [13] and gene therapy [14].

We have previously shown that human bone marrow (BM) mesenchymal stem cells (MSCs) can be cultured on CHACC [9, 10]. Human umbilical cord matrix (UCM) is a relatively new source of MSCs which has several advantages over BM including an abundant supply obtained noninvasively; it does not induce donor site morbidity and avoids ethical restrictions. Moreover, UCM MSCs have a higher proliferation rate, can be expanded further without loss of differentiation potential, and exhibit reduced immunogenicity for clinical use [15]. Osteogenesis of UCM-MSCs has been observed in both monolayer culture systems [16] and 3D culture systems, for example, on a demineralised bone [17] and polycaprolactone tricalcium phosphate [18]. Few studies have compared UCM MSC to BM MSC in 3D culture systems [16, 19].

Therefore, the aim of this study was to (1) confirm that MSCs could adhere to, proliferate on, and undergo osteogenic differentiation on 200–300 μm CHACC particles to form 3D organoids and (2) to evaluate the osteogenic potential of UCM MSCs compared to BM MSCs. MSCs were isolated from BM and UCM and characterised by flow cytometry. CHACC was crushed into 200–300 μm particles onto which MSCs were seeded and cultured in osteogenic differentiation medium. The resulting organoids were characterised by brightfield and scanning electron microscopy, alkaline phosphatase staining, and immunocytochemistry and PCR for key osteogenic markers.

2. Materials and Methods

2.1. Preparation of Human Bone Marrow. This study was approved by the South West Wales Research Ethics Committee (12/WA/0029) and all patients gave informed written consent. Exclusion criteria included preexisting conditions (e.g., connective tissue disease, diabetes, and malignancy) or medication (e.g., steroids and cytotoxic agents). BM aspirates were harvested from the iliac crest of two females (aged 25 and 29 years) and two males (aged 22 and 36 years) undergoing surgery to the pelvic ring or acetabulum using a BM aspiration needle (Mana-Tech Ltd., Burton-on-Trent, UK). Samples were collected in heparinised aspiration needles, transported at room temperature, and processed within 120 min.

Mononuclear cells (MNC) were isolated from the BM aspirate using Histopaque-1077 according to the manufacturer's instructions (Sigma-Aldrich, Poole, UK). Up to 40×10^6 MNCs were seeded into 75 cm^2 tissue culture flasks (CellSTAR, Greiner Bio-One, Stonehouse, UK) in 10 ml Minimum Essential Eagle Alpha Modification media with 10% fetal calf serum (Biosera, Uckfield, UK) and 1% Antibiotic-Antimycotic (100x, Life Technologies, Paisley, UK) and incubated for 7 days at 37°C under 5% CO_2 in air. The media were changed every 3-4 days to remove contaminating nonadherent haematopoietic cells, and the adherent MSCs were cultured until 70% confluent. Cells were detached using Accutase according to the manufacturer's instructions (Sigma-Aldrich) and either propagated at a seeding density of 3×10^5 per 75 cm^2 culture flask or cryopreserved in 10% dimethyl sulfoxide (DMSO) (Sigma-Aldrich) in 90% FBS in liquid nitrogen for future use.

2.2. Preparation of Human Umbilical Cord Matrix. Human umbilical cords and placentas were collected from full-term births after elective caesarean section delivery of four mothers aged 30–35 and processed within 120 min. This study was approved by the South West Wales Research Ethics Committee and all mothers gave informed written consent. Inclusion criteria included mothers aged 18–50 who were at least 37 weeks pregnant. Exclusion criteria included preexisting health conditions (e.g., HIV, hepatitis C, or immunology complications), stillborn babies, or twins. A 3 cm section of the umbilical cord proximal to the placenta was dissected and the vasculature was carefully removed. The remaining matrix was finely diced using a scalpel. The diced tissue was placed in 25 cm^2 flasks with 0.5 ml FBS. After 24 hours, 1 ml Dulbecco's modified Eagle's medium (DMEM, Life Technologies, Paisley, UK) supplemented with 10% FBS and 1% Antibiotic-Antimycotic was added. After 72 hours, an additional 3 ml DMEM was added. Cultures were subsequently fed twice weekly until 70% confluent at which point they were harvested and either propagated or cryopreserved *as above.* Cryopreserved UCM MSCs and BM MSCs were simultaneously used in the experiments for the assessment on CHACC.

2.3. Characterisation by Flow Cytometry. The following antibodies were used to phenotype the cells based on the International Society for Cellular Therapy (ISCT) criteria [20]: CD14-APC-eFluor780 (clone 61D3), CD34-eFluor450 (clone 4H11), CD73-FITC (clone AD2), CD90-APC (clone eBio5E10), CD105-PE (clone SN6) (eBioscience, Hatfield, Ireland, UK), CD19-PE-Cy7 (clone J3-119), and CD45-Krome Orange (clone J.33) (Beckman Coulter, High Wycombe, UK). All antibodies were mouse isotype IgG1, κ. Unstained cells were used as controls. Gating was performed on the forward and side scatter (FSC versus SSC) profile to remove debris and doublets based on scatter. Cells (3×10^5) in 100 μl FACS buffer (Dulbecco's PBS, Life Technologies; 0.2% BSA and 0.05% sodium azide, Sigma-Aldrich) were incubated on ice in the dark for 30 min with predetermined titrations of antibody. The cells were washed in FACS buffer and resuspended in 200 μl FACS buffer for analysis.

The stained cells were analysed within 2 hours using a BD FACS Aria I flow cytometer with FACS Diva 6.1.3 software (BD Bioscience, Oxford, UK). The instrument was turned on for at least 1 hour prior to each run to allow the lasers to warm up, and Cytometer Setup & Tracking Beads (BD Bioscience) were used to check instrument performance. 10,000 cell events were recorded for each antibody. Voltages were set on unstained samples [21]. The FCS files were analysed in Kaluza 1.2 (Beckman Coulter) and the median fluorescent intensity (MFI) was displayed on logicle (biexponential) axes [22]. To convey information as to the density of events, contour density plots with visualised outliers were chosen as the standard plot [23].

2.4. Preparation of Coralline Hydroxyapatite/Calcium Carbonate Microscaffolds. CHACC (Affiliated Hospital, Hainan Medical College, Haikou, People's Republic of China) was crushed with a mortar and pestle and subsequently sieved through a 300 μm followed by a 200 μm sieve to capture only 200–300 μm particles. The sieved CHACC were then autoclaved for sterilisation. 10 μl of complete organoid medium (α-MEM supplemented with 10% FBS and 1% Antibiotic-Antimycotics), and three CHACC particles were placed into each well of a Terasaki microplate (Greiner Bio-One, Stonehouse, UK) and incubated for 24 hours at 37°C under 5% CO_2 in air.

2.5. Formation and Differentiation of Organoids. 3000 MSCs (P3-5) per 10 μl organoid medium were added to the previously prepared scaffold particles in the Terasaki microplates to produce organoids. The next day, the organoids were transferred to a 100 mm petri dish (Fisher Scientific, Loughborough, UK) and swirled to allow the particles to come into contact with each other, enabling a larger scaffold conglomerate to be created. The organoids were treated with either plain organoid medium (control) or organoid medium supplemented with 100 nM dexamethasone, 10 mM β-glycerol phosphate, and 100 μM 2-phosphate-ascorbic acid to stimulate osteogenic differentiation.

2.6. Characterisation by Microscopy and Live/Dead Assay. The organoids were analysed by brightfield and scanning electron microscopy (SEM). The samples were analysed on days 1, 7, 14, and 21 during differentiation. For SEM, the samples were cut to 1 mm diameter, fixed in 4% glutaraldehyde (Sigma-Aldrich), and then gradually dehydrated through an ethanol series, using sequentially higher concentrations of ethanol (70%, 80%, 90%, 95%, and 100%) for 10 min each. Finally, samples were further dehydrated in 50% hexamethyldisilazane (Sigma-Aldrich) diluted with ethanol for 10 min, followed by full immersion in absolute hexamethyldisilazane, and left to evaporate overnight in a fume cupboard. Control scaffold particles (no cells) were also incubated for 7 days in organoid medium, at 37°C under 5% CO_2 in air, before being fixed and dehydrated. SEM was carried out using a Hitachi S-4800 II SEM with an accelerating voltage of 1 kV at 110x and 5000x. Samples were mounted onto SEM stubs using a double-coated carbon conductive tape (Acros Organics, supplied by Fisher Scientific).

Cell viability was also assessed after 14 and 21 days using Live/Dead assay kit (Life Technologies, Paisley, UK), in which cells were stained with calcein acetoxymethyl (0.1 μg/ml) and propidium iodide (1 μg/ml) and viewed by fluorescence microscopy.

2.7. Assessing Differentiation by Immunocytochemistry. At 21 days differentiation, organoids were washed in PBS and orientated within a large droplet of Bright Cryo-M-Bed embedding compound which was snap frozen on dry ice. 10 μm sections were then cut using a Leica CM1900 and melted onto slides for staining. Slides were fixed in 10% neutral buffered formalin (Sigma-Aldrich), permeabilised in PBS : 0.1% Triton X-100 (Sigma-Aldrich), and incubated in PBS : 0.5% bovine serum albumin (BSA) (Sigma-Aldrich) for 30 min to block nonspecific binding. The organoids were stained with preoptimised concentrations of monoclonal mouse primary antibodies targeting Runx2 (3 μg/ml) (R&D Systems, Abingdon, UK), osteocalcin (10 μg/ml), or polyclonal rabbit primary antibody targeting type I collagen (10 μg/ml) (Abcam, Cambridge, UK) overnight in a humidified environment at +4°C. Unbound primary antibody was removed by washing in PBS and the slides were incubated for 1 hour in the dark at room temperature with a secondary NL557-conjugated anti-mouse or NL493-conjugated anti-rabbit antibody (1 : 200) (R&D Systems). Slides were washed in PBS and stained with 0.1% 4′,6-diamidino-2-phenylindole (DAPI, Life Technologies) for 1 min at room temperature. Each sample was washed in PBS and imaged using a confocal microscope (Zeiss LSM710, Oberkochen, Germany). Negative (no primary antibody) and blank (scaffold without cells) controls were included.

2.8. Alkaline Phosphatase Staining. The slides were fixed in ice cold 70% ethanol (Fisher Scientific) for 10 min after sectioning and washed in PBS, before being immersed in ALP substrate kit (Vector Laboratories, Peterborough, UK) according to the manufacturer's instructions. Slides were stained in 0.1% DAPI (Life Technologies) for 1 min at room temperature to stain nuclei and imaged using a confocal microscope.

2.9. Real-Time PCR Analysis. Key markers of osteogenesis (Runx2, ALP, and type I collagen) were assessed using real-time PCR. 21 days post differentiation, RNA was isolated from the cells using the MasterPure kit (Cambio, Cambridge, UK) according to the manufacturer's instructions. In brief, samples were lysed in 300 μl of tissue and cell lysis solution at 65°C for 30 min. Protein was precipitated out of solution using 150 μl of protein precipitation reagent. After centrifugation, the supernatant was collected and incubated for 1 hour at 37 °C with deoxyribonuclease to remove DNA. This process was then repeated. RNA was collected by precipitation using 2-propanol and centrifugation. 1 μg of RNA was reverse transcribed into cDNA using RETROscript® Kit (Life Technologies) in a reaction volume of 20 μl. Real-time PCR reactions were run at 50°C for 2 min and 95°C for 2 min, as

TABLE 1: Primer sequences used in real-time PCR.

Gene	Forward primer (5′-3′)	Reverse primer (5′-3′)
Glyceraldehyde-3-phosphate dehydrogenase	TCA TTG ACC TCA ACT ACA TGG T	TCT CGC TCC TGG AAG ATG GTG
RUNX2	CCT AGG CGC ATT TCA GGT GCT T	CTG AGG TGA CTG GCG GGG TGT
Type I collagen	ATG TTC AGC TTT GTG GAC CTC CGG	CGC AGG TGA TTG GTG GGA TGT CT
Alkaline phosphatase	GAC CCT TGA CCC CCA CAA T	GCT CGT ACT GCA TGT CCC CT

an initial denaturation step, followed by 40 cycles at 95°C for 15 secs to denature and 60°C for 30 secs to anneal using SsoFast EvaGreen Supermix and the 2005 MyiQ real-time PCR detection system (Bio-Rad Laboratories, Hemel Hempstead, UK). Amplification of each gene included 10 μl of SsoFast EvaGreen®, 0.6 μl forward primers, 0.6 μl reverse primers, 6.8 μl of nuclease free water, and 2 μl of diluted cDNA (1 : 10 with nuclease-free water). This was followed by a melt curve analysis. The cycle threshold (CT) of amplification for each gene of interest (Table 1) was normalised against the housekeeping gene GAPDH in all samples, and relative gene expression level was determined by the 2^(GAPDH CT-Test CT) method.

2.10. Statistical Analysis. All experiments were repeated at least once until consistent results were obtained. Nonparametric tests were used to analyse statistical data (Statistica Version 6, StatSoft Ltd., UK). All data are expressed as mean ± standard error.

3. Results

3.1. Characterisation by Flow Cytometry. UCM and BM MSC demonstrated the traditional MSC phenotype [20] showing positive expression for CD73, CD90, and CD105 and negative expression for the haematopoietic markers CD14, CD19, CD34, and CD45 (Figure 1).

3.2. Morphology Characterised by Bright Field and Scanning Electron Microscopy. Bright field (Figure 2) and SEM images (Figure 3) were taken on days 1, 7, 14, and 21 of the differentiation process and compared to a control image taken at day 21 with no addition of osteogenic supplement. Bright field images (Figure 2) showed large gaps in between particles devoid of UCM MSCs (Figure 2(A4), white arrow) until day 21. In contrast, BM MSCs (Figure 2(B)) were observed to proliferate and rapidly occupy the spaces between particles as early as day 7 and did not change in appearance after this time point. SEM images (Figure 3) showed over time the surface of the organoids to become smoother due increasing cell density and deposition of extracellular matrix, which bound the CHACC particles together forming a larger conglomerate. Smoother surfaces were exhibited using BM MSCs (Figure 3(B3)) at day 14, whereas UCM MSCs (Figure 3(A4)) did not cover the entire surface until day 21. The addition of osteogenic supplement was not observed to have any significant impact on organoid morphology in relation to the control images at 21 days.

Cell viability was also assessed after 14 and 21 days using Calcein acetoxymethyl (0.1 μg/ml) and propidium iodide (1 μg/ml) and viewed by fluorescence microscopy. Dead cells were barely observed on CHACC using UCM or BM MSCs, which demonstrated that the cell viability was not affected by CHACC microparticles.

3.3. Osteogenesis Characterised by Immunocytochemistry and Alkaline Phosphatase Staining. UCM and BM MSCs were observed throughout the organoid by 21 days of differentiation. Excluding UCM MSCs grown in control α-MEM that did not label for ALP (Figure 4(a), A1), osteogenically induced and noninduced organoids were positive for ALP (Figure 4(a), A2–A4), Runx2 (Figure 4(b), B1–B4), type I collagen, and osteocalcin (Figure 4(c), C1–C4). ALP was active within the MSC's cytoplasm. Runx2 was largely found within the nucleus of MSCs and appeared purple due to blending with the nuclear stain DAPI. Type I collagen and osteocalcin were found within the extracellular matrix on the surface of the organoid.

ALP (Figure 4(a), A5), Runx2 (Figure 4(b), B5), and type I collagen (Figure 4(c), C5) were also assessed by real-time PCR. Osteogenically induced BM MSCs were shown to have significantly more ALP (Figure 4(a), A5) and Runx2 (Figure 4(b), B5) mRNA than osteogenically induced UCM MSCs, relative to the housekeeping gene, GAPDH. However, control BM MSCs were also shown to have significantly more Runx2 mRNA compared to UCM MSC. Nonosteogenically induced UCM MSCs showed high type I collagen mRNA and protein expression but low ALP and Runx2.

4. Discussion

Novel biomaterials for bone regeneration are desired as they do not have inherent disadvantages of autografts (blood loss, infection and morbidity risks, and limited supply). However, they need to match the gold standard of autografts in bone replacement surgery. CHACC has been shown to have excellent properties to function as a bone graft, but it lacks the key component required for autografts: living cells with osteogenic capacity.

In this study, UCM and BM MSCs were incorporated with CHACC microparticles to form organoids and their *in vitro* osteogenic potential was assessed and compared. Human UCM MSCs have been proven to differentiate down the osteogenic lineage and share common surface markers to BM MSCs [15]. CHACC is already used as a bone graft. Therefore, it was expected to provide a 3D structure for UCM and BM MSC attachment, proliferation, and

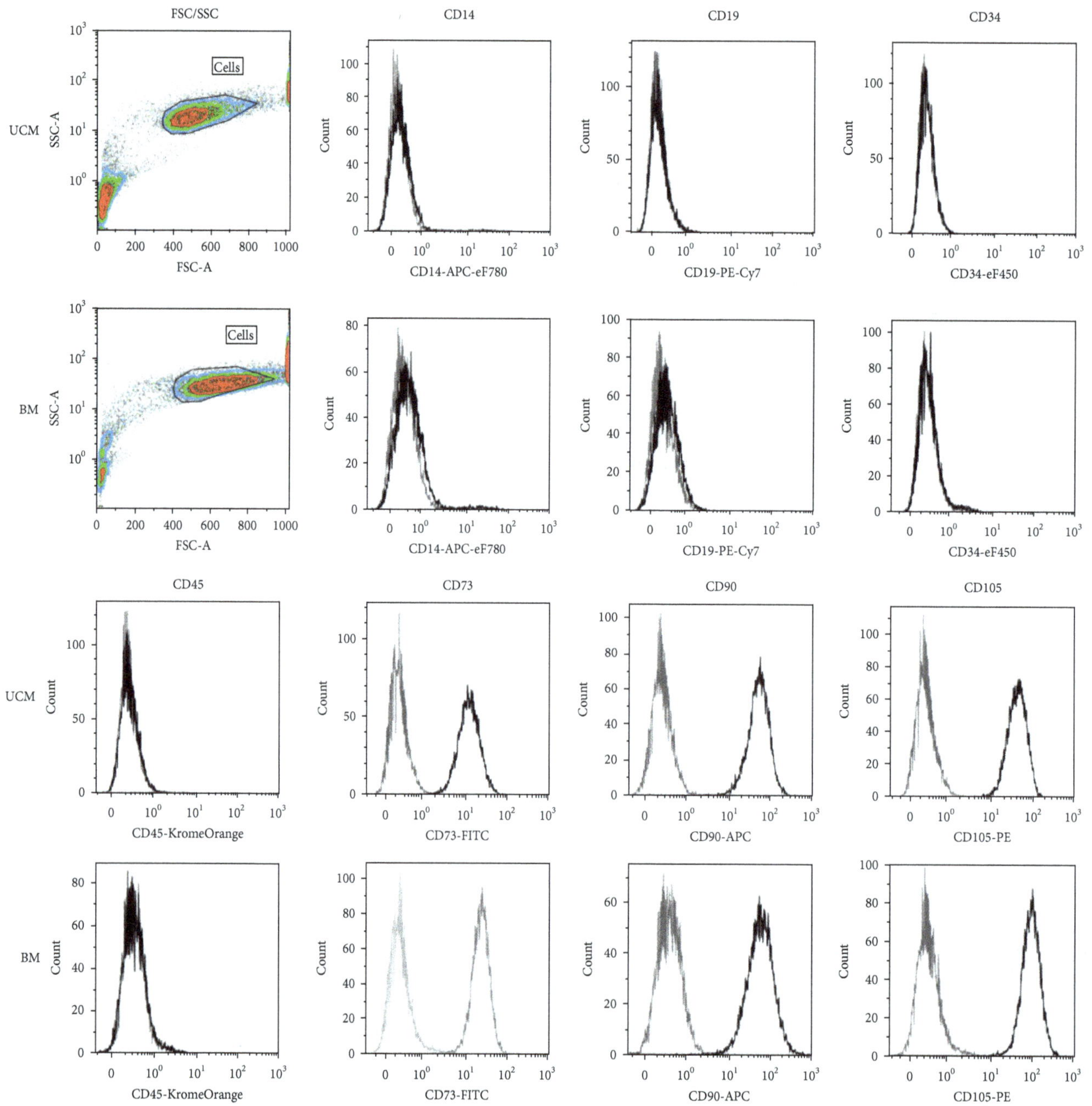

FIGURE 1: Human UCM and BM MSCs single stained with antibodies against surface markers. MSCs were CD14-CD19-CD34-CD45-CD73+CD90+ and CD105+, correlating with an MSC phenotype defined by ISCT. Grey: unstained; black: stained.

differentiation. Organoids can result in increased cell numbers compared to the cell suspension method [24], and the hydroxyapatite layer on CHACC should accelerate the differentiation of cells and consequently mineralisation [24–26].

Although both BM and UCM MSCs were able to attach to CHACC microparticles, form organoids, proliferate, and differentiate down the osteogenic lineage, as expected, the BM MSCs showed higher levels of osteogenic differentiation than UCM MSCs. BM MSCs showed a dramatic increase in cell proliferation indicating that they entered into the first stage of osteogenic differentiation [27] before UCM MSCs. Increased osteogenic differentiation in BM MSCs was further evidenced by increased expression of runx2 and ALP and the labelling of osteocalcin in immunocytochemistry [25]. Other researchers have also found BM MSCs to have superior osteogenic potential compared to UCM MSCs [28]. Similar to our study, Schneider et al. found BM MSCs to express more ALP but less type I collagen than UCM MSCs [29]. Zhang et al. compared MSCs on 3D scaffolds derived from different sources and found BM MSCs to form more bone than UCM MSC [18]. Reduced osteogenic potential of UCM MSCs maybe explained by the anatomical origins that they

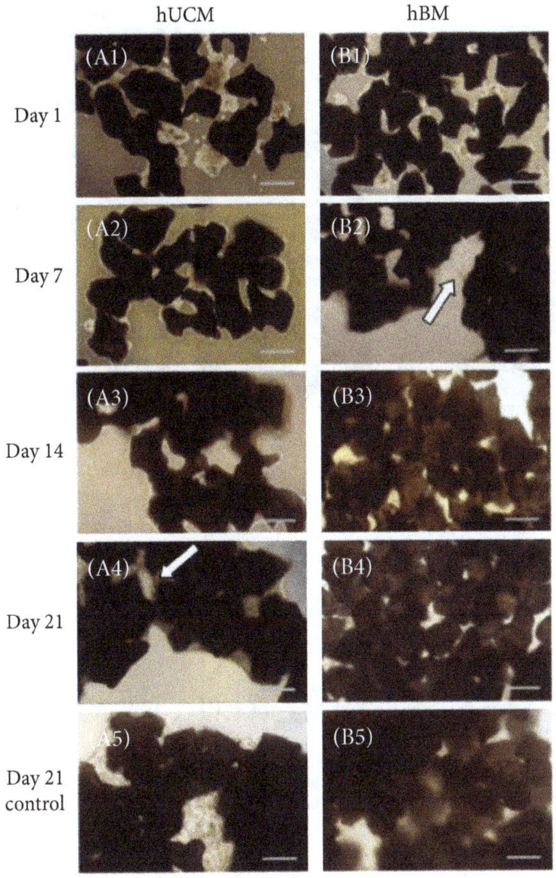

Figure 2: Bright field images of organoids with UCM (A) and BM (B) MSCs during the process of osteogenesis. Images were taken on days 1 (A1, B1), 7 (A2, B2), 14 (A3, B3), and 21 (A4, B4) of the differentiation process and compared to a control (α-MEM) image at day 21 (A5, B5). BM MSCs were observed to proliferate into the voids created by the numerous coral particles by day 7 and UCM MSCs by day 7 (white arrows). SP: scaffold particle. Scale bars: 250 μm.

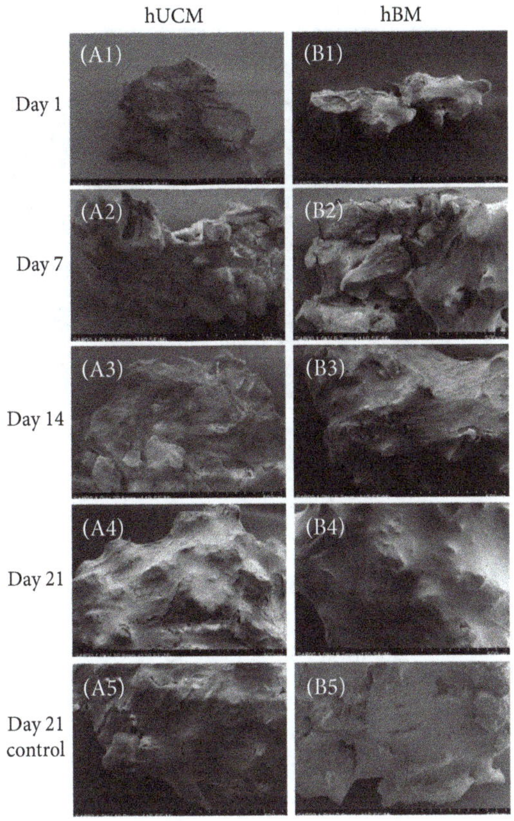

Figure 3: SEM images of organoids with UCM (A) and BM (B) MSCs during the process of osteogenesis. Images were taken on days 1 (A1, B1), 7 (A2, B2), 14 (A3, B3), and 21 (A4, B4) of the differentiation process and compared to a control (α-MEM) image at day 21 (A5, B5). Over time, the voids within the organoid were filled with MSCs and associated extracellular matrix which formed a smoother surface that covered CHACC surfaces. Significant coverage was exhibited using BM MSCs at day 14 (B3), whereas UCM MSCs did not cover surfaces until day 21 (A4). Scale bars: 500 μm.

were derived from. Panepucci et al. found higher levels of genes related to osteogenesis in BM MSCs compared to umbilical cord vein MSCs [30]. Umbilical cord vein MSCs expressed genes more related to matrix remodelling via metalloproteinases and angiogenesis. Consequently, UCM MSCs could be less committed to osteogenesis but instead committed to angiogenesis.

Interestingly, Zhang et al. also showed that UCM MSCs could differentiate down the osteogenic lineage better than BM MSCs if they were cultured in monolayer [18]. Based on this study, future work should investigate differentiating UCM MSCs in monolayer first and then seed these cells onto 3D scaffolds. Although ectopic bone formation using UCM MSCs has been proven to be inferior compared to BM MSCs in vivo, the angiogenic nature of UCMs has been utilised to improve bone regeneration. Todeschi et al. showed that UCM MSCs implanted orthotopically caused a similar amount of new bones to form compared to BM MSCs by recruiting host osteogenic cells [31]. Chen et al. also utilised the angiogenic nature of umbilical cord mesenchymal stem cells by coculturing them with human umbilical cord vein endothelial cells. They found that a similar amount of new bone formation could be achieved in vivo compared to coculturing human umbilical cord vein endothelial cells with BM MSCs [32].

There are a number of limitations to this study; immunocytochemistry and real-time PCR only assess a narrow spectrum of markers, meaning MSCs could be differentiating down a lineage not being specifically looked at. Furthermore, quantitative PCR only gives a snap shot of RNA expression at the day it is extracted and has a very short half-life of approximately 9 hours [33] meaning expression levels could be missed. Cell attachment and growth was limited to arbitrary qualitative assessment via bright field and SEM images.

Future work is expected to overcome the inferior osteogenic capacity of UCM MSCs, such as to initiate the osteogenic differentiation at 2D culture stage, and the osteogenic gene and protein expression will be assessed at more time points to show the full spectrum of differentiation over the three-week period or longer to assess the full potential of UCM MSCs. Also, to utilise the angiogenic nature of UCM, MSCs with CHACC should be explored as well.

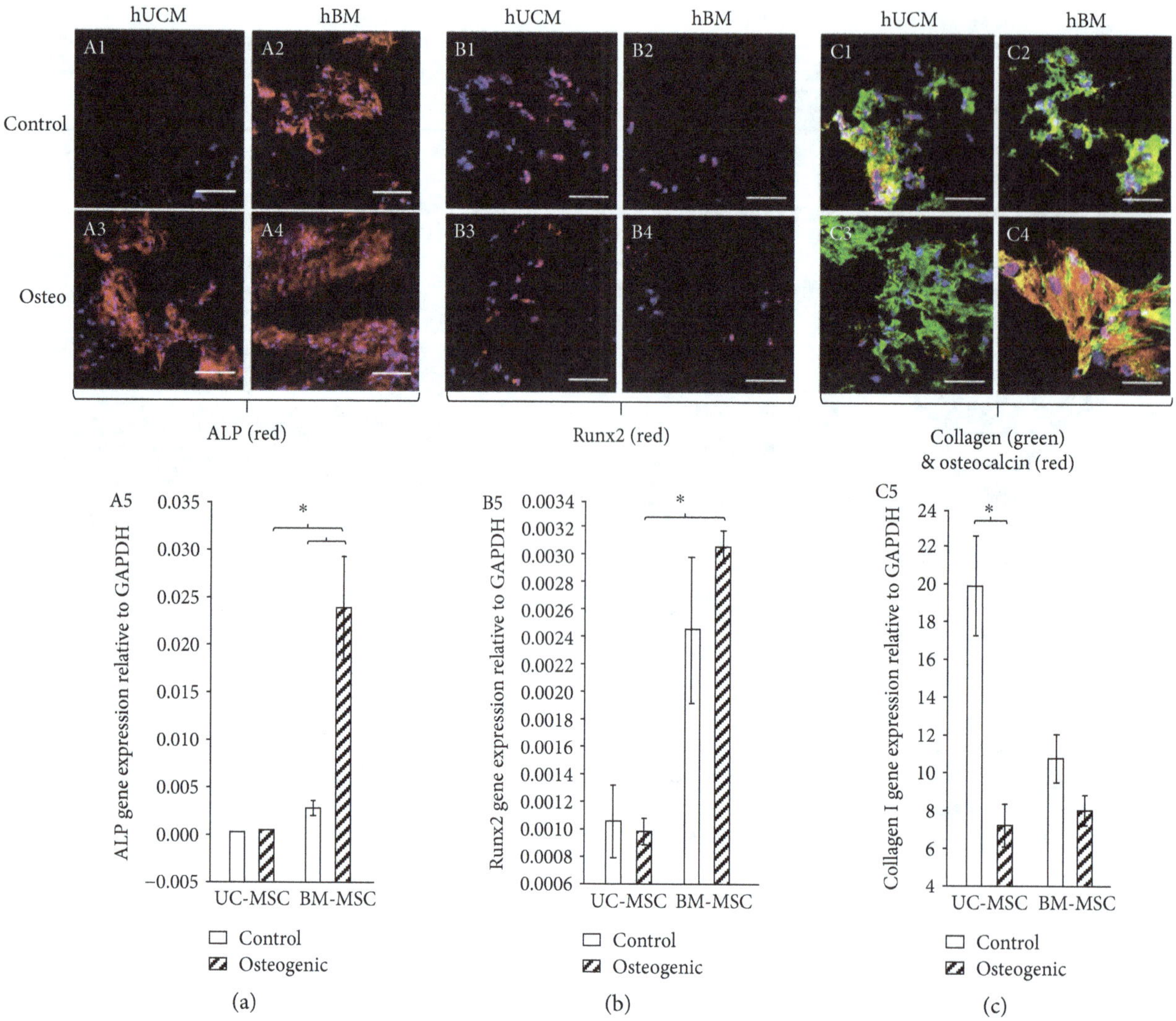

Figure 4: On day 21, control and osteogenically induced organoids were cryosectioned (10 μm) and stained for alkaline phosphatase (ALP) (a), Runx2 (b), collagen type I, and osteocalcin (c). Real-time PCR was used to assess mRNA levels of ALP (A5), Runx2 (B5), and collagen type I (C5) in UCM and BM MSCs lysed directly from the control and osteogenically induced scaffolds at 21 days. MSCs derived from UCM expressed good collagen I mRNA and protein production but poor ALP and Runx2 in relation to MSCs derived from BM. $n = 4$ ($^*p < 0.05$).

5. Conclusion

This study has shown that 200–300 μm CHACC granules can be a suitable carrier for human MSC proliferation and differentiation *in vitro*, for the purpose of injectable delivery opening up the use of CHACC for new applications within maxillofacial surgery and dentistry. In addition, UCM MSCs show inferior osteogenic capacity when cultured as CHACC organoids compared to BM MSCs. Therefore, further research is required to optimise the osteogenicity of UCM MSCs to release their full potential as a readily available, accessible, and abundant tissue source for bone tissue engineering.

Acknowledgments

The authors would like to thank the Newborn Immunity Group for providing antibodies and umbilical cord collections and Professor Ian Pallister and the Dept. of Trauma and Orthopaedics at Morriston Hospital, Swansea, for bone marrow collections. They thank Dr. David Guy, Dr. Chris Wright, Dr. Sam Webster, Dr. Jo Bishop, and Professor Cathy Thornton for their support and advice for this research project. This project was supported by the European Regional Development Fund (ERDF), Hainan International S&T Cooperation Project (GJXM201101), National Natural Science Foundation of China (NSFC 81260271), Osseo Regenerative Technologies (UK) LTD., and Knowledge Economy Skills Scholarships (KESS).

References

[1] G. E. Friedlaender, "Bone-Banking," *The Journal of Bone & Joint Surgery*, vol. 64, no. 2, pp. 307–311, 1982.

[2] P. D. Costantino and C. D. Friedman, "Synthetic bone graft substitutes," *Otolaryngologic Clinics of North America*, vol. 27, no. 5, pp. 1037–1074, 1994.

[3] N. Shibuya and D. C. Jupiter, "Bone graft substitute: allograft and xenograft," *Clinics in Podiatric Medicine and Surgery*, vol. 32, no. 1, pp. 21–34, 2015.

[4] D. J. Sartoris, R. E. Holmes, R. W. Bucholz, V. Mooney, and D. Resnick, "Coralline hydroxyapatite bone-graft substitutes in a canine diaphyseal defect model: radiographic-histometric correlation," *Investigative Radiology*, vol. 22, no. 7, pp. 590–596, 1987.

[5] S. Koëter, S. J. Tigchelaar, P. Farla, L. Driessen, A. van Kampen, and P. Buma, "Coralline hydroxyapatite is a suitable bone graft substitute in an intra-articular goat defect model," *Journal of Biomedical Materials Research Part B: Applied Biomaterials*, vol. 90B, no. 1, pp. 116–122, 2009.

[6] K. Fu, Q. Xu, J. Czernuszka, G. R. G. Russell, and J. T. Triffitt, "Characterisation, osteogenic potential and clinical performance of a South China Sea coralline hydroxyapatite/calcium carbonate," *Calcified Tissue International*, vol. 83, no. 1, pp. 20–20, 2008.

[7] R. Vago, D. Plotquin, A. Bunin, I. Sinelnikov, D. Atar, and D. Itzhak, "Hard tissue remodeling using biofabricated coralline biomaterials," *Journal of Biochemical and Biophysical Methods*, vol. 50, no. 2-3, pp. 253–259, 2002.

[8] J. S. Thalgott, Z. Klezl, M. Timlin, and J. M. Giuffre, "Anterior lumbar interbody fusion with processed sea coral (coralline hydroxyapatite) as part of a circumferential fusion," *Spine*, vol. 27, no. 24, pp. E518–E525, 2002.

[9] K. Fu, Q. Xu, J. Czernuszka, J. T. Triffitt, and Z. Xia, "Characterization of a biodegradable coralline hydroxyapatite/calcium carbonate composite and its clinical implementation," *Biomedical Materials*, vol. 8, no. 6, article 065007, 2013.

[10] K. Fu, Q. Xu, J. Czernuszka et al., "Prolonged osteogenesis from human mesenchymal stem cells implanted in immunodeficient mice by using coralline hydroxyapatite incorporating rhBMP2 microspheres," *Journal of Biomedical Materials Research. Part A*, vol. 92, no. 4, pp. 1256–1264, 2010.

[11] J. Michel, M. Penna, J. Kochen, and H. Cheung, "Recent advances in hydroxyapatite scaffolds containing mesenchymal stem cells," *Stem Cells International*, vol. 2015, Article ID 305217, 13 pages, 2015.

[12] Y. Sambuy and I. De Angelis, "Formation of organoid structures and extracellular matrix production in an intestinal epithelial cell line during long-term in vitro culture," *Cell Differentiation*, vol. 19, no. 2, pp. 139–147, 1986.

[13] A. Astashkina and D. W. Grainger, "Critical analysis of 3-D organoid in vitro cell culture models for high-throughput drug candidate toxicity assessments," *Advanced Drug Delivery Reviews*, vol. 69-70, pp. 1–18, 2014.

[14] N. Eliopoulos, A. al-Khaldi, M. Crosato, K. Lachapelle, and J. Galipeau, "A neovascularized organoid derived from retrovirally engineered bone marrow stroma leads to prolonged in vivo systemic delivery of erythropoietin in nonmyeloablated, immunocompetent mice," *Gene Therapy*, vol. 10, no. 6, pp. 478–489, 2003.

[15] A. Can and S. Karahuseyinoglu, "Concise review: human umbilical cord stroma with regard to the source of fetus-derived stem cells," *Stem Cells*, vol. 25, no. 11, pp. 2886–2895, 2007.

[16] Y. Diao, Q. Ma, F. Cui, and Y. Zhong, "Human umbilical cord mesenchymal stem cells: osteogenesis *in vivo* as seed cells for bone tissue engineering," *Journal of Biomedical Materials Research Part A*, vol. 91A, no. 1, pp. 123–131, 2009.

[17] S. Honsawek, D. Dhitiseith, and V. Phupong, "Effects of demineralized bone matrix on proliferation and osteogenic differentiation of mesenchymal stem cells from human umbilical cord," *Journal of the Medical Association of Thailand= Chotmaihet thangphaet*, vol. 89, Supplement 3, pp. S189–S195, 2006.

[18] Z.-Y. Zhang, S. H. Teoh, M. S. K. Chong et al., "Superior osteogenic capacity for bone tissue engineering of fetal compared with perinatal and adult mesenchymal stem cells," *Stem Cells*, vol. 27, no. 1, pp. 126–137, 2009.

[19] L. Wang, M. Singh, L. F. Bonewald, and M. S. Detamore, "Signalling strategies for osteogenic differentiation of human umbilical cord mesenchymal stromal cells for 3D bone tissue engineering," *Journal of Tissue Engineering and Regenerative Medicine*, vol. 3, no. 5, pp. 398–404, 2009.

[20] M. Dominici, K. le Blanc, I. Mueller et al., "Minimal criteria for defining multipotent mesenchymal stromal cells. The International Society for Cellular Therapy position statement," *Cytotherapy*, vol. 8, no. 4, pp. 315–317, 2006.

[21] H. T. Maecker and J. Trotter, "Flow cytometry controls, instrument setup, and the determination of positivity," *Cytometry Part A*, vol. 69A, no. 9, pp. 1037–1042, 2006.

[22] L. A. Herzenberg, J. Tung, W. A. Moore, L. A. Herzenberg, and D. R. Parks, "Interpreting flow cytometry data: a guide for the perplexed," *Nature Immunology*, vol. 7, no. 7, pp. 681–685, 2006.

[23] D. F. Alvarez, K. Helm, J. DeGregori, M. Roederer, and S. Majka, "Publishing flow cytometry data," *American Journal of Physiology. Lung Cellular and Molecular Physiology*, vol. 298, no. 2, pp. L127–L130, 2010.

[24] F. Langenbach, C. Naujoks, A. Laser et al., "Improvement of the cell-loading efficiency of biomaterials by inoculation with stem cell-based microspheres, in osteogenesis," *Journal of Biomaterials Applications*, vol. 26, no. 5, pp. 549–564, 2010.

[25] K. Jähn, R. G. Richards, C. W. Archer, and M. J. Stoddart, "Pellet culture model for human primary osteoblasts," *European Cells and Materials*, vol. 20, pp. 149–161, 2010.

[26] M. Kabiri, B. Kul, W. B. Lott et al., "3D mesenchymal stem/stromal cell osteogenesis and autocrine signalling," *Biochemical and Biophysical Research Communications*, vol. 419, no. 2, pp. 142–147, 2012.

[27] S. J. Roberts, Y. Chen, M. Moesen, J. Schrooten, and F. P. Luyten, "Enhancement of osteogenic gene expression for the differentiation of human periosteal derived cells," *Stem Cell Research*, vol. 7, no. 2, pp. 137–144, 2011.

[28] S. Kargozar, M. Mozafari, S. J. Hashemian et al., "Osteogenic potential of stem cells-seeded bioactive nanocomposite scaffolds: a comparative study between human mesenchymal stem cells derived from bone, umbilical cord Wharton's jelly, and adipose tissue," *Journal of Biomedical Materials Research Part B: Applied Biomaterials*, vol. 106, no. 1, pp. 61–72, 2016.

[29] R. K. Schneider, A. Puellen, R. Kramann et al., "The osteogenic differentiation of adult bone marrow and perinatal umbilical mesenchymal stem cells and matrix remodelling in three-dimensional collagen scaffolds," *Biomaterials*, vol. 31, no. 3, pp. 467–480, 2010.

[30] R. A. Panepucci, J. L. C. Siufi, W. A. Silva Jr et al., "Comparison of gene expression of umbilical cord vein and bone marrow-

derived mesenchymal stem cells," *Stem Cells*, vol. 22, no. 7, pp. 1263–1278, 2004.

[31] M. R. Todeschi, R. el Backly, C. Capelli et al., "Transplanted umbilical cord mesenchymal stem cells modify the in vivo microenvironment enhancing angiogenesis and leading to bone regeneration," *Stem Cells and Development*, vol. 24, no. 13, pp. 1570–1581, 2015.

[32] W. Chen, X. Liu, Q. Chen et al., "Angiogenic and osteogenic regeneration in rats via calcium phosphate scaffold and endothelial cell co-culture with human bone marrow mesenchymal stem cells (MSCs), human umbilical cord MSCs, human induced pluripotent stem cell-derived MSCs and human embryonic stem cell-derived MSCs," *Journal of Tissue Engineering and Regenerative Medicine*, vol. 12, no. 1, pp. 191–203, 2018.

[33] B. Schwanhäusser, D. Busse, N. Li et al., "Corrigendum: global quantification of mammalian gene expression control," *Nature*, vol. 495, no. 7439, pp. 126-127, 2013.

9

Therapeutic Effect of Human Umbilical Cord Mesenchymal Stem Cells at Various Passages on Acute Liver Failure in Rats

Yongting Zhang,[1,2] Yuwen Li,[3] Wenting Li,[4] Jie Cai,[1] Ming Yue,[1] Longfeng Jiang,[1] Ruirui Xu,[1] Lili Zhang,[1] Jun Li,[1] and Chuanlong Zhu[1]

[1]*Department of Infectious Disease, The First Affiliated Hospital of Nanjing Medical University, Nanjing 210029, China*
[2]*Department of Pediatrics, The Affiliated Hospital of Yangzhou University, Yangzhou 225000, China*
[3]*Department of Pediatrics, The First Affiliated Hospital of Nanjing Medical University, Nanjing 210029, China*
[4]*Third Liver Unit, Department of Infectious Disease, The First Affiliated Hospital of Science and Technology of China, Hefei 230001, China*

Correspondence should be addressed to Chuanlong Zhu; chuanlong@yahoo.com

Guest Editor: Yuchen Xia

Recent studies have described beneficial effects of an infusion of mesenchymal stem cells (MSCs) derived from Wharton's jelly tissue, for the treatment of acute liver failure (ALF). However, data on the therapeutic potential of culture-expanded MSCs are lacking. We examined the therapeutic potential of passage five (P5) and ten (P10) human umbilical cord- (hUC-) MSCs via their transplantation into Sprague-Dawley (SD) rats with D-galactosamine (D-GalN) and LPS-induced acute liver failure (ALF). SD rats were randomly divided into three groups: control group, P5 hUC-MSCs group, and P10 hUC-MSCs group. After transplantation, P5 hUC-MSCs provided a significant survival benefit. The analysis of aspartate aminotransferase (AST), alanine aminotransferase (ALT), and total bilirubin (TBIL) levels showed that transplantation with P5 hUC-MSCs was more effective than treatment with P10 hUC-MSCs. P5 hUC-MSCs also successfully downregulated the hepatic activity index (HAI) scores. Compared to P10 hUC-MSCs *in vivo*, P5 hUC-MSCs significantly enhanced the regeneration and inhibited the apoptosis of hepatocytes. CM-Dil-labeled hUC-MSCs were found to engraft within the recipient liver, whereas the homing of cells to the recipient liver in the P10 hUC-MSCs group was less effective compared to the P5 hUC-MSCs group. Previous studies have shown that the concentration of hepatocyte growth factor (HGF) in the injured liver was significantly increased. HGF is commonly known as the ligand of c-Met. The level of c-Met in hUC-MSCs as detected by Western blotting indicated that at a higher passage number, there is a decrease in c-Met. These data suggest that direct transplantation of P5 hUC-MSCs can more efficiently home to an injured liver. Subsequently, the P5 hUC-MSCs can rescue ALF and repopulate the livers of rats through the stimulation of endogenous liver regeneration and inhibition of hepatocellular apoptosis for compensated liver function, which is dependent on the higher level of c-Met than P10 hUC-MSCs.

1. Introduction

Liver failure is a clinical syndrome characterized by jaundice, ascites, hepatic encephalopathy, and a bleeding tendency due to the impaired liver function. The syndrome can be caused by a variety of factors such as viral hepatitis, autoimmune hepatitis, drug-induced liver injuries, metabolic diseases, and circulatory disturbances [1].

To date, the only therapeutic option for liver failure is orthotopic liver transplantation. Reasons for failure to receive transplantation have included lack of available organs, high expense, and the requirement for lifelong immunosuppressive medication. Other treatment strategies include bioartificial livers that are short of liver cells and medical management [2]. Consequently, there is an urgent need for novel therapeutic options. Saunders et al. suggested that liver failure results from the catastrophic consequences of liver loss and the regeneration of remnant hepatocytes fails to repair in a timely manner, resulting in higher mortality rates [3]. Cell-based therapy in regenerative medicine shows considerable promise. Mesenchymal stem cells (MSCs) have a number of advantages, including their self-renewal, proliferation, and differentiation properties. MSCs were originally found in bone marrow and can also be isolated from the umbilical cord, adipose tissue, dental pulp, and amniotic fluid [4, 5]. MSCs, which are easily acquired and devoid of any ethical contentions, are preferred for autografts, especially cells from the bone marrow (BM). The moderate efficacy of autologous BM-MSCs is thought to be due to their aging and deficiency in vitality [6].

Recently, several studies reported that human umbilical cord mesenchymal stem cells (hUC-MSCs) are another promising source, as they are free from aging and are unlimited in their supply. They are also characterized by lower immunogenic potency, higher proliferative activity, and multipotency [7]. Gholamrezanezhad et al. [8] have shown that there was no significant improvement in liver function after a 1-month period of follow-up because the homing ability of BM-MSCs into the liver occurred in only a limited number of infused cells. Peng et al. also reported that the homing ability of MSCs is the main reason why autologous MSC transplantation did not achieve acceptable long-term effects on the prognosis of a patient [9]. The lingering problem pertaining to cell-based therapies is whether the delivered cells home to the injured sites and how to improve their homing ability.

Hepatocyte growth factor (HGF), which is the most effective mitogen for hepatocytes, functions via a receptor termed the cellular mesenchymal to epithelial transition factor (c-Met) [10]. The HGF-c-Met axis has been extensively examined, as it is crucial for MSC homing during liver injury [11]. Our primary experiment found that levels of HGF in the liver significantly increased and peaked at 24 h and 48 h, respectively, post-D-GalN/LPS injection. Meanwhile, overexpressed c-Met in BM-MSCs improved the homing efficacy to the injured liver and improved the liver function [12]. Furthermore, freshly isolated MSCs lose ligands or receptors, which respond to migratory signals during expansion [13].

In this study, we aimed to investigate the effect of CM-Dil-labeled hUC-MSCs on liver failure and the underlying mechanism of homing among various passages in hUC-MSCs.

2. Materials and Methods

2.1. Animals. Male Sprague-Dawley rats weighing 220 to 250 g were purchased from the Animal Laboratory Center of Nanjing Medical University (Nanjing, China). All procedures were performed in strict accordance with the recommendations in the Guide for the Care and Use of Laboratory Animals of Nanjing Medical University. All experimental protocols were approved by the Animal Ethical and Welfare Committee of Nanjing Medical University (Nanjing, China).

2.2. hUC-MSCs. P2 hUC-MSCs were purchased from Cyagen. The cell pellet was cultured in an expansion medium composed of the human umbilical cord mesenchymal stem cell basal medium (HUXUC-01001, Cyagen, China), supplemented with 10% human umbilical cord mesenchymal stem cell cell-qualified fetal bovine serum, 1% glutamine, and 1% penicillin-streptomycin (Cyagen), at 37°C, with 5% carbon dioxide in a fully humidified environment.

Native hUC-MSCs (at P5) were suspended at a concentration of 1×10^6 cells/mL, washed twice in phosphate-buffered saline (PBS), and then incubated for 30 min at 4°C in the dark with the following anti-human antibodies conjugated with fluorescein isothiocyanate (FITC) or phycoerythrin (PE): anti-CD31-PE (303105), anti-CD45-PE (368509), anti-CD34-PE (343605), anti-CD44-FITC (338803), anti-CD90-FITC (328107), and anti-CD105-FITC (328107; all from BioLegend). After 30 min, cells were washed and resuspended in 300 mL Cell Fix (BD). PE-conjugated IgG1 and FITC-conjugated IgG1 were used as isotype controls (R&D Systems Inc. and Santa Cruz Biotechnology Inc.). Immunophenotyping of hUC-MSCs was performed by flow cytometry.

2.3. Animal Model and Cell Transplantation. The animal model used was described in a previous study [14]. D-galactosamine (D-GalN, 1000 mg/kg body weight, Sigma) and lipopolysaccharide (LPS, 10 μg/kg body weight; Sigma) were dissolved in PBS and simultaneously administered to animals intraperitoneally. Cells were transplanted under 10% chloral hydrate injection anesthesia, 24 h after the administration of D-GalN/LPS. SD rats were randomly divided into three groups: group A, rats that received 1 mL of normal saline via tail vein as the control ($n = 12$); group B, rats that received 1 mL of P5 hUC-MSCs (1×10^7 cells/kg) via tail vein ($n = 12$); and group C, rats that received P10 hUC-MSCs (1×10^7 cells/kg) via tail vein ($n = 12$). Blood samples were collected at 24 h, 48 h, and 72 h after the injection of D-GalN/LPS, and finally, entire livers were collected, fixed, then prepared for further analysis.

2.4. Serum Transaminase Levels. Serum samples were stored at −80°C until the time of analysis. Serum aspartate aminotransferase (AST), total bilirubin (TBil), and alanine aminotransferase (ALT) levels in the rat blood were measured according to the manufacturer's directions with a kit from the Nanjing Jiancheng Bioengineering Institute (Nanjing, China).

2.5. Liver Histology. Formalin-fixed, paraffin-embedded liver samples were sectioned at a thickness of 4 μm and stained with hematoxylin & eosin (H&E). Histological assessment was performed using the hepatic activity index (HAI) and was graded following guidelines previously described [15].

2.6. Cell Labeling. Before labeling, the P5 and P10 hUC-MSCs in plates were trypsinized for cell counting. CM-Dil (Invitrogen, USA) was then directly added to the culture medium to label cells in the working solution (2 μg/mL) for 5 minutes at 37°C, and then for an additional 15 minutes at 4°C. Following labeling, the medium was discarded, and the cells were washed three times with PBS to eliminate residual fluorescent-conjugated antibodies. At 24 h after the injection of D-GalN/LPS, the labeled P5 and P10 hUC-MSCs (1×10^6 cells in 1 mL of normal saline) were transplanted into the rats, and the control rats received 1 mL of normal saline. After an additional 24 h, the rats were killed so the livers could be removed. The frozen sections were examined by fluorescence microscope and analyzed by Image-Pro Plus.

2.7. Immunohistochemistry. The sections of formalin-fixed tissue were left for 1 hour at 60°C before deparaffinized, rehydrated, and blocked in 3% hydrogen peroxide in ethanol for 15 minutes. For proliferating cell nuclear antigen (PCNA) immunohistochemistry, sections were blocked with 1.5% bovine serum albumin (BSA) for 30 minutes and incubated with anti-mouse PCNA (Google biology, Wuhan) overnight at 4°C. Sections were washed and incubated with a rabbit anti-human IgG secondary antibody (K5007, DAKO, Denmark) for 50 minutes at room temperature. The sections were then added to a newly prepared DAB kit (DAKO, Denmark). The positive nucleus is indicated with brown and yellow colors. Sections were counterstained with hematoxylin for 3 minutes and 1% of hydrochloric acid for several seconds. Finally, the sections were observed under a Nikon light microscope after being dehydrated. For terminal deoxynucleotidyl transferase-mediated nick-end labeling (TUNEL) staining, we used the In Situ Cell Death Detection Kit (Roche, Switzerland) according to the vendor's instructions.

2.8. Western Blot Analysis of c-Met Protein. To detect the level of c-Met, the total protein samples in the same quantity for P3, P5, P8, and P10 hUC-MSCs were extracted. Proteins were identified based on instructions provided with the BCA Kit (Thermo Scientific, USA) and then separated by sodium dodecyl sulfate-polyacrylamide gel electrophoresis (SDS-PAGE) and transferred onto nitrocellulose membranes. The membranes were incubated with mouse monoclonal anti-c-Met antibody (Santa Cruz Biotechnology, Santa Cruz, USA) at a 1 : 500 dilution overnight at 4°C and then incubated with a sheep anti-mouse immunoglobulin G secondary antibody (GE Healthcare Biosciences, USA) for 60 minutes at room temperature. The results were detected using an enhanced chemiluminescence (ECL) kit (GE Healthcare Biosciences, USA) and visualized under an imaging system.

2.9. Statistics. The data are expressed as mean ± standard deviation (SD) using SPSS version 16.0 (Chicago, IL, USA). Statistical significance was determined via a one-way analysis of the variance (ANOVA) and the log-rank test for survival analysis among the three groups. A P value of <0.05 was considered to be statistically significant.

3. Results

3.1. Identification of Cultured hUC-MSCs. After resuscitation and cultivation for 5–7 days, cells started to present a fibroblast-like phenotype. After 14 days, the number of cells increased and grew in a parallel arrangement. After serial passage, they proliferated rapidly *in vitro*, without significant changes in morphology. Flow cytometry revealed that these cells were negative for the expression of hematopoietic markers such as CD45, CD34, and CD31. However, they were positive for CD105, CD90, and CD44, which are generally considered to be markers of MSCs. This indicated that these cells were hUC-MSCs (Figure 1).

3.2. Improved Survival Rate and Liver Function of ALF Rats That Received Transplanted hUC-MSCs. All rats in the control group died between 48 h and 96 h after the saline injection. The survival rate was 37.5% in the P10 hUC-MSCs group, with three rats surviving after a week. Rats treated with the P5 hUC-MSCs had a survival rate of 62.5% at 7 days, and only three rats died. A significantly higher survival rate was observed for the P5 hUC-MSCs group (Figure 2(a)).

As shown in Figures 2(b)–2(d), the serum ALT, AST, and TBil levels in the P5 hUC-MSCs group decreased 24 h after transplantation (165.50 ± 22.73 U/L, 254.69 ± 22.89 U/L, and 27.03 ± 2.92 μmol/L, respectively), while the liver function of the P10 hUC-MSCs group still increased (312.13 ± 14.98 U/L, 382.70 ± 23.48 U/L, and 35.98 ± 2.10 μmol/L, respectively). 48 h after transplantation, the serum levels in the P10 hUC-MSCs group were also dramatically decreased (ALT: 269.50 ± 24.16 U/L, AST: 325.07 ± 33.38 U/L, and TBil: 35.98 ± 2.10 μmol/L), with indicators of liver injury that were still lower than those of the rats that received the P5 hUC-MSCs (ALT: 118.56 ± 23.05 U/L, AST: 114.47 ± 23.06 U/L, and TBil: 18.67 ± 2.33 μmol/L). Moreover, significant differences in serum levels of ALT, AST, and TBil between the P5 hUC-MSCs group and P10 hUC-MSCs group were observed at 48 h and 72 h post-D-GalN/LPS injection ($P < 0.01$). No significant differences were observed at 24 h after the D-GalN/LPS coinjection.

3.3. hUC-MSCs Therapy Improves Gross and Microscopic Liver Histopathology and Reduces Inflammatory Cell Infiltration. To evaluate whether treatment with P5 hUC-MSCs regenerated the injured liver to a greater extent than with P10 hUC-MSCs, we further assessed the liver histology with H&E staining. H&E-stained sections revealed massive necrosis and hepatic lobule damage in the control group at 72 h, but hepatocyte necrosis was suppressed in both the P5 hUC-MSC and P10 hUC-MSC groups (Figure 3(a)). While microscopic evaluation of the H&E-stained liver sections revealed significant cytoplasmic vacuolization and severe inflammatory cell infiltration at 48 h post-P10 hUC-MSC transplantation, the sections from rats that received P5 hUC-MSC transplantation demonstrated moderate periportal inflammatory cell infiltration and hepatocyte edema at 48 h after P5 hUC-MSC transplantation (Figure 3(a)). Furthermore, HAI scores randomly assessed by expert pathologists were significantly different between necrosis and inflammatory cell infiltration ($P < 0.05$; Figure 3(b)), indicating that there was less necrosis and milder inflammatory reactions in the P5 hUC-MSC group compared to the P10 hUC-MSC group.

3.4. hUC-MSCs Inhibit Hepatocellular Apoptosis In Vivo. To determine whether different passages of hUC-MSCs have an impact on hepatocellular apoptosis, the number of

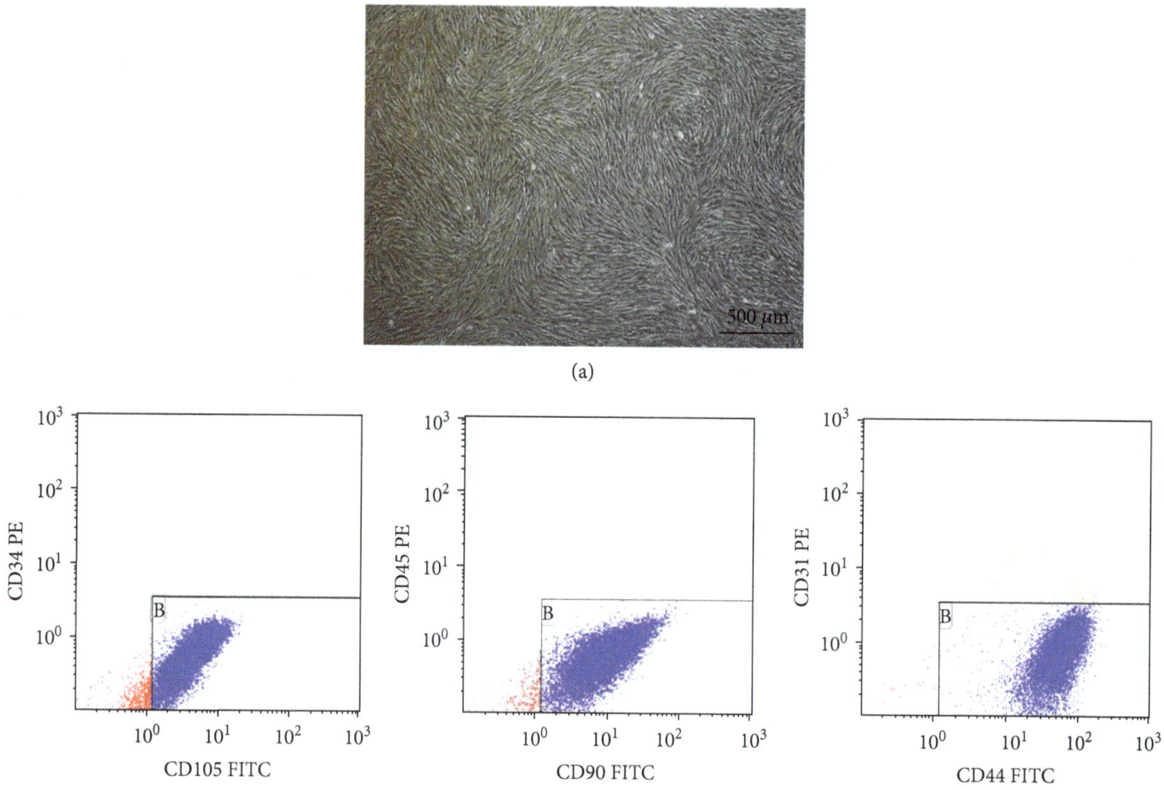

(b)

Figure 1: Characterization of hUC-MSCs. (a) Morphology of passage 3 hUC-MSC identification of human umbilical cord mesenchymal stem cells. (b) Flow cytometric analysis showing the immunophenotype of the passage 5hUC-MSCs. The cells were positive for CD105 (96.4%), CD44 (99.6%), and CD90 (97.6%), but negative for CD34, CD31, and CD45.

TUNEL-reactive hepatocyte nuclei in liver sections was determined. Four 400x fields were randomly selected from the three groups, and the number of accumulated apoptotic cells was counted using Image-Pro Plus software. Many apoptotic hepatocytes were observed in the control samples (NS: 24.0 ± 4.8), while a significant reduction was present with hUC-MSC treatment (P10: 14.0 ± 3.4; P5: 7.4 ± 1.8; Figure 4(a)). Quantification of TUNEL revealed that P5 hUC-MSC treatment effectively reduces hepatocellular death post coinjection of D-GalN and LPS when compared with P10 hUC-MSCs (Figure 4(b)).

3.5. hUC-MSCs Enhance Liver Regeneration. To evaluate whether hUC-MSCs promoted liver regeneration, the number of PCNA-positive hepatocytes was quantified and compared with control saline-treated animals. Few PCNA-positive hepatocytes were observed in the control, while many were seen after hUC-MSC administration (Figure 5(a)). In the P5 hUC-MSC group, a significant increase in the number of proliferating cells (IOD: 24604.99 ± 1132.43) was found, compared to the control (IOD: 13929.3 ± 813.7). In addition, the number of PCNA-positive cells in the P10 hUC-MSC group also increased slightly (IOD: 188550.99 ± 1654.58). These results provide evidence that infusion with MSCs enhances liver regeneration programs during ALF (Figure 5(b)).

3.6. CM-Dil-Labeled hUC-MSCs In Vivo. The administration of P5 hUC-MSCs to rats with injured livers is more effective than P10 hUC-MSCs. Importantly, primary MSCs lose ligands or receptors that respond to migratory signals during *in vitro* expansion [16]. Therefore, we assessed the homing efficacy of P5 and P10 hUC-MSCs with regard to injured livers. To investigate the homing efficacy, CM-Dil-labeled P5 and P10 hUC-MSCs (1×10^6 cells) were engrafted via tail vein 24 h after the injection with D-GalN/LPS. As shown in Figure 6(a), the engrafted cells mainly distributed around the central vein and in the sinusoids. After P5 hUC-MSC administration, the number of cells with fluorescence (120 ± 14) was higher than for P10 hUC-MSC administration (77 ± 12) in the liver (Figure 6(b)). These data suggested that P5 hUC-MSCs migrated more efficiently to the injured livers.

3.7. c-Met Expression in hUC-MSCs. Our primary experiment found that levels of HGF in the liver significantly increased and peaked at 24 h and 48 h, respectively, post-D-GalN/LPS injection. In addition, overexpressed c-Met in BM-MSCs improved the homing efficacy to injured livers and improved liver function. Furthermore, freshly isolated MSCs lose ligands or receptors that respond to migratory signals during expansion [13, 16]. The c-Met protein levels in hUC-MSCs of P3, P5, P8, and P10 generations were analyzed via Western

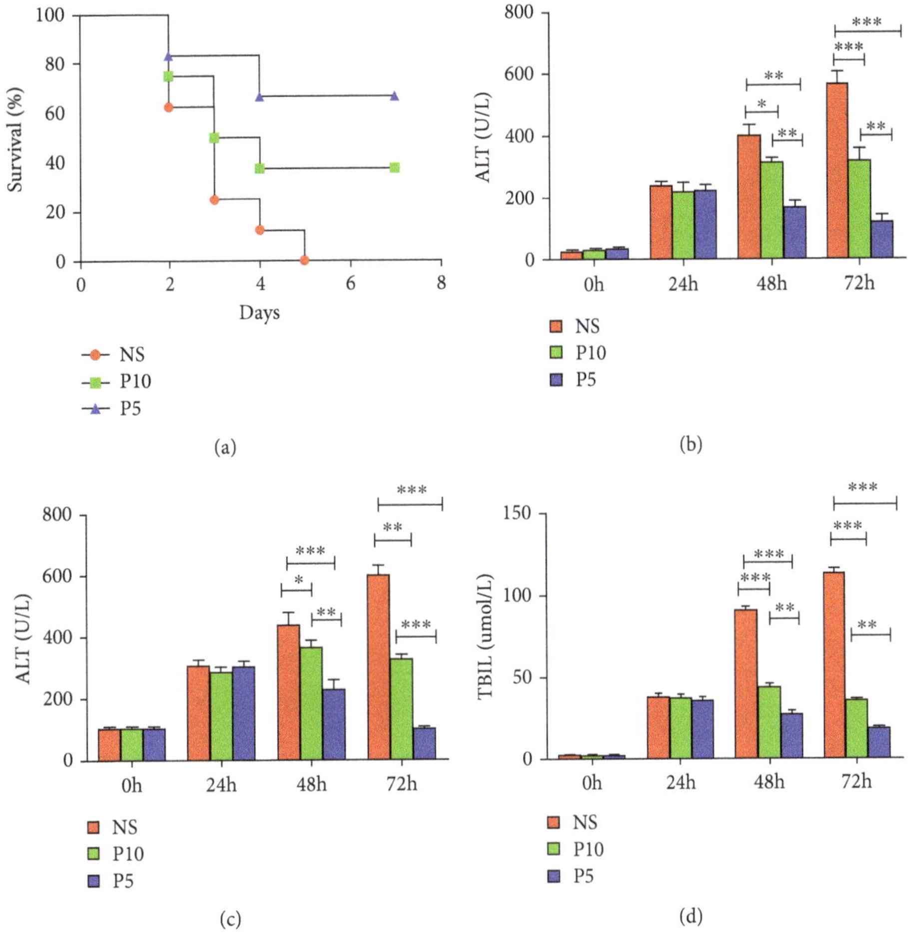

FIGURE 2: Effects of hUC-MSC transplantation on the survival rates and liver function in ALF rats. A total of 36 rats were randomly divided into three groups: P5 hUC-MSCs group, P10 hUC-MSCs group, and NS group ($n = 12$ per group). D-GalN/LPS were administered to rats intraperitoneally to induce ALF. 24 h later, the P5 hUC-MSCs and P10 hUC-MSCs (dose: 1.0×10^7 cells/kg/mL) were transplanted, respectively, while the NS group was given 1 mL normal saline. The blood samples were collected at 0 h, 24 h, 48 h, and 72 h post-D-GalN/LPS injection. (a) The survival rate in the P5 hUC-MSCs, P10 hUC-MSCs, and NS groups. Levels of serum (b) alanine transferase (ALT), (c) aspartate aminotransferase (AST), and (d) total bilirubin (TBil) in treatment of ALF rats. Data were expressed as mean ± SD. $^{*}P < 0.05$, $^{**}P < 0.01$, $^{***}P < 0.001$. hUC-MSCs, human umbilical cord-derived mesenchymal stem cells; D-GalN, D-galactosamine; LPS, lipopolysaccharide.

blotting. As the number of cell passages increased, the c-Met expression level of hUC-MSCs gradually decreased. There was a significant difference in the expression of c-Met between P5 and P8 hUC-MSCs, while c-Met expression in P10 hUC-MSCs could barely be measured (Figure 7). These results seem to be indicative of the better homing efficacy of the P5 hUC-MSCs, and the enhanced homing efficacy of the P5 hUC-MSC transplantation noticeably improves liver function.

4. Discussion

With the capacity of self-renewal and multipotency, MSCs have been increasingly used in tissue engineering and regenerative medicine [17]. BM-MSCs have been thoroughly characterized [18, 19]. However, their acquisition can be harmful, and their differentiation capability decreases with age [20].

In a previous study, UC-MSCs were successfully isolated and cultivated [21]. Due to the ease of accessibility, low immunogenicity, and higher differentiation capacity, hUC-MSCs have been investigated as an ideal clinical source of MSCs for cell therapy [21, 22]. The present study was conducted to validate the characteristics of hUC-MSCs. The cells formed a morphologically homogeneous population of fibroblast-like cells, when cultured in vitro. Flow cytometry indicated that the cells were positive for CD105, CD90, and CD44, but negative for CD34, CD31, and CD45. The results suggest that these cells have a mesenchymal origin, which is consistent with previous reports [23, 24]. During P5 hUC-MSC transplantation, the mortality of rats with ALF was effectively reduced by 62.5%, compared with the control. Furthermore, the serum levels of AST, ALT, and TBil were significantly decreased after treatment with P5 hUC-MSCs, which was superior to P10 hUC-MSC transplantation. Liver histopathology

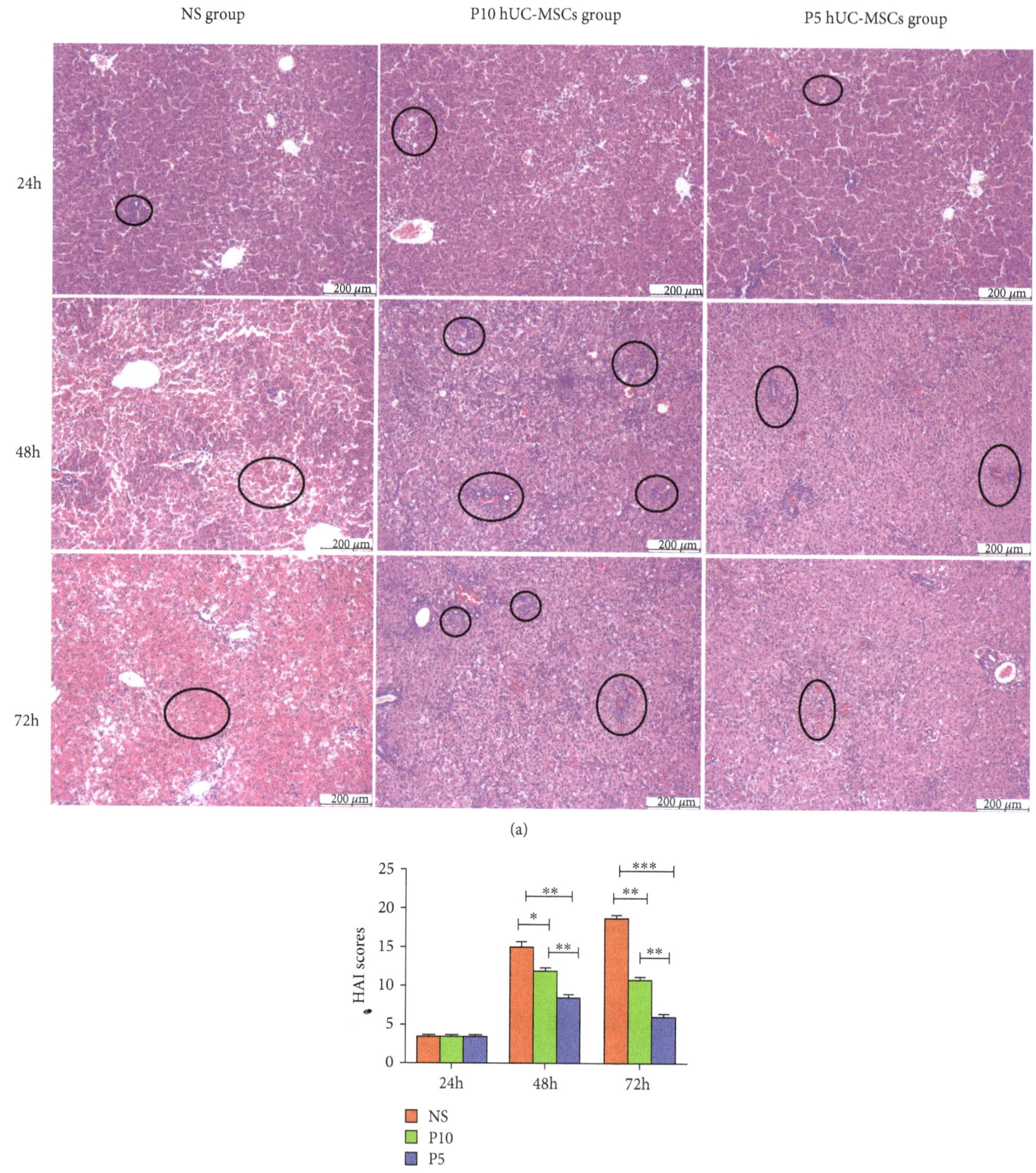

FIGURE 3: Histopathological recovery of D-GaIN/LPS-induced ALF transplanted with hUCMSCs at 24 h, 48 h, and 72 h. (a) H&E staining showed that there were massive necrosis and hepatic lobule damage in the NS group. In contrast, hepatocyte necrosis was suppressed in both P5 hUC-MSCs group and P10 hUC-MSCs group after transplantation. hUC-MSCs treatment also reduces the number of inflammatory infiltration. The black circles represent the hepatocyte necrosis and severe inflammatory cell infiltration. Bar = 200 μm. (b) Histopathological grading of necrosis and inflammation of the liver sections. Data are presented as mean ± SD. $^{*}P < 0.05$, $^{**}P < 0.01$, $^{***}P < 0.001$. D-GalN, D-galactosamine; HAI, hepatic activity index; IP, intraperitoneal; LPS, lipopolysaccharide; NS, normal saline.

and pathological scores were assessed to evaluate the effectiveness of hUC-MSC transplantation. Histological evaluation of the liver tissue after cell administration provided initial insights into the cellular targets of this therapy. The results suggest that hUC-MSCs may reconstitute liver tissue.

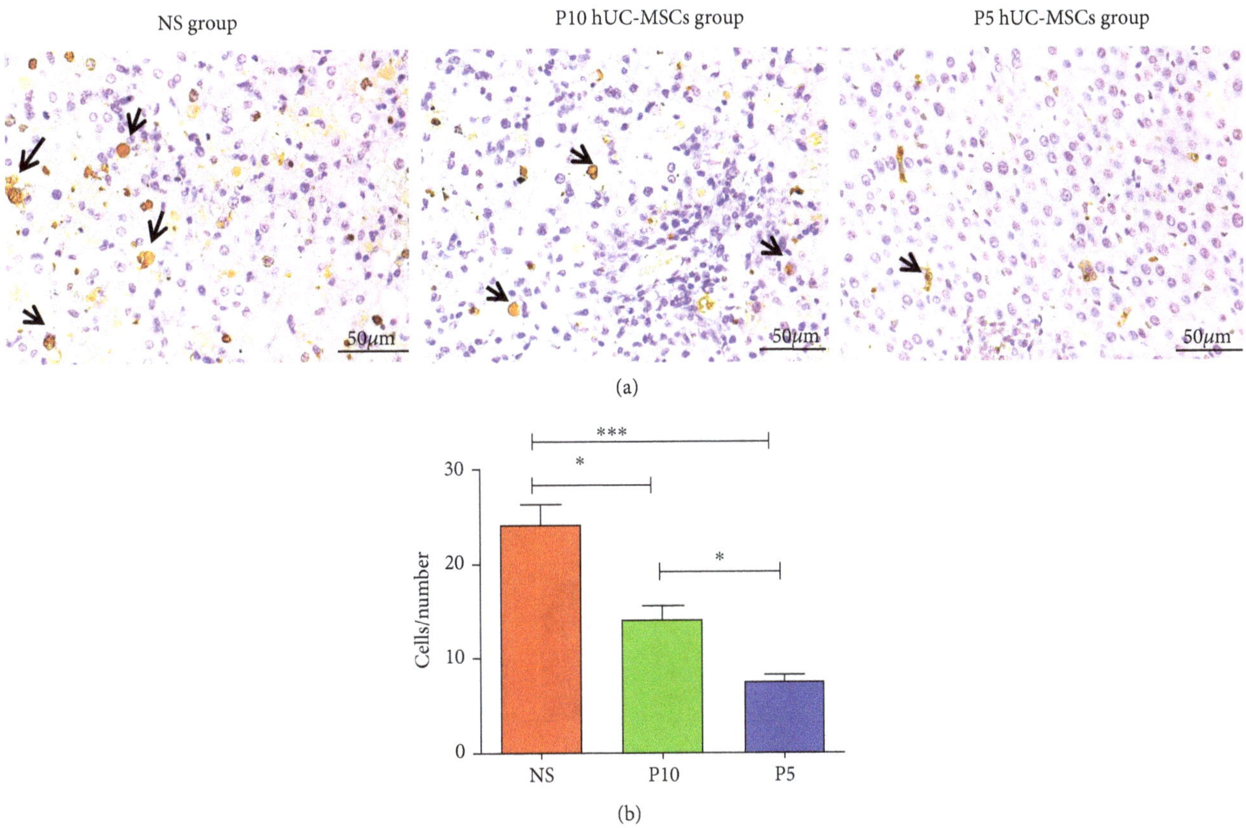

Figure 4: Infusion of hUC-MSCs decreases levels of apoptosis in livers D-GaIN/LPS-induced ALF. (a) Liver sections were stained by TUNEL (dark brown nuclei). Representative images from NS-treated, P10 hUC-MSC-treated, and P5 hUC-MSC-treated rats. Bar = 50 μm. (b) Quantification of TUNEL-positive hepatocyte-nuclei by digital image analysis. Data are reported as mean ± SD. $^{*}P < 0.05$, $^{***}P < 0.001$. TUNEL, terminal deoxynucleotidyl transferase-mediated nick-end labeling.

ALF is typically associated with progressive, massive hepatocellular necrosis [25]. Although UC-MSCs can differentiate into hepatocytes *in vivo*, the proportion of hepatocytes derived from hUC-MSCs was <1% of the total hepatocytes. The data suggested that the differentiated hepatocytes may not compensate for the recovery of liver function [26]. Stimulation of endogenous regeneration represents another potential mechanism of an MSC-based therapeutic effect, previously described in models of myocardial infarction [27]. Our results demonstrated that the delivery of hUC-MSCs can increase the number of proliferating hepatocytes. The P5 hUC-MSC therapy increased PCNA nearly twofold compared to the control group, while the P10 hUC-MSCs had a more moderate increase. Furthermore, inhibition of cell death is one therapeutic basis of MSC therapy that has been observed in models of myocardial infarction and stroke [28, 29]. In this study, we also provided evidence that the delivery of hUC-MSCs has the potential to reduce hepatocyte apoptosis. This correlated with observations in previous studies involving CCL4-induced liver injuries, where hUC-MSC therapy inhibited hepatocellular apoptosis and stimulated liver regeneration *in vivo* [30]. It is generally known that MSCs secrete trophic factors and cytokines, acting in a paracrine role as a mediator, involving antiapoptotic factors (HGF and insulin-like growth factor-1 (IGF-1)), angiogenetic factors (vascular endothelial growth factor (VEGF)), and mitogenetic factors (epidermal growth factor (EGF) and HGF) [31]. Recently, it has been recognized that MSCs release numerous extracellular vesicles (EVs) that participate in tissue regeneration via transferring information to damaged cells or tissue and exert biological activity similar to the MSCs [31]. Tan et al. showed that MSC-EVs increased hepatocyte regeneration by upregulating proteins associated with proliferation such as PCNA and cyclin D1 and the antiapoptosis gene Bcl-xL [32]. Moreover, Tamura et al. evaluated that MSC-EVs inhibited the secretion of proinflammatory cytokines and also increased the release of anti-inflammatory cytokines and the level of regulatory T cells [33]. In addition, MSC-EVs modulated the inflammatory response and activated antiapoptotic pathways via specific RNAs [34].

Most reports describe cell transplantation as the primary mode of MSC therapy, but the therapeutic effect of MSCs depends on the homing efficacy to the injured sites. HGF is the most effective mitogen in hepatocyte regeneration during tissue injury, and its biological effects rely on tyrosine kinase receptors and on c-Met. The HGF-c-Met axis played a crucial role in the homing of MSCs during liver injury [11].

Our primary experiment demonstrated that the highest concentration of HGF was observed in the liver at 24 h post-DGalN/LPS coinjection. Meanwhile, overexpressed c-

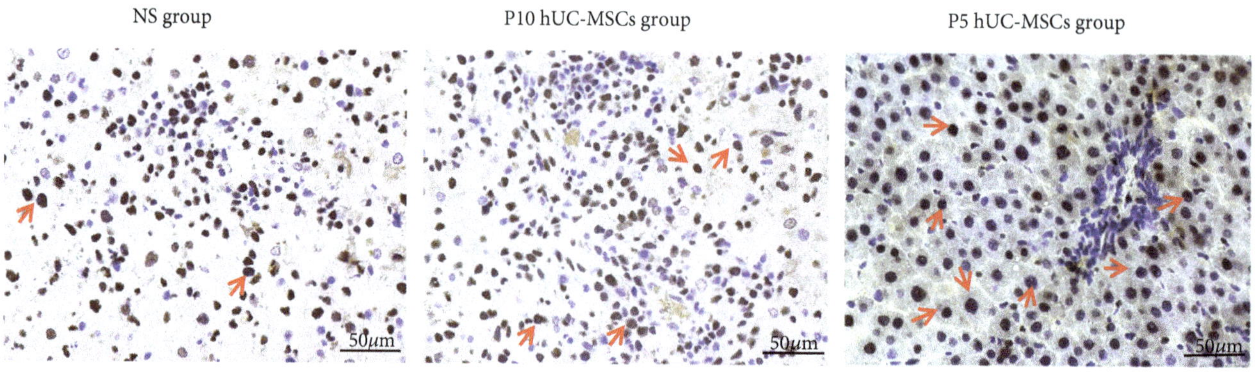

(a)

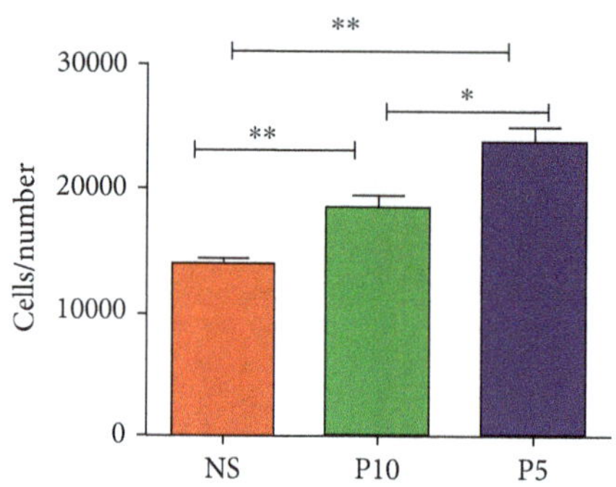

(b)

FIGURE 5: Infusion of hUC-MSCs enhances liver regeneration in livers D-GaIN/LPS-induced ALF at 48 h. (a) Liver sections were stained for PCNA (dark brown nuclei). Representative images from NS-treated, P10 hUC-MSC-treated, and P5hUC-MSC-treated rats. Bar = 50 μm. (b) Quantification of PCNA-positive hepatocyte-nuclei by Image-Pro Plus software. Data are reported as mean ± SD. $^{*}P < 0.05$, $^{**}P < 0.01$, $^{***}P < 0.001$. PCNA, proliferating cell nuclear antigen.

Met in BM-MSCs improved the homing efficacy to the injured liver [12].

In addition, during expansion, primary MSCs lose ligands or receptors that respond to migratory signals [13, 16]. Our results suggested that P5 hUC-MSCs migrate more efficiently to the injured liver, compared to P10 hUC-MSCs. In addition, our results showed that the c-Met expression was dependent on the cell passage number. Higher levels of c-Met may correlate with the better homing efficacy of P5 hUC-MSCs when compared to P10 hUC-MSCs. Despite higher c-Met expression in P3 hUC-MSCs, the limited number of P3 hUC-MSCs collected cannot achieve the required number for delivery. Even if the required number of MSCs for treatment could be achieved, the economic costs also need to be taken into account. As a result, P5 hUC-MSCs may be the ideal alternative for cell therapy. Furthermore, G. Wang and P. Wang demonstrated that hypoxia plays an important role in the increase of c-Met expression and the invasiveness of human prostatic carcinomas. Invasion of DU 145 cells (human prostate cells) in hypoxic conditions correlates with the expression level of c-Met [35]. Whether hypoxia promotes the c-Met expression in P5 hUC-MSCs needs to be further verified.

Migration within the injured tissues is influenced by multiple factors. Administration of the MSCs via the portal vein or hepatic artery shows homing efficacy less than 5% and 20–30%, respectively [36, 37]. Moreover, hypoxia induces the expression of leptin, which augments the recruitment of MSCs to the liver [38]. Meanwhile, more than 60 different microRNAs in MSCs have recently been described, and some of them are involved in migration, including let7, microRNA-10b, microRNA-27b, microRNA-335, and microRNA-886-3b [39]. Moreover, the loss of SH3, ICAM, and integrin-1 has been reported in the production of extracellular molecules accompanied with the culture of primary human MSCs [40].

5. Conclusions

Recent studies have detailed the potential benefit of hUC-MSC infusion for the treatment of ALF. The administration shows that systemic hUC-MSC therapy has profound inhibitory effects on hepatocellular apoptosis and stimulates liver regeneration for compensated liver function and also improves survival rates in rats with D-GalN/LPS-induced ALF. Furthermore, our results suggested that P5 hUC-MSCs migrate more efficiently to the injured liver, compared with P10 hUC-MSCs. The primary mechanism seems to be the regulation of homing molecules on MSCs during incubation *in vitro*, such as chemokine receptors or adhesion molecules, which has also been shown to affect the homing of HSCs [41, 42]. However, we can only presume that the rapid decrease in MSC homing efficiency *in vivo* is dependent on the level of c-Met.

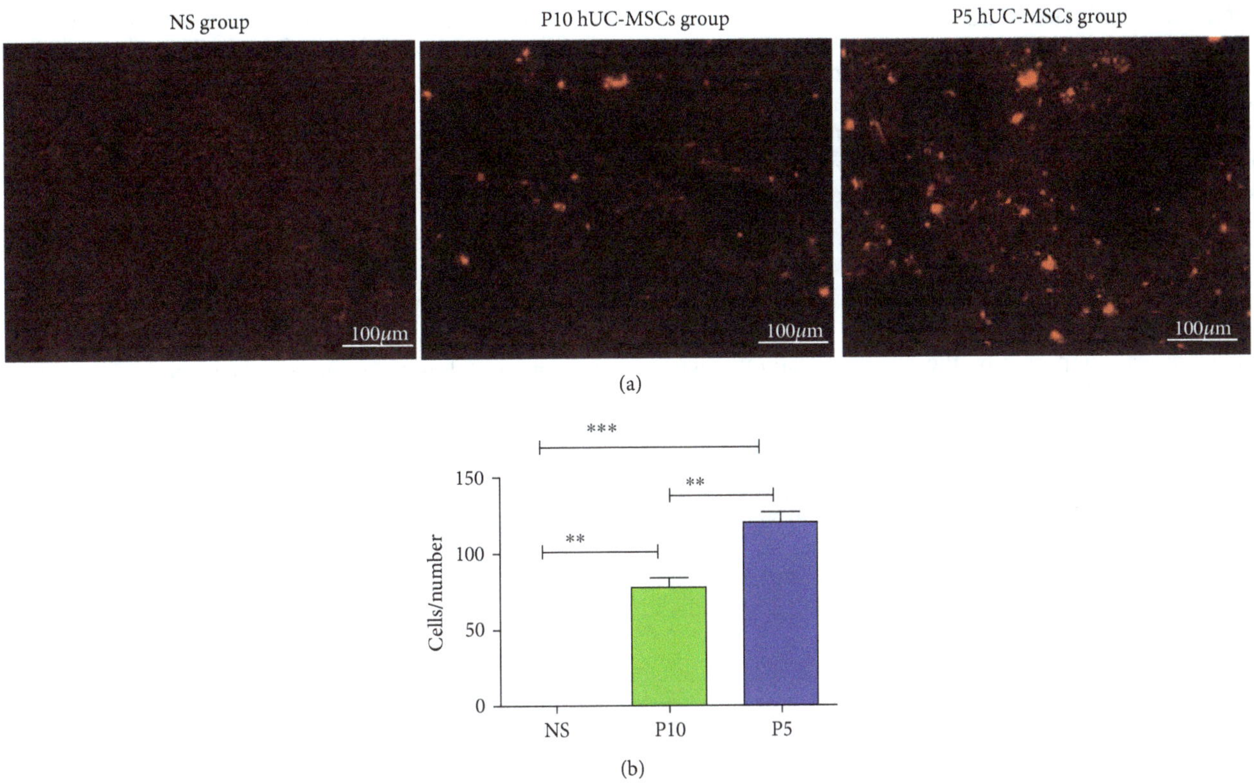

FIGURE 6: Infusion of CM-Dil-labeled hUC-MSCs enhances homing to livers D-GalN/LPS-induced ALF at 48 h. (a) Liver sections were observed by fluorescence microscope. Representative images from NS-treated, P10 hUC-MSC-treated, and P5 hUC-MSC-treated rats. Bar = 100 μm. (b) Quantification of the accumulated hUC-MSCs by Image-Pro Plus software. Data are reported as mean ± SD of the mean. $^{*}P < 0.05$, $^{**}P < 0.01$, $^{***}P < 0.001$.

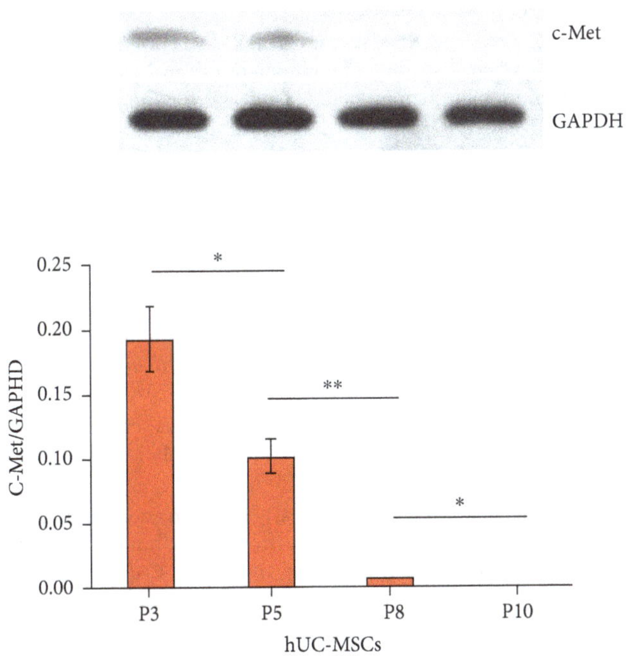

FIGURE 7: The protein levels of c-Met were analyzed by Western blotting in P3, P5, P8, and P10 hUC-MSCs. Data are presented as mean ± SD. $^{*}P < 0.05$, $^{**}P < 0.01$.

Thus, hUC-MSCs may be a potential alternative source for cell therapy of ALF and may additionally mitigate the shortage of hepatocytes.

Abbreviations

MSCs:	Mesenchymal stem cells
hUC-MSCs:	Human umbilical cord mesenchymal stem cells
ALF:	Acute liver failure
D-GalN:	D-galactosamine
HGF:	Hepatocyte growth factor
C-Met:	Cellular mesenchymal to epithelial transition factor
AST:	Aspartate aminotransferase
TBil:	Total bilirubin
ALT:	Alanine aminotransferase
EVs:	Extracellular vesicles
PCNA:	Proliferating cell nuclear antigen
TUNEL:	Terminal deoxynucleotidyl transferase-mediated nick-end labeling
IGF-1:	Insulin-like growth factor-1
VEGF:	Vascular endothelial growth factor
EGF:	Epidermal growth factor.

Authors' Contributions

YZ, YL, JL, and CZ conceived and designed the experiments. YZ, YL, WL, JC, LJ, and RX performed the experiments. MY and LZ conducted the statistical analysis. YZ and CZ drafted the manuscript. All authors read and approved the final manuscript. Yongting Zhang and Yuwen Li contributed equally to this article.

Acknowledgments

This work was supported by the National Natural Science Foundation of China (No. 81770591, No. 81800778), the Gilead Sciences Research Scholars Program in Liver Disease-Asia, the Key Medical Talents Fund of Jiangsu Province (ZDRCA2016007), the Medjaden Academy & Research Foundation for Young Scientists (MJR20160021), the Medical Innovation Team Project of Jiangsu Province (CXTDA2017023), and the Chinese National Thirteenth Five Years Project in Science and Technology (2017ZX10202201).

References

[1] Y. Cai, Z. Zou, L. Liu et al., "Bone marrow-derived mesenchymal stem cells inhibits hepatocyte apoptosis after acute liver injury," *International Journal of Clinical & Experimental Pathology*, vol. 8, no. 1, pp. 107–116, 2015.

[2] S. Basto, C. A. Villela-Nogueira, B. R. Tura et al., "Risk factors for long term mortality in a large cohort of waitlisted patients for liver transplantation in Brazil," *Liver Transplantation*, vol. 17, no. 9, pp. 1013–1020, 2011.

[3] S. J. Saunders, R. Hickman, R. Macdonald, and J. Terblanche, "The treatment of acute liver failure," *Progress in Liver Diseases*, vol. 4, pp. 333–344, 1972.

[4] P. Bianco, P. G. Robey, and P. J. Simmons, "Mesenchymal stem cells: revisiting history, concepts, and assays," *Cell Stem Cell*, vol. 2, no. 4, pp. 313–319, 2008.

[5] C. K. Rebelatto, A. M. Aguiar, M. P. Moretão et al., "Dissimilar differentiation of mesenchymal stem cells from bone marrow, umbilical cord blood, and adipose tissue," *Experimental Biology and Medicine*, vol. 233, no. 7, pp. 901–913, 2008.

[6] T. Schubert, D. Xhema, S. Vériter et al., "The enhanced performance of bone allografts using osteogenic differentiated adipose-derived mesenchymal stem cells," *Biomaterials*, vol. 32, no. 34, pp. 8880–8891, 2011.

[7] D. Baksh, R. Yao, and R. S. Tuan, "Comparison of proliferative and multilineage differentiation potential of human mesenchymal stem cells derived from umbilical cord and bone marrow," *Stem Cells*, vol. 25, no. 6, pp. 1384–1392, 2007.

[8] A. Gholamrezanezhad, S. Mirpour, M. Bagheri et al., "In vivo tracking of 111In-oxine labeled mesenchymal stem cells following infusion in patients with advanced cirrhosis," *Nuclear Medicine and Biology*, vol. 38, no. 7, pp. 961–967, 2011.

[9] L. Peng, D. Y. Xie, B. L. Lin et al., "Autologous bone marrow mesenchymal stem cell transplantation in liver failure patients caused by hepatitis B: short-term and long-term outcomes," *Hepatology*, vol. 54, no. 3, pp. 820–828, 2011.

[10] L. Trusolino, A. Bertotti, and P. M. Comoglio, "MET signalling: principles and functions in development, organ regeneration and cancer," *Nature Reviews. Molecular Cell Biology*, vol. 11, no. 12, pp. 834–848, 2010.

[11] J. Liu, G. Pan, T. Liang, and P. Huang, "HGF/c-Met signaling mediated mesenchymal stem cell-induced liver recovery in intestinal ischemia reperfusion model," *International Journal of Medical Sciences*, vol. 11, no. 6, pp. 626–633, 2014.

[12] K. Wang, Y. Li, T. Zhu et al., "Overexpression of c-Met in bone marrow mesenchymal stem cells improves their effectiveness in homing and repair of acute liver failure," *Stem Cell Research & Therapy*, vol. 8, no. 1, p. 162, 2017.

[13] S. S. Fatimah, G. C. Tan, K. Chua, M. M. N. Fariha, A. E. Tan, and A. R. Hayati, "Stemness and angiogenic gene expression changes of serial-passage human amnion mesenchymal cells," *Microvascular Research*, vol. 86, no. 3, pp. 21–29, 2013.

[14] S. Zheng, J. Yang, Y. Tang et al., "Effect of bone marrow mesenchymal stem cells transplantation on the serum and liver HMGB1 expression in rats with acute liver failure," *International Journal of Clinical and Experimental Pathology*, vol. 8, no. 12, pp. 15985–15992, 2015.

[15] N. D. Theise, "Liver biopsy assessment in chronic viral hepatitis: a personal, practical approach," *Modern Pathology*, vol. 20, pp. S3–S14, 2007.

[16] W. J. C. Rombouts and R. E. Ploemacher, "Primary murine MSC show highly efficient homing to the bone marrow but lose homing ability following culture," *Leukemia*, vol. 17, no. 1, pp. 160–170, 2003.

[17] A. Mobasheri, C. Csaki, A. L. Clutterbuck, M. Rahmanzadeh, and M. Shakibaei, "Mesenchymal stem cells in connective tissue engineering and regenerative medicine: applications in cartilage repair and osteoarthritis therapy," *Histology and histopathology*, vol. 24, no. 3, pp. 347–366, 2009.

[18] P. Charbord, "Bone marrow mesenchymal stem cells: historical overview and concepts," *Human Gene Therapy*, vol. 21, no. 9, pp. 1045–1056, 2010.

[19] O. K. Lee, T. K. Kuo, W. M. Chen, K. D. Lee, S. L. Hsieh, and T. H. Chen, "Isolation of multipotent mesenchymal stem cells from umbilical cord blood," *Blood*, vol. 103, no. 5, pp. 1669–1675, 2004.

[20] K. Stenderup, J. Justesen, C. Clausen, and M. Kassem, "Aging is associated with decreased maximal life span and accelerated senescence of bone marrow stromal cells," *Bone*, vol. 33, no. 6, pp. 919–926, 2003.

[21] X. Li, J. Bai, X. Ji, R. Li, Y. Xuan, and Y. Wang, "Comprehensive characterization of four different populations of human mesenchymal stem cells as regards their immune properties, proliferation and differentiation," *International Journal of Molecular Medicine*, vol. 34, no. 3, pp. 695–704, 2014.

[22] H. S. Wang, S. C. Hung, S. T. Peng et al., "Mesenchymal stem cells in the Wharton's jelly of the human umbilical cord," *Stem Cells*, vol. 22, no. 7, pp. 1330–1337, 2004.

[23] H. Zhang, B. Zhang, Y. Tao et al., "Isolation and characterization of mesenchymal stem cells from whole human umbilical cord applying a single enzyme approach," *Cell Biochemistry and Function*, vol. 30, no. 8, pp. 643–649, 2012.

[24] A. K. Batsali, M.-C. Kastrinaki, H. A. Papadaki, and C. Pontikoglou, "Mesenchymal stem cells derived from Wharton's jelly of the umbilical cord: biological properties and emerging clinical applications," *Current Stem Cell Research & Therapy*, vol. 8, no. 2, pp. 144–155, 2013.

[25] W. Bernal, G. Auzinger, A. Dhawan, and J. Wendon, "Acute

liver failure," *Lancet*, vol. 376, no. 9736, pp. 190–201, 2010.

[26] S. Zhang, L. Chen, T. Liu et al., "Human umbilical cord matrix stem cells efficiently rescue acute liver failure through paracrine effects rather than hepatic differentiation," *Tissue Engineering Part A*, vol. 18, no. 13-14, pp. 1352–1364, 2012.

[27] K. E. Hatzistergos, H. Quevedo, B. N. Oskouei et al., "Bone marrow mesenchymal stem cells stimulate cardiac stem cell proliferation and differentiation," *Circulation Research*, vol. 107, no. 7, pp. 913–922, 2010.

[28] M. Gnecchi, H. He, O. D. Liang et al., "Paracrine action accounts for marked protection of ischemic heart by Akt-modified mesenchymal stem cells," *Nature Medicine*, vol. 11, no. 4, pp. 367-368, 2005.

[29] Y. Li, J. Chen, X. G. Chen et al., "Human marrow stromal cell therapy for stroke in rat: neurotrophins and functional recovery," *Neurology*, vol. 59, no. 4, pp. 514–523, 2002.

[30] Y. Yan, W. Xu, H. Qian et al., "Mesenchymal stem cells from human umbilical cords ameliorate mouse hepatic injury in vivo," *Liver International*, vol. 29, no. 3, pp. 356–365, 2009.

[31] A. I. Caplan and J. E. Dennis, "Mesenchymal stem cells as trophic mediators," *Journal of Cellular Biochemistry*, vol. 98, no. 5, pp. 1076–1084, 2006.

[32] C. Y. Tan, R. C. Lai, W. Wong, Y. Y. Dan, S.-K. Lim, and H. K. Ho, "Mesenchymal stem cell-derived exosomes promote hepatic regeneration in drug-induced liver injury models," *Stem Cell Research & Therapy*, vol. 5, no. 3, p. 76, 2014.

[33] R. Tamura, S. Uemoto, and Y. Tabata, "Immunosuppressive effect of mesenchymal stem cell-derived exosomes on a concanavalin A-induced liver injury model," *Inflammation and Regeneration*, vol. 36, no. 1, p. 26, 2016.

[34] H. Haga, I. K. Yan, K. Takahashi, A. Matsuda, and T. Patel, "Extracellular vesicles from bone marrow-derived mesenchymal stem cells improve survival from lethal hepatic failure in mice," *Stem Cells Translational Medicine*, vol. 6, no. 4, pp. 1262–1272, 2017.

[35] G. Wang and P. Wang, "Effects of hypoxia on the expression of c-met and in vasiveness of DU145 prostatic carcinoma cell line," *Chinese Journal of Cancer Prevention and Treatment*, vol. 18, no. 6, pp. 416–419, 2011.

[36] J. Puppi, S. C. Strom, R. D. Hughes et al., "Improving the techniques for human hepatocyte transplantation: report from a consensus meeting in London," *Cell Transplantation*, vol. 21, no. 1, pp. 1–10, 2012.

[37] A. A. Khan, M. V. Shaik, N. Parveen et al., "Human fetal liver-derived stem cell transplantation as supportive modality in the management of end-stage decompensated liver cirrhosis," *Cell Transplantation*, vol. 19, no. 4, pp. 409–418, 2010.

[38] X. Hu, R. Wu, Z. Jiang et al., "Leptin signaling is required for augmented therapeutic properties of mesenchymal stem cells conferred by hypoxia preconditioning," *Stem Cells*, vol. 32, no. 10, pp. 2702–2713, 2014.

[39] E. A. Clark, S. Kalomoiris, J. A. Nolta, and F. A. Fierro, "Concise review: microRNA function in multipotent mesenchymal stromal cells," *Stem Cells*, vol. 32, no. 5, pp. 1074–1082, 2014.

[40] P. A. Conget and J. J. Minguell, "Phenotypical and functional properties of human bone marrow mesenchymal progenitor cells," *Journal of Cellular Physiology*, vol. 181, no. 1, pp. 67–73, 1999.

[41] V. M. Berrios, G. J. Dooner, G. Nowakowski et al., "The molecular basis for the cytokine induced defect in homing and engraftment of hematopoietic stem cells," *Experimental Hematology*, vol. 29, no. 11, pp. 1326–1335, 2001.

[42] M. Ramirez, J. C. Segovia, I. Benet et al., "Ex vivo expansion of umbilical cord blood (UCB) CD34(+) cells alters the expression and function of alpha 4 beta 1 and alpha 5 beta 1 integrins," *British Journal of Haematology*, vol. 115, no. 1, pp. 213–221, 2001.

10

Tendon-Derived Stem Cell Differentiation in the Degenerative Tendon Microenvironment

Chang Liu,[1,2] Jing-wan Luo,[1] Ke-ke Zhang,[1] Long-xiang Lin,[1] Ting Liang,[3] Zong-ping Luo,[3] Yong-qing Zhuang,[4] and Yu-long Sun[1]

[1]*Center for Translational Medicine Research and Development, Shenzhen Institute of Advanced Technology, Chinese Academy of Sciences, Shenzhen 518000, China*
[2]*Central Laboratory, Dalian Municipal Central Hospital, Dalian 116033, China*
[3]*Institute of Orthopaedics, Soochow University, Suzhou 215007, China*
[4]*Shenzhen People's Hospital, Shenzhen, Guangdong, China*

Correspondence should be addressed to Yu-long Sun; sunyulong@yahoo.com

Academic Editor: Stan Gronthos

Tendinopathy is prevalent in athletic and many occupational populations; nevertheless, the pathogenesis of tendinopathy remains unclear. Tendon-derived stem cells (TDSCs) were regarded as the key culprit for the development of tendinopathy. However, it is uncertain how TDSCs differentiate into adipocytes, chondrocytes, or osteocytes in the degenerative microenvironment of tendinopathy. So in this study, the regulating effects of the degenerative tendon microenvironment on differentiation of TDSCs were investigated. TDSCs were isolated from rat Achilles tendons and were grown on normal and degenerative (prepared by stress-deprived culture) decellularized tendon slices (DTSs). Immunofluorescence staining, H&E staining, real-time PCR, and Western blot were used to delineate the morphology, proliferation, and differentiation of TDSCs in the degenerative microenvironment. It was found that TDSCs were much more spread on the degenerative DTSs than those on normal DTSs. The tenocyte-related markers, COL1 and TNMD, were highly expressed on normal DTSs than the degenerative DTSs. The expression of chondrogenic and osteogenic markers, COL2, SOX9, Runx2, and ALP, was higher on the degenerative DTSs compared with TDSCs on normal DTSs. Furthermore, phosphorylated FAK and ERK1/2 were reduced on degenerative DTSs. In conclusion, this study found that the degenerative tendon microenvironment induced TDSCs to differentiate into chondrogenic and osteogenic lineages. It could be attributed to the cell morphology changes and reduced FAK and ERK1/2 activation in the degenerative microenvironment of tendinopathy.

1. Introduction

Tendinopathy is common in athletes and people in many occupations involving repetitive work. It is associated with focal tendon tenderness, activity-related pain, and decrease of strength and movement in the affected position. The pathogenesis of tendinopathy remains elusive. There still is a big challenge to prevent tendinopathy and to develop effective treatment for it [1].

Kannus and Jozsa analyzed the histological changes in tendon tissue of 891 tendinopathy patients in 1991 [2]. It was found that over 97 percent of injured tendon tissues had degenerative changes including tendolipomatosis, proteoglycan accumulation, and calcifying tendinopathy, which implied the presence of adipocytes, chondrocytes, or even osteocytes in tendinopathy. However, it was unclear where these nontendinous cells came from. Tendon-derived stem cells (TDSCs) were discovered in tendon tissues in 2007 [3]. Similar to other multipotent stem cells, TDSCs were positive for stem cell-related surface markers such as CD44, CD90, and CD146 and negative for CD34, CD45, and CD106 [3]. They were able to self-renew and had adipogenic, chondrogenic, and osteogenic differentiation potentials. Therefore, the adipocytes, chondrocytes, and osteocytes in tendinopathy were considered to be differentiated from TDSCs [4, 5]. TDSCs could be the culprit for degenerative tendinopathy by undergoing aberrant nontenocyte differentiation into fatty-like, cartilage-like, and bone-like tissues in tendons that compromise tendon structures [6, 7].

Repetitive mechanical loading has generally been considered to be the etiology of tendinopathy [8]. In vivo and in vitro studies performed by Zhang and Wang confirmed that TDSCs differentiated into adipocytes, chondrocytes, and osteocytes when large mechanical stretching was applied [9]. It was found that the microenvironment, where stem cells reside in, regulates the differentiation of stem cells [10, 11]. Nevertheless, nontenocyte differentiation of TDSCs into adipocytes, chondrocytes, and osteocytes in the degenerative microenvironment within tendinopathy has remained unrevealed. Therefore, this study investigated the effects of degenerative tendon microenvironment on the differentiation of TDSCs in vitro to further clarify how TDSCs played their roles in the development of tendinopathy.

Recent discoveries confirmed that complete removal of external stress, also known as stress deprivation, could lead to the degeneration of tendons as well [12–14]. Clinical observations from bedridden patients to astronauts all support this point of view [15]. In addition, when microinjuries in the tendon result from repetitive loading, the unloaded portion of the tendon was stress deprived [16]. And it has been hypothesized that the subsequent stress deprivation conditions resulted from the preconditioned overload are responsible for the development of tendinopathy [16, 17]. Thus, stress deprivation is a relevant model, which simulates some effects of clinical tendinopathy.

In recent years, an extracellular matrix (ECM) from decellularized tendons was isolated, which harbors the biochemical cues of tissue microenvironment including growth factors, proteins, glycosylaminoglycans, and proteoglycans. Besides, they maintain the native ultrastructure and mechanical strength of the tendon tissue to the greatest extent, which provide ideal scaffolds for in vitro study [9, 18, 19].

2. Materials and Methods

2.1. Isolation of Tendon-Derived Stem Cells (TDSCs). Approval was obtained from the Institutional Animal Care and Use Committee of Shenzhen Institutes of Advanced Technology, Chinese Academy of Sciences, prior to performing the study. Achilles tendons were harvested from Sprague-Dawley rats (4–6 weeks, male, 160–180 g) (Vital River Laboratory Animal Technology Co., Beijing, China). After the tendon sheaths were removed, the core portions were minced into small pieces. Then the pieces were digested with 4 mg/ml dispase (Sigma-Aldrich, St. Louis, MO, USA) and 3 mg/ml collagenase I (Sigma-Aldrich, St. Louis, MO, USA) in phosphate-buffered saline (PBS) (HyClone, Logan, Utah, USA) solution for 3 hours at 37°C. After adding Dulbecco's Modified Eagle's Medium (DMEM) (HyClone, Logan, Utah, USA) supplemented with 10% FBS (Thermo Fisher Scientific, Pittsburgh, PA, USA), cell suspension was centrifuged at 300*g* for 15 minutes to obtain cell pellets. After cell counting, the cells were inoculated in a 25 cm^2 culture flask with the density of 500 cells/cm^2 in DMEM supplement with 10% FBS, 100 U/ml penicillin (HyClone, Logan, Utah, USA), and 100 mg/ml streptomycin (HyClone, Logan, Utah, USA). Approximately 10 days later, TDSC colonies were formed and were isolated by local digestion with 0.25% trypsin (HyClone, Logan, Utah, USA).

2.2. Fluorescence-Activated Cell Sorting (FACS) Analysis. To verify the stemness of the cells, TDSCs at passage 2 were incubated with FITC-CD44 (1 : 1000) (BioLegend, San Diego, CA, USA), FITC-CD90 (1 : 8000) (BioLegend), FITC-CD45 (1 : 1000) (BioLegend), and PE-CD106 (1 : 1000) (BioLegend) in the dark at 4°C for 20 minutes. After being washed three times with PBS, TDSCs were analyzed by a BD FACSCanto II flow cytometer (BD Biosciences, San Jose, CA, USA).

2.3. Multidifferentiation Potential of TDSCs. TDSCs were inoculated in a six-well plate with 500 cells/cm^2 density, and adipogenic, chondrogenic, and osteogenic induction media (Thermo Scientific, Pittsburgh, PA, USA) were added. The media were changed every other day. Two weeks later, TDSCs were fixed with 4% paraformaldehyde (Sigma-Aldrich, St. Louis, MO, USA) at room temperature for 15 minutes. After being washed with deionized water, cells were stained with Oil Red O (Solarbio Life Science, Beijing, China), Safranin O (Solarbio life science), and Alizarin Red S (Solarbio Life Science). The stained cells were verified by inverted light microscope (CKX41, Olympus, Tokyo, Japan).

2.4. Stress-Deprived Tendon Model Construction. Rat Achilles tendons were harvested and maintained under stress-deprived conditions, based on a previously reported study with some modifications [13]. In brief, the fresh Achilles tendons were cultured in DMEM supplemented with 10% FBS, 100 U/ml penicillin, and 100 mg/ml streptomycin and incubated at 37°C in a humidified atmosphere of 5% CO_2 in air for up to 4 weeks. The medium was changed every other day. The stress-deprived tendons were collected as degenerative tendons hereafter in this study.

2.5. Live/Dead Staining. Normal and degenerative tendons were stained with live/dead staining working solution (Life Technologies, Pittsburgh, PA, USA) composed of 2 μM calcein AM and 4 μM ethidium homodimer-1 at 37°C for 0.5 h. After being washed with PBS, the cells within the depth of 70 μm of the tissue surface were observed using confocal laser scanning microscopy (LSM 880, Zeiss, Oberkochen, Germany).

2.6. H&E Staining. Normal and degenerative tendons were fixed with 4% paraformaldehyde, dehydrated with 30% sucrose and embedded with OCT (Sakura Finetek, Torrance, CA, USA), and frozen at −80°C before section. Cryosections were cut at 5 μm thickness and stained with hematoxylin and eosin (Sakura Finetek, Torrance, CA, USA) to observe cell morphology and cell number. Histological samples were imaged using an upright microscope (BX53, Olympus, Tokyo, Japan).

2.7. Preparation of Decellularized Tendon Slices (DTSs). DTSs were prepared according to the published protocols with some modifications [18]. In brief, normal and degenerative tendon tissues were embedded with OCT, frozen at −80°C, fixed to the cutting base plate of a cryostat (CM1950, Leica, Nussloch, Germany), and longitudinally cut into slices with a thickness of 100 μm. After removing the OCT by washing with PBS 3 times for 30 minutes, tendon slices were frozen in liquid nitrogen for 2 minutes and thawed in normal saline for 10 minutes at 37°C for 5 cycles. Then the tendon slices were incubated in 200 μg/ml RNase and 400 μg/ml DNase (Sigma-Aldrich, St. Louis, MO, USA) for 4 hours at 37°C, followed by washing with PBS at room temperature with gentle agitation. Finally, each side of the DTSs was sterilized with UV radiation for 2 hours for further usage.

2.8. DNA Staining and Extraction. Normal and degenerative DTSs were incubated with DAPI at room temperature for 15 minutes, followed by washing with PBS 3 times. The cell nucleus was observed by an inverted fluorescence microscope (Eclipse, Nikon, Tokyo, Japan). Total DNA of normal and degenerative DTSs was extracted by TIANamp Genomic DNA Kit (TIANGEN Biotech Co., Beijing, China) following the manufacturer's instructions. DNA content was measured with an ultraviolet spectrophotometer (NanoDrop 2000, Thermo Fisher Scientific, Pittsburgh, PA, USA).

2.9. Elastic Modulus of Normal and Degenerative DTSs. The elastic modulus of normal and degenerative DTSs was measured by atomic force microscope (AFM) (Dimension ICON, Bruker, Billerica, Massachusetts, USA). Oxide-sharpened, square-based pyramidal silicon-nitride tips with a borosilicate glass sphere at a radius of 5 μm glued onto the V-shaped silicon-nitride cantilevers with a nominal spring constant of 0.06 N/m were employed. Cyclic load-displacement curves were recorded at 6 different sites on the sample surface. In all cases, the DTSs were immersed into pH 7.4 PBS solution.

2.10. Cell Viability Analysis. Cell viability was detected using a Cell Counting Kit-8 (CCK8) assay (Dojindo Laboratories, Kumamoto, Japan), according to the manufacturer's instructions. Briefly, TDSCs were inoculated on normal and degenerative DTSs with a density of 1000 cells/cm^2. At selected time points, TDSCs were incubated with DMEM plus 10% (v/v) CCK8 at 37°C for 2 h, then 200 μl supernatant was used to measure the absorbance. The absorbance at 450 nm with a reference wavelength of 630 nm was recorded using a microplate reader (FC, Thermo Fisher Scientific, Pittsburgh, PA, USA).

2.11. F-Actin Staining. TDSCs on normal and degenerative DTSs were fixed with 4% paraformaldehyde at room temperature for 15 minutes, followed by washing with PBS 3 times, then treated with PBS containing 0.1% Tween-20 (Sigma) and 1% goat serum (Thermo) for 15 minutes, and washed with PBS 3 times. Finally, the TDSs were incubated with Flash Phalloidin Green 488 (1 : 20) (BioLegend) and DAPI (Sigma) at 4°C in the dark for 30 minutes. Photos were taken by an inverted fluorescence microscope (Eclipse, Nikon).

2.12. Quantitative Real-Time Reverse Transcription-Polymerase Chain Reaction. Total RNA was isolated using an RNA purification kit (Corning, New York, USA) according to the manufacturer's instructions. Reverse transcription (RT) was performed using a PrimeScript RT Reagent Kit (TaKaRa, Shiga, Japan). Real-time polymerase chain reaction (PCR) was carried out with SYBR Premix Ex Taq (Perfect Real Time) (Takara). PCR amplification and fluorescence detection were performed using a LightCycler® 96 System (Roche, Basel, Switzerland). The primers used in this study were listed in Table S. GAPDH was used as an internal control. The results were presented as the calculated comparative expression ratios of the target sample to control group for each sample using the C_T method ($2^{-\Delta\Delta C_T}$).

2.13. Western Blot. TDSCs were lysed in lysis buffer containing protease and phosphatase inhibitors (Keygentec, Nanjing, China). Protein concentration was quantified by BCA kit (Keygentec), and an equal amount of protein was loaded in each lane. Constant voltage electrophoresis was carried out with 10% polyacrylamide gels. Then the proteins were transferred to polyvinylidene fluoride (PVDF) membranes (Merck, Massachusetts, USA). PVDF membranes were blocked with 3% BSA (Sigma) and hybridized with ERK1/2 (Santa Cruz Biotechnology, Dallas, TX, USA), phospho-ERK1/2 (Thr202/Tyr204) (Santa Cruz Biotechnology), FAK (Santa Cruz Biotechnology), phospho-FAK (Tyr397) (Santa Cruz Biotechnology), and β-actin (Santa Cruz Biotechnology) primary antibodies overnight at 4°C. After being washed with TBST (Keygentec), the PVDF membranes were incubated with secondary antibodies (ZSGB-bio, Beijing, China) at room temperature for 30 minutes, followed by washing with TBST. Finally, the PVDF membranes were covered with 3,3-diaminobenzidine (DAB) for the display of specific protein bands.

2.14. Statistical Analysis. All individual experiments were performed at least three times, with three replicates. Data were expressed as means ± standard deviation (SD). The significance of differences between two groups were determined using unpaired Student's t-tests. Differences among more than two experimental groups were evaluated by one-way ANOVA. Differences were considered significant at $P < 0.05$.

3. Results

3.1. Characterization of TDSCs. TDSCs, from rat Achilles tendon, showed cobblestone-shaped morphology (Figure 1(a)) and had clone-forming ability (Figure 1(b)). In addition, the flow cytometric analysis showed that 95.3% of cells were positive for CD44 (Figure 1(c)) and 99.6% of cells were positive for CD90 (Figure 1(d)), which are stem cell-related markers. In addition, TDSCs were negative for leukemia cell marker CD45 and endothelial cell marker CD106 (Figures 1(e) and 1(f)). Furthermore, the multilineage differentiation assay confirmed that TDSCs were able to differentiate into adipocytes, chondrocytes, and osteocytes,

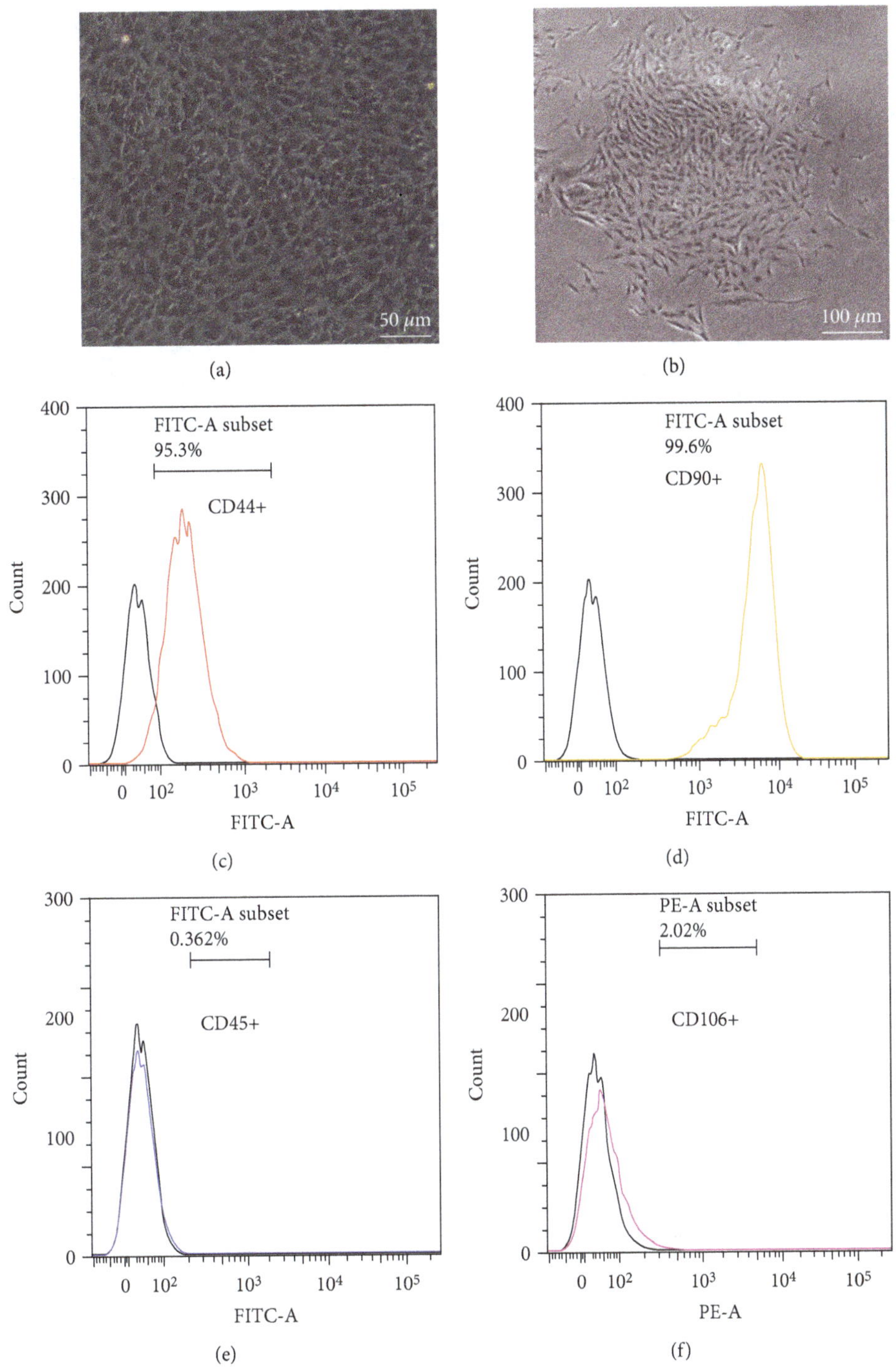

FIGURE 1: The morphology and stemness characteristics of TDSCs: (a) morphology and (b) colon-formation ability of TDSCs and flow cytometric analysis of (c) CD44, (d) CD90, (e) CD45, and (f) CD106 expression of TDSCs.

which were demonstrated by Oil Red O (Figures 2(a) and 2(b)), Safranin O (Figures 2(c) and 2(d)), and Alizarin Red S (Figures 2(e) and 2(f)) staining, respectively, after induction.

3.2. Degenerative Tendon Construction. The degenerative tendon was produced by stress-deprived culture of rat Achilles tendons ex vivo for 4 weeks. Live/dead staining showed that almost all cells have good viability within a fresh tendon (Figure 3(a)); however, a large number of cells in the stress-deprived tendon died (Figure 3(b)). H&E staining confirmed that tendon cells had elongated morphology in the normal tendon (Figures 3(c) and 3(d)). While in the degenerative tendon, more rounded cells, a loose collagen structure, and increased gaps between the collagen fibers were observed (Figures 3(e) and 3(f)). In addition, the number of cells decreased significantly in the degenerative tendon compared with the normal tendon (Figures 3(e) and 3(f)). Higher

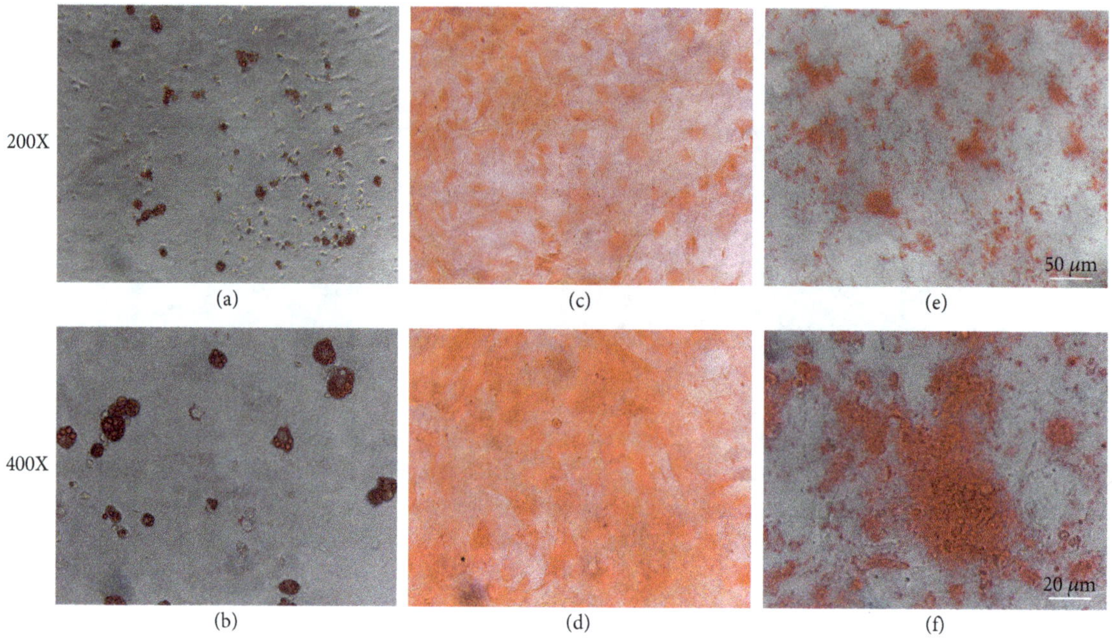

Figure 2: Multidifferentiation potential of TDSCs: (a-b) Oil Red O staining, (c-d) Safranin O staining, and (e-f) Alizarin Red S staining.

expressions of matrix metalloproteinase (MMP), such as MMP 1 and MMP 2, were found in the tendinopathic tendons. MMP 1 is one of the collagenases with proteolytic activity in type I collagen, the most abundant collagen in tendons. This study found that TDSCs on the degenerative tendon tissues expressed significantly higher levels of MMP 1 and MMP 2 compared to those on normal tendons. It suggested the degradation of type I collagen in the degenerative tendon (Figure 3(g)). The above results indicated the degeneration occurred in the Achilles tendon under stress-deprived culture.

3.3. Preparation of Decellularized Tendon Slices (DTSs). A repetitive freeze/thaw procedure with nuclease treatment on normal and degenerative tendon tissues was applied to remove the resident cells and to produce extracellular matrix scaffolds of normal and degenerative tendons. After decellularization, the number of cells in normal (Figures 4(a) and 4(b)) and degenerative (Figures 4(c) and 4(d)) tendons deceased significantly. Furthermore, DNA content in normal and degenerative tendons were significantly lower after decellularization (Figure 4(e)).

3.4. Matrix Stiffness of Normal and Degenerative DTSs. The compressive elastic modulus can be used to represent the matrix stiffness of tendon tissue. The matrix stiffness of degenerative DTS was 20.98 ± 9.57 kPa, significantly lower than that of normal DTS (36.79 ± 7.39 kPa) (Figure 4(f)), which indicated that the degeneration was associated with the lower stiffness of tendon microenvironment.

3.5. Cell Viability and Proliferation of TDSCs. During the culture period of 14 days, TDSCs were well attached to the surfaces and maintained good viability on normal (Figures 5(a)–5(c)) and degenerative (Figures 5(d)–5(f)) DTSs. From the 7th day, TDSCs started to show elongated spindle morphology and were aligned along the direction of collagen fibers on normal DTSs (Figures 5(b) and 5(c)). However, the shape of TDSCs on degenerative DTSs was more spread out (Figures 5(e) and 5(f)). Similar to the microscopic observation, the CCK8 assay revealed that during the culture period of 14 days, the viability of TDSCs on normal and degenerative DTSs was significantly increased (Figure 5(g)). The proliferation of TDSCs had the same trend on normal and degenerative DTSs. However, TDSCs on normal DTSs showed higher viability since day 7, and the difference was significant on day 10 (Figure 5(g)).

3.6. F-Actin Fiber Formation and Distribution. F-actin staining was performed to investigate the alteration of TDSC cytoskeleton organization between normal and degenerative DTSs. TDSCs were aligned, with disorganized actin filaments on normal DTSs (Figures 6(a)–6(f)). However, TDSCs adopted polygonal shapes with bundled actin fibers on degenerative DTSs (Figures 6(g)–6(l)).

3.7. TDSC Differentiation on DTSs. In order to understand the effects of degenerative tendon microenvironment on the differentiation of TDSCs, the expressions of tenogenic, chondrogenic, and osteogenic markers were detected. Tenocyte markers, COL1, SCX, and TNMD, were highly expressed on normal DTSs than on degenerative DTSs, especially COL1 and TNMD (Figure 7). On the contrary, chondrogenic markers COL2 and SOX9 and osteogenic markers Runx2 and ALP were expressed at higher levels on degenerative DTSs than normal DTSs (Figure 7). The results indicated that a normal tendon matrix tended to induce the differentiation of TDSCs into tenocytes. However, TDSCs in the degenerative microenvironment had a tendency to differentiate into chondrocytes and osteocytes.

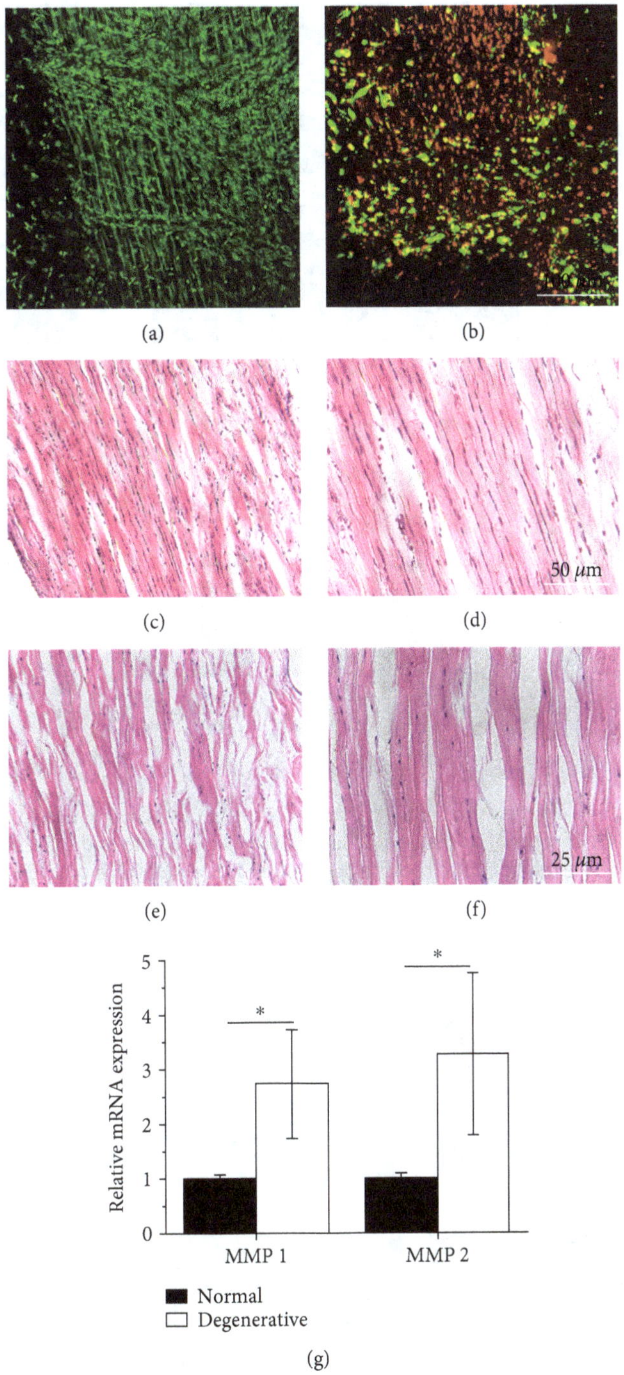

FIGURE 3: Live/dead, H&E staining, and MMP expressions of normal and degenerative tendons. Live/dead staining of (a) normal and (b) degenerative tissues. H&E staining of (c-d) normal and (e-f) degenerative tendons. (g) Comparison of expressions of MMP 1 and MMP 2 in normal and degenerative tendons ($n = 8$). $^*P < 0.05$, compared with normal tendons.

3.8. Expression of Integrin β1, FAK, and ERK. The expression of FAK and ERK1/2 was evaluated both at gene and protein levels. It was found that the expression of integrin β1, FAK, and ERK at the mRNA level was lower on degenerative DTSs than on normal ones, and the differences of integrin β1 and FAK were significant (Figure 8(a)). In addition, phosphorylated FAK on Tyr397 and phosphorylated ERK1/2 on Thr202 and Tyr204 were significantly decreased on degenerative DTSs than on normal DTSs (Figure 8(b)).

4. Discussion

It was hypothesized that the erroneous differentiation of TDSCs to chondrocytes or osteoblasts leads to chondrometaplasia and ossification in tendinopathy [20]. However, it is unclear what factors induce TDSCs to differentiate into the tenogenic, adipogenic, chondrogenic, and osteogenic phenotypes. In this study, an in vitro degenerative tendon model, which was constructed by stress deprivation, was used to

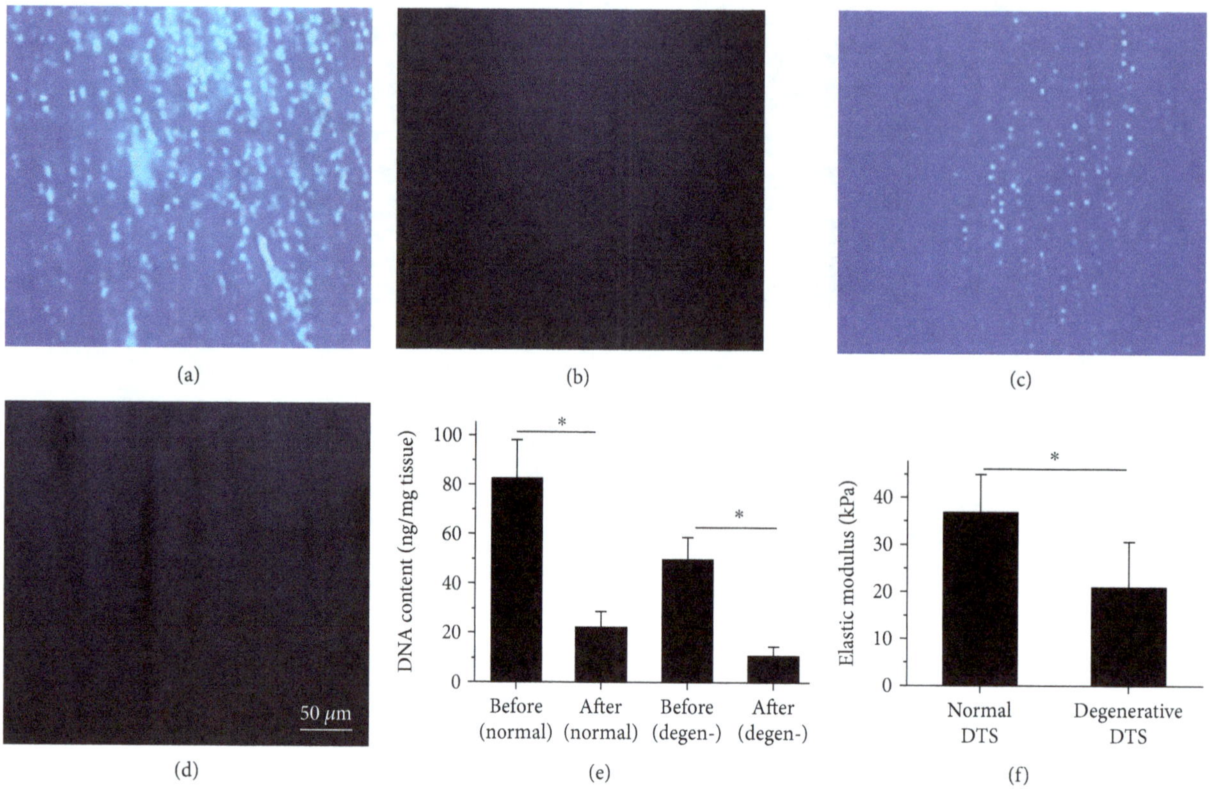

FIGURE 4: Decellularization of normal and degenerative tendons. DAPI staining of (a-b) normal and (c-d) degenerative DTSs before and after decellularization, respectively. (e) DNA content of normal and degenerative DTSs before and after decellularization. $^*P < 0.05$, compared with the after decellularization group. The error bars represent the standard deviation of measurements for 5 separated samples ($n = 5$). (f) Elastic modulus of normal and degenerative DTSs. $^*P < 0.05$, compared with normal DTSs. The error bars represent the standard deviation of measurements for 6 points in 3 separated samples ($n = 18$).

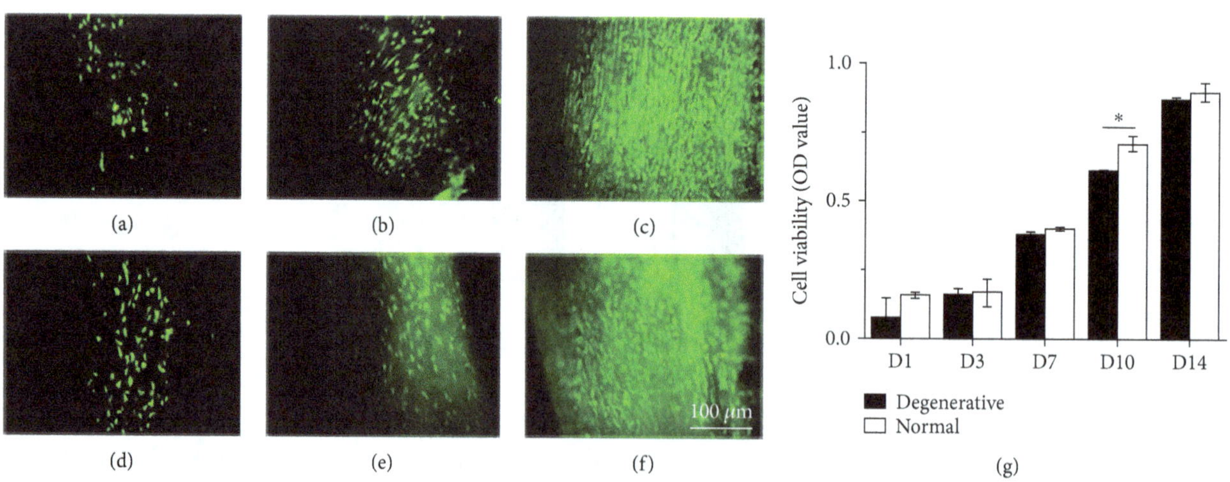

FIGURE 5: Live/dead staining and proliferative ability of TDSCs on normal and degenerative DTSs. Live/dead staining of TDSCs on normal DTSs at (a) day 1, (b) day 7, and (c) day 14. And live/dead staining of TDSCs on degenerative DTSs at (d) day 1, (e) day 7, and (f) day 14. (g) Proliferative ability assessment of TDSCs on normal and degenerative DTSs. $^*P < 0.05$, compared with normal DTSs. The error bars represent the standard deviation of measurements for 3 replicates of 3 separated samples ($n = 9$).

investigate the tenogenic and nontenogenic differentiation of TDSCs in the degenerative microenvironment.

Mechanical loading is essential for maintaining the homeostasis of tendons. However, when the microinjuries occurred in tendons, the partially unloaded area, which was stress deprived, was created at the same time. Stress deprivation has been confirmed to lead to the degeneration of tendons, including changes in collagen organization and mechanical properties similar to the effects of tendinopathy [21, 22]. So, at least to some extent, the degenerative tendon

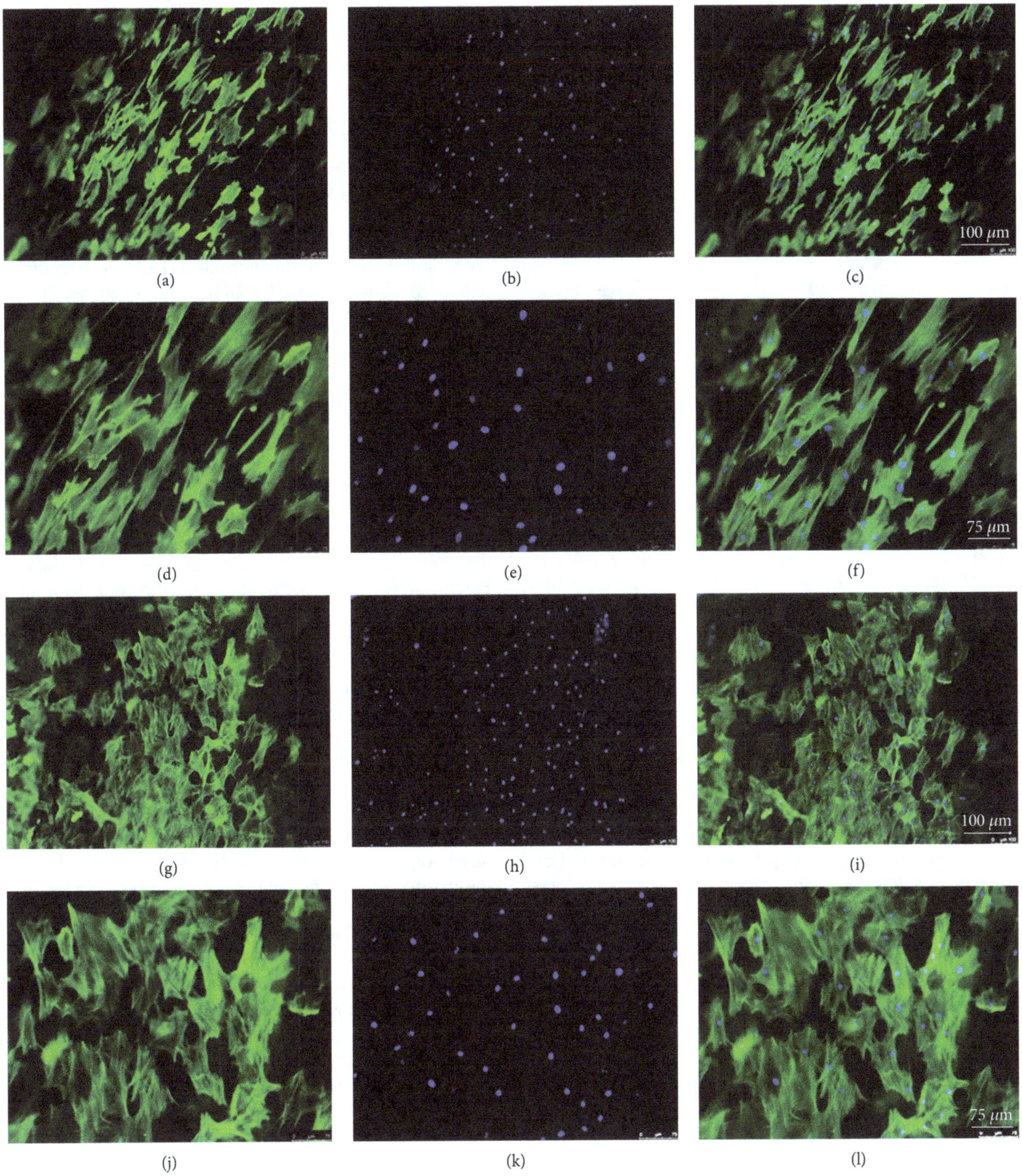

FIGURE 6: F-actin (labeled with Alexa488-phalloidin) and nucleus (labeled with DAPI) staining and merged images of TDSCs. TDSCs on (a–f) normal and (g–l) degenerative DTSs magnified 100 and 200 times, respectively.

model produced by stress-deprived culture could mimic the degenerative microenvironment of tendinopathy.

Shi et al. [23] found that elongated TDSCs exhibited enhanced gene expression of tenogenic markers compared with the cells which were spread out. However, the elongated cell shape inhibited chondrogenic and osteogenic differentiation of TDSCs. Our results were in accordance with the previous study; on normal DTSs, TDSCs adopted elongated shape and expressed a significantly higher level of tenogenic markers. On the contrary, on degenerative DTSs, TDSCs were more spread and significantly enhanced the expression of chondrogenic and osteogenic markers. These results indicated that in the degenerative microenvironment, TDSCs tended to be spread and differentiated toward chondrogenic

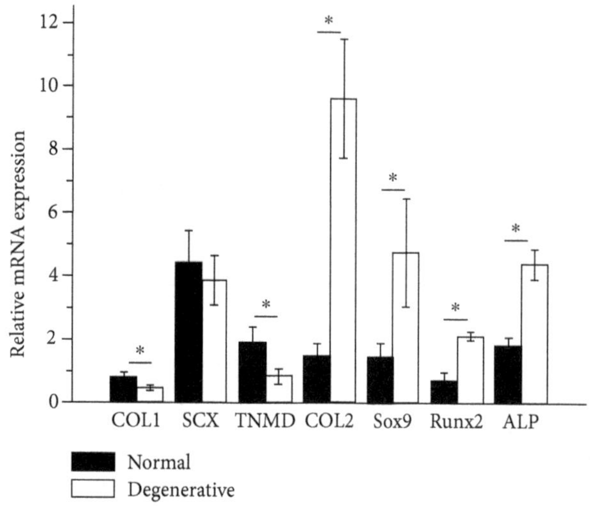

FIGURE 7: The differentiation of TDSCs toward tenogenic, chondrogenic, and osteogenic lineages. Relative gene expression of tenocyte markers COL1, SCX, and TNMD, chondrocyte markers COL2 and SOX9, and osteocyte markers Runx2 and ALP. The results were represented as the calculated comparative expression ratios of normal and degenerative DTS groups to the culture dish group. $^*P < 0.05$, compared with normal DTSs. The error bars represent the standard deviation of measurements for 2 replicates of 8 separated samples ($n = 16$).

and osteogenic phenotypes other than the tenogenic phenotype, which might lead to calcification or even ossification identified in tendinopathy.

Matrix stiffness, a biophysical cue in the cell microenvironment, played important roles in stem cell differentiation [24–26]. Mesenchymal stem cells (MSCs) [27], adipose-derived stem cells (ADSCs) [28], and umbilical cord mesenchymal stem cells (UCMSCs) [11], which were cultured on substrates with different stiffness, have been shown to possess diverse lineage commitments. MSCs would differentiate toward bone, muscle, or neuronal lineages as they grew on substrates with high, medium, or low stiffness, respectively [29]. The mechanical strength of the injured tendon tissues decreased significantly [30, 31]. The tissue stiffness would decline from 185 kPa to 60.3 kPa [31]. In this study, we found that the matrix stiffness of degenerative DTSs was significantly lower than the normal ones. So the matrix stiffness could be involved in the regulation of TDSC differentiation.

Matrix stiffness was sensed by integrin $\beta1$ on the cell membrane, which mediated the interaction between cell and ECM [32]. It was shown that TDSCs on normal DTSs had a higher expression level of integrin $\beta1$ compared with that on degenerative DTSs. Similar findings were shown by Gershlak and Black, in which the MSCs growing on the collagen I-coated PA gels displayed a general increase in the average number of the $\beta1$ integrin subunit with increasing stiffness [32].

Focal adhesion kinase (FAK) plays an important role in mediating mechanotransduction pathways. It mediates the interactions between cell-cell and cell-matrix. Furthermore, FAK affects intracellular signals through the extracellular signals. Extracellular signal-regulated kinase 1/2 (ERK1/2) is a well-known downstream signaling molecular of FAK and a force-activated protein kinase [33]. The FAK-ERK1/2 signaling pathway was confirmed to be involved in many cell activities including cell proliferation and cell differentiation [34]. Shih et al. [35] found that when FAK or ERK1/2 activation was inhibited, the differentiation of MSCs toward the osteogenic lineage was blocked. However, Wang et al. obtained an opposite result: the phosphorylated activation of ERK1/2 leads to the inhibition of osteogenic differentiation of MSCs [36]. In this study, similar results with Wang's were found: TDSCs on normal DTSs had significantly enhanced phosphorylated ERK1/2 expression, while osteogenic lineage-related markers Runx2 and ALP were lower expressed. However, TDSCs on degenerative DTSs expressed reduced phosphorylated ERK1/2, but osteogenic markers were highly expressed.

The morphology of cells was determined by the cytoskeleton, a structure subject to extracellular stress. The cytoskeleton connects with the ECM through focal adhesions (FA). Therefore, the actin cytoskeleton is continuously stabilized and destabilized by FAK-regulated processes. Several studies showed that when ADSCs or MSCs grew on substrates of different stiffness, the spreading area increased and more F-actin stress fibers formed on the substrate with higher stiffness [26, 28]. Nevertheless, in this study, it was found that the degenerative DTSs with lower stiffness enhanced the formation of F-actin stress fibers. There was evidence that F-actin fiber formation was promoted when FAK-ERK1/2 signaling was inhibited in liver cancer stem cells [33]. Our results were in accordance with theirs that the phosphorylation of FAK and ERK1/2 were reduced on degenerative DTSs, so that F-actin formation was increased compared with the normal DTSs with higher stiffness.

Mechanical loading constantly acts on tendons under physiological conditions. The differentiation of TDSCs toward tenocytes and nontenocytes was reported to be affected by the mechanical loading. When loaded with a 4% stretch, TDSCs highly expressed tenocyte-related markers COL1 and TNMD, while nontenocyte markers LPL, Sox9, Runx2, and Osterix were not affected [9]. However, as TDSCs were exposed to 8% stretching, both tenocyte- and nontenocyte-related genes were upregulated [9]. This study only focused on the different behaviors of TDSCs on degenerative DTSs without mechanical loading. The mechanical loading will be included in the future study.

Finally, besides the biophysical cues, the degenerative tendon experienced a series of biochemical changes, including the growth factor or ECM protein loss during the stress-deprived culture period. Tuan et al. found that the soluble fraction of tendon ECM could enhance the differentiation of ADSCs into tenogenic lineage [37], which indicated that the soluble ECM was also important for tenogenic differentiation. We cannot exclude that the observed differences were influenced by the ECM protein loss in the degenerative tendon microenvironment in this study. We will investigate the effect of biochemical changes in the degenerative tendon on the differentiation of TDSCs in the following study. Nevertheless, the results we found in this study would provide evidence that the degenerative

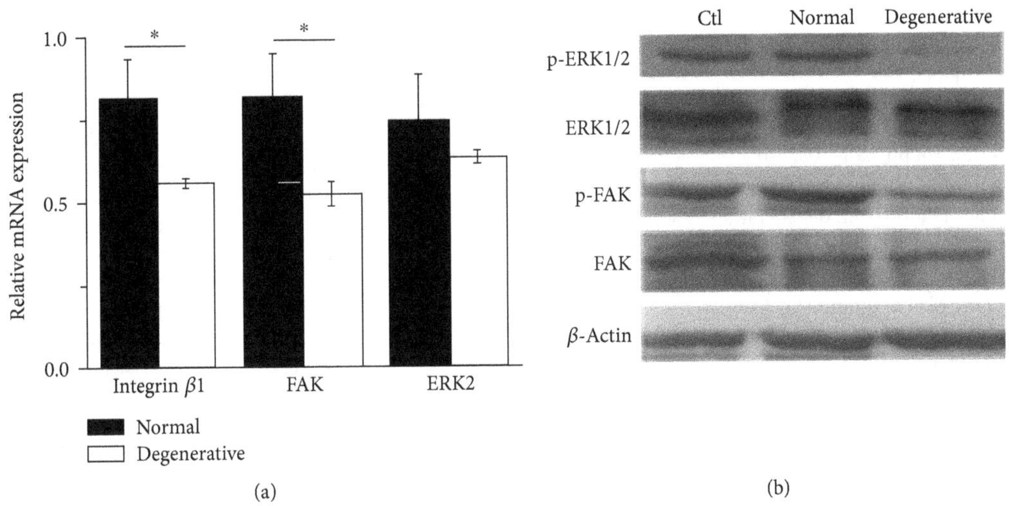

Figure 8: Gene and protein expression of FAK and ERK: (a) Relative gene expressions of integrin β1, FAK, and ERK and (b) Western blot from whole-cell lysates showing expressions of phosphorylated FAK^{Tyr397} and phosphorylated ERK1/2$^{Thr202/Tyr204}$ in TDSCs on a culture dish (as the control) and normal and degenerative DTSs. $^*P < 0.05$, compared with normal DTSs. The error bars represent the standard deviation of measurements for 2 replicates of 8 separated samples ($n = 16$).

microenvironment could induce TDSCs to differentiate into chondrogenic and osteogenic lineages. The regulating effect might be attributed to the cell morphology change and the reduced FAK and ERK1/2 activation in the degenerative microenvironment with reduced matrix stiffness.

5. Conclusions

It is important to understand the role of TDSCs in the pathogenesis of tendinopathy and the mechanisms contributing to their erroneous differentiation for the management of tendinopathy. This study demonstrated that TDSCs undergo erroneous differentiation toward chondrogenic and osteogenic lineages on degenerative DTSs. The underlying mechanism might be attributed to the degenerative microenvironment with the decrease of matrix stiffness, which resulted in the change of cell morphology and the reduced activation of FAK and ERK1/2.

Acknowledgments

This study was supported by the Shenzhen Science and Technology Innovation Committee [Grant nos. JCYJ20170818155915362, GJHS20160331171605415, GJHS20170314153933234, and GJHZ20170314154914747] and "Hundred Talents Program" of the Chinese Academy of Sciences.

References

[1] J. H. C. Wang, M. I. Iosifidis, and F. H. Fu, "Biomechanical basis for tendinopathy," *Clinical Orthopaedics and Related Research*, vol. 443, pp. 320–332, 2006.

[2] P. Kannus and L. Jozsa, "Histopathological changes preceding spontaneous rupture of a tendon—a controlled-study of 891 patients," *The Journal of Bone & Joint Surgery*, vol. 73, no. 10, pp. 1507–1525, 1991.

[3] Y. M. Bi, D. Ehirchiou, T. M. Kilts et al., "Identification of tendon stem/progenitor cells and the role of the extracellular matrix in their niche," *Nature Medicine*, vol. 13, no. 10, pp. 1219–1227, 2007.

[4] J. Zhang and J. H. Wang, "Mechanobiological response of tendon stem cells: implications of tendon homeostasis and pathogenesis of tendinopathy," *Journal of Orthopaedic Research*, vol. 28, no. 5, pp. 639–643, 2010.

[5] J. Zhang and J. H. Wang, "Production of PGE_2 increases in tendons subjected to repetitive mechanical loading and induces differentiation of tendon stem cells into non-tenocytes," *Journal of Orthopaedic Research*, vol. 28, no. 2, pp. 198–203, 2010.

[6] J. Zhang and J. H. Wang, "PRP treatment effects on degenerative tendinopathy—an in vitro model study," *Muscle, Ligaments and Tendons Journal*, vol. 4, no. 1, pp. 10–17, 2014.

[7] J. H. C. Wang and I. Komatsu, "Tendon stem cells: mechanobiology and development of tendinopathy," *Advances in Experimental Medicine and Biology*, vol. 920, pp. 53–62, 2016.

[8] E. M. Spiesz, C. T. Thorpe, S. Chaudhry et al., "Tendon extracellular matrix damage, degradation and inflammation in response to in vitro overload exercise," *Journal of Orthopaedic Research*, vol. 33, no. 6, pp. 889–897, 2015.

[9] J. Zhang and J. H. C. Wang, "The effects of mechanical loading on tendons—an in vivo and in vitro model study," *PLoS One*, vol. 8, no. 8, article e71740, 2013.

[10] A. M. Cozzolino, V. Noce, C. Battistelli et al., "Modulating the substrate stiffness to manipulate differentiation of resident liver stem cells and to improve the differentiation state of hepatocytes," *Stem Cells International*, vol. 2016, Article ID 5481493, 12 pages, 2016.

[11] J. Xu, M. Sun, Y. Tan et al., "Effect of matrix stiffness on the proliferation and differentiation of umbilical cord mesenchymal stem cells," *Differentiation*, vol. 96, pp. 30–39, 2017.

[12] G. M. Thornton, X. Shao, M. Chung et al., "Changes in mechanical loading lead to tendonspecific alterations in mmp and timp expression: influence of stress deprivation and intermittent cyclic hydrostatic compression on rat supraspinatus and Achilles tendons," *British Journal of Sports Medicine*, vol. 44, no. 10, pp. 698–703, 2010.

[12] G. M. Thornton, X. Shao, M. Chung et al., "Changes in mechanical loading lead to tendonspecific alterations in mmp and timp expression: influence of stress deprivation and intermittent cyclic hydrostatic compression on rat supraspinatus and Achilles tendons," *British Journal of Sports Medicine*, vol. 44, no. 10, pp. 698–703, 2010.

[13] T. Wang, Z. Lin, M. Ni et al., "Cyclic mechanical stimulation rescues Achilles tendon from degeneration in a bioreactor system," *Journal of Orthopaedic Research*, vol. 33, no. 12, pp. 1888–1896, 2015.

[14] S. P. Arnoczky, M. Lavagnino, M. Egerbacher, O. Caballero, and K. Gardner, "Matrix metalloproteinase inhibitors prevent a decrease in the mechanical properties of stress-deprived tendons," *The American Journal of Sports Medicine*, vol. 35, no. 5, pp. 763–769, 2017.

[15] N. D. Reeves, C. N. Maganaris, G. Ferretti, and M. V. Narici, "Influence of 90-day simulated microgravity on human tendon mechanical properties and the effect of resistive countermeasures," *Journal of Applied Physiology*, vol. 98, no. 6, pp. 2278–2286, 2005.

[16] M. Lavagnino, S. P. Arnoczky, M. Egerbacher, K. L. Gardner, and M. E. Burns, "Isolated fibrillar damage in tendons stimulates local collagenase mRNA expression and protein synthesis," *Journal of Biomechanics*, vol. 39, no. 13, pp. 2355–2362, 2006.

[17] D. Rowson, M. M. Knight, and H. R. C. Screen, "Zonal variation in primary cilia elongation correlates with localized biomechanical degradation in stress deprived tendon," *Journal of Orthopaedic Research*, vol. 34, no. 12, pp. 2146–2153, 2016.

[18] L. J. Ning, Y. J. Zhang, Y. Zhang et al., "The utilization of decellularized tendon slices to provide an inductive microenvironment for the proliferation and tenogenic differentiation of stem cells," *Biomaterials*, vol. 52, pp. 539–550, 2015.

[19] Z. Yin, X. Chen, T. Zhu et al., "The effect of decellularized matrices on human tendon stem/progenitor cell differentiation and tendon repair," *Acta Biomaterialia*, vol. 9, no. 12, pp. 9317–9329, 2013.

[20] Y. Rui, P. Lui, L. Chan, K. M. Chan, S. C. Fu, and G. Li, "Does erroneous differentiation of tendon-derived stem cells contribute to the pathogenesis of calcifying tendinopathy?," *Chinese Medical Journal*, vol. 124, no. 4, pp. 606–610, 2011.

[21] N. Yamamoto, K. Ohno, K. Hayashi, H. Kuriyama, K. Yasuda, and K. Kaneda, "Effects of stress shielding on the mechanical properties of rabbit patellar tendon," *Journal of Biomechanical Engineering*, vol. 115, no. 1, pp. 23–28, 1993.

[22] E. Yamamoto, K. Hayashi, and N. Yamamoto, "Effects of stress shielding on the transverse mechanical properties of rabbit patellar tendons," *Journal of Biomechanical Engineering*, vol. 122, no. 6, pp. 608–614, 2000.

[23] Y. Shi, K. Zhou, W. Zhang et al., "Microgrooved topographical surface directs tenogenic lineage specific differentiation of mouse tendon derived stem cells," *Biomedical Materials*, vol. 12, no. 1, article 015013, 2017.

[24] J. H. Hwang, M. R. Byun, A. R. Kim et al., "Extracellular matrix stiffness regulates osteogenic differentiation through MAPK activation," *PLoS One*, vol. 10, no. 8, article e0135519, 2015.

[25] Y. Navaro, N. Bleich-Kimelman, L. Hazanov et al., "Matrix stiffness determines the fate of nucleus pulposus-derived stem cells," *Biomaterials*, vol. 49, pp. 68–76, 2015.

[26] J. S. Park, J. S. Chu, A. D. Tsou et al., "The effect of matrix stiffness on the differentiation of mesenchymal stem cells in response to TGF-β," *Biomaterials*, vol. 32, no. 16, pp. 3921–3930, 2011.

[27] A. Islam, T. Mbimba, M. Younesi, and O. Akkus, "Effects of substrate stiffness on the tenoinduction of human mesenchymal stem cells," *Acta Biomaterialia*, vol. 58, pp. 244–253, 2017.

[28] T. Zhang, S. Lin, X. Shao et al., "Regulating osteogenesis and adipogenesis in adipose-derived stem cells by controlling underlying substrate stiffness," *Journal of Cellular Physiology*, vol. 233, no. 4, pp. 3418–3428, 2018.

[29] A. J. Engler, S. Sen, H. L. Sweeney, and D. E. Discher, "Matrix elasticity directs stem cell lineage specification," *Cell*, vol. 126, no. 4, pp. 677–689, 2006.

[30] C. Helland, J. Bojsen-Møller, T. Raastad et al., "Mechanical properties of the patellar tendon in elite volleyball players with and without patellar tendinopathy," *British Journal of Sports Medicine*, vol. 47, no. 13, pp. 862–868, 2013.

[31] T. Dirrichs, V. Quack, M. Gatz, M. Tingart, C. K. Kuhl, and S. Schrading, "Shear wave elastography (SWE) for the evaluation of patients with tendinopathies," *Academic Radiology*, vol. 23, no. 10, pp. 1204–1213, 2016.

[32] J. R. Gershlak and L. D. Black III, "Beta 1 integrin binding plays a role in the constant traction force generation in response to varying stiffness for cells grown on mature cardiac extracellular matrix," *Experimental Cell Research*, vol. 330, no. 2, pp. 311–324, 2015.

[33] J. Sun, Q. Luo, L. Liu, X. Yang, S. Zhu, and G. Song, "Salinomycin attenuates liver cancer stem cell motility by enhancing cell stiffness and increasing F-actin formation via the FAK-ERK1/2 signalling pathway," *Toxicology*, vol. 384, pp. 1–10, 2017.

[34] I. Takahashi, K. Onodera, Y. Sasano et al., "Effect of stretching on gene expression of $\beta 1$ integrin and focal adhesion kinase and on chondrogenesis through cell-extracellular matrix interactions," *European Journal of Cell Biology*, vol. 82, no. 4, pp. 182–192, 2003.

[35] Y. R. V. Shih, K. F. Tseng, H. Y. Lai, C. H. Lin, and O. K. Lee, "Matrix stiffness regulation of integrin-mediated mechanotransduction during osteogenic differentiation of human mesenchymal stem cells," *Journal of Bone and Mineral Research*, vol. 26, no. 4, pp. 730–738, 2011.

[36] Y. Wang, J. Li, Y. Wang et al., "Effects of hypoxia on osteogenic differentiation of rat bone marrow mesenchymal stem cells," *Molecular and Cellular Biochemistry*, vol. 362, no. 1-2, pp. 25–33, 2012.

[37] G. Yang, B. B. Rothrauff, H. Lin, S. Yu, and R. S. Tuan, "Tendon-derived extracellular matrix enhances transforming growth factor-$\beta 3$-induced tenogenic differentiation of human adipose-derived stem cells," *Tissue Engineering. Part A*, vol. 23, no. 3-4, pp. 166–176, 2017.

11

Amniotic Epithelial Cells Accelerate Diabetic Wound Healing by Modulating Inflammation and Promoting Neovascularization

Yongjun Zheng,[1] Shiqing Zheng,[1,2] Xiaoming Fan,[1] Li Li,[3] Yongqiang Xiao,[1] Pengfei Luo,[1] Yingying Liu,[1] Li Wang,[1] Zhenci Cui,[1] Fei He,[1] Yuhuan Liu,[3] Shichu Xiao,[1] and Zhaofan Xia[1]

[1]*Burns Center, Changhai Hospital, Second Military Medical University, Shanghai, China*
[2]*No. 73051 Troop of the Chinese People's Liberation Army, Xiamen, China*
[3]*Department of Obstetrics and Gynecology, Changhai Hospital, Second Military Medical University, Shanghai, China*

Correspondence should be addressed to Yuhuan Liu; 13651968369@163.com, Shichu Xiao; huangzhuoxiao@sohu.com, and Zhaofan Xia; xiazhaofan_smmu@163.com

Yongjun Zheng, Shiqing Zheng, Xiaoming Fan, and Li Li contributed equally to this work.

Academic Editor: Isotta Chimenti

Human amniotic epithelial cells (hAECs) are nontumorigenic, highly abundant, and low immunogenic and possess multipotent differentiation ability, which make them become ideal alternative stem cell source for regenerative medicine. Previous studies have demonstrated the therapeutic potential of hAECs in many tissue repairs. However, the therapeutic effect of hAECs on diabetic wound healing is still unknown. In this study, we injected hAECs intradermally around the full-thickness excisional skin wounds of db/db mice and found that hAECs significantly accelerated diabetic wound healing and granulation tissue formation. To explore the underlying mechanisms, we measured inflammation and neovascularization in diabetic wounds. hAECs could modulate macrophage phenotype toward M2 macrophage, promote switch from proinflammatory status to prohealing status of wounds, and increase capillary density in diabetic wounds. Furthermore, we found that the hAEC-conditioned medium promoted macrophage polarization toward M2 phenotype and facilitated migration, proliferation, and tube formation of endothelial cells through in vitro experiments. Taken together, we first reported that hAECs could promote diabetic wound healing, at least partially, through paracrine effects to regulate inflammation and promote neovascularization.

1. Introduction

Diabetic ulcers are a severe, resistant complication of diabetes mellitus (DM), and about one fourth of DM patients endure diabetic lower extremity ulcers during their whole lives [1]. Diabetic wounds tend to heal slowly and be frequently recurrent, not only leading to increasing cost of medical care but also seriously impairing the quality of life in diabetic patients. Current standard treatments in clinics such as debridement, moist dressings, infection control, or wound offloading have not achieved the satisfactory results. Therefore, we urgently need more effective therapeutic approaches to promote diabetic wound healing.

Stem cells have shown great potential in repairing damaged tissue. Mesenchymal stem cell (MSC) is one of the most widely studied stem cells for wound healing, and several studies have demonstrated inspiring preclinical results through animal models [2–5]. Nonetheless, several arguments still exist against the widely use of MSC in clinics, including the probability of tumorigenesis and low cell production from MSC harvesting. Human amniotic epithelial cells (hAECs) are derived from the amniotic membrane and demonstrate a potential source of stem cells. These cells are nontumorigenic and low immunogenic and possess multipotent differentiation ability [6–8]. Furthermore, hAECs are highly plentiful, and about 1.5×10^8 cells could be separated from each amniotic membrane, which is plenty for using hAECs directly in clinics without amplification in vitro [9]. In this regard, the use of hAECs for regenerative medicine holds great promise.

Recently, the beneficial effects of hAECs in many tissue repairs are reported [10–13]. Although studies have shown that hAECs play their beneficial roles through preventing inflammatory responses, the exact mechanisms of hAECs for promoting tissue repairs remain unclear [11, 14]. A common feature of refractory healing wound is persistent inflammation, impaired vascularization, and decreased expression of growth factors [15]. Whether hAECs play a role in diabetic wound healing associated with inflammation and neovascularization is still unknown.

In this study, we determined whether hAEC transplantation could promote diabetic wound healing by injecting hAECs intradermally around the full-thickness excisional skin wounds of db/db mice. We further explored related mechanisms through in vivo and in vitro experiments, mainly focusing on inflammation and neovascularization.

2. Materials and Methods

2.1. Cell Isolation and Culture. All research proposals were permitted by the Ethics Committee of Changhai Hospital, Shanghai, China. We first obtained informed consent from parturients and then got placentas directly from parturients immediately after cesarean section. All donors had no human hepatitis B and C, syphilis, and HIV verified by serological tests. Collection and isolation of hAECs was performed as described previously [9]. hAECs were cultured in a high-glucose DMEM supplemented with 10% FBS (complete medium), and hAECs at passage 2-3 were used.

Mouse macrophages were separated from bone marrow of wild-type C57BL/6 mice and cultured in a complete medium, and primary-cultured macrophages were used for further cell experiments as previously described [16]. Human umbilical vein endothelial cells (HUVECs) were purchased from ScienCell (San Diego, USA) and cultured in the endothelial cell medium (ECM, Gibco, Life Technologies) supplemented with 10% FBS, and HUVECs between passages 2 and 4 were used for further in vitro experiments. To assess the effects of the hAEC-conditioned medium (hAEC-CM) on macrophage phenotype switch in vitro, we used IFN-γ and TNF-α (20 ng/ml each, R&D Systems) to stimulate the macrophages for 24 hours with or without hAEC-CM. Complete medium without TNF-α and IFN-γ was used as control.

2.2. Preparation of the hAEC-Conditioned Medium (hAEC-CM). We prepared hAEC-CM using a method analogous to the one described previously [17]. In brief, hAECs were digested with trypsin and then 2×10^6 hAECs were cultured in a 100 mm plate overnight. We changed the complete culture medium into a 10 ml serum-free high-glucose DMEM and cultured for another 24 hours. The supernatant was collected and concentrated to 10 times the concentration of the collected hAEC-CM as the final hAEC-CM by using Amicon Ultra-15 ultrafiltration conical tubes (Millipore, 3 kDa).

2.3. Animal Model and Treatment. All animal protocols were complied with the rules of the animal use and care committee of Changhai Hospital, Shanghai, China. The db/db mouse was a widely accepted animal model of type 2 diabetes. We purchased the male and 8–12 weeks old db/db mouse (C57BL/KsJ, leptin receptor-deficient diabetes) from SLAC Laboratory Animal Co. Ltd., Shanghai, China. Only mice with a >300 mg/dl blood glucose level were included for further animal experiments. Mice were anesthetized, and then two symmetric splint wounds (10 mm diameter) with full-thickness skin defect were made on the back of each mouse based on the previous study [18]. We divided the mice equally into 2 groups: hAEC group and blank group (PBS group). 1×10^6 cells suspended in 100 μl PBS were injected intradermally around the wound. Photographs of wounds were taken regularly, and then, the wound healing rate was figured by Image-Pro Plus software.

2.4. Skin Histological Analysis and Immunohistochemistry. The wounds with the margins were excised at day 10 after wounding, fixed in 10% formalin, and then embedded in paraffin for hematoxylin and eosin (H&E) staining and immunohistochemistry staining. We measured the wound bed area of each section stained with H&E using Image-Pro Plus software. Angiogenesis in day 10 wounds was observed by immunohistochemistry using CD31 (Santa Cruz, USA) as the primary antibody and then stained with DAB (Thermo, USA). For evaluation the number of M1 and M2 macrophages in day 10 wounds, we counterstained the sections by immunofluorescence with CD68 (Abcam) and iNOS (Abcam) to calculate M1 macrophages and with CD68 and CD206 (Abcam) to calculate M2 macrophages. All sections were finally stained with DAPI.

2.5. ELISA. Wounds with the margins at day 10 were excised with a skin biopsy punch and homogenized in cold PBS by a Dounce homogenizer. After being sonicated, the homogenates were centrifuged at 4°C (10,000 rpm, 20 minutes). Supernatants were collected, and expression levels of IL-6, IL-1β, TNF-α, VEGF, TGF-β1, and IGF-1 were calculated by ELISA. All ELISA kits were purchased from R&D Systems and used according to the manufacturer's instruction.

2.6. HUVEC Proliferation Assay. Proliferation of HUVECs was evaluated by a CCK-8 Kit (Liankebio, China) in conformity to the instruction of the manufacturer. In brief, HUVECs were digested with trypsin, and 5×10^3 cells were plated into each well of a 96-well plate (BD Falcon). After being cultured in a complete medium for 24 hours, the cells were then cultured in hAEC-CM for another 72 hours. Complete medium was treated as a positive control medium, and serum-free high-glucose DMEM was used as a negative control medium.

2.7. HUVEC Tube Formation Assay. We performed the tube formation assay in conformity to the instructions of the manufacturer. Matrigel (BD Biosciences, USA) was diluted with serum-free DMEM to 5 mg/ml, and 50 μl gel was plated into each well of a 96-well plate. 4×10^4 HUVECs suspended in 100 μl hAEC-CM were plated into each well. After

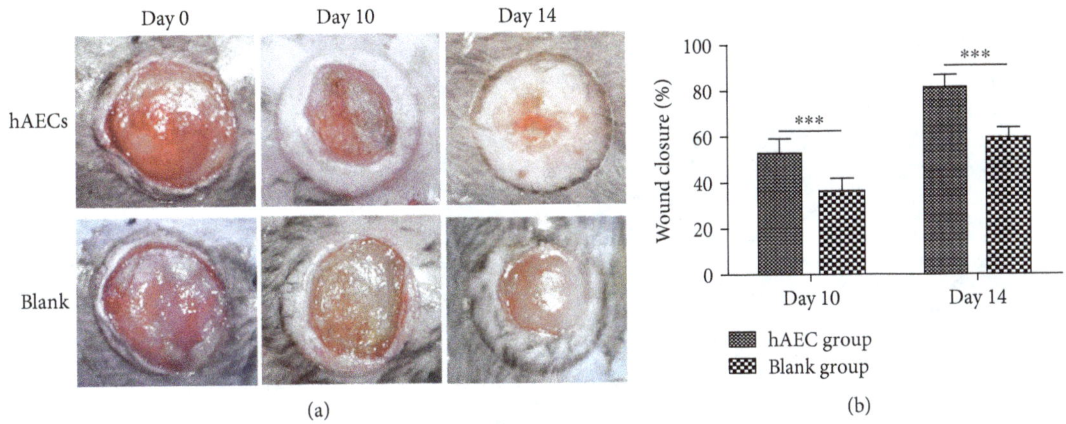

FIGURE 1: Topical administration of hAECs accelerated diabetic wound healing. (a) Diabetic wounds were treated with hAECs or PBS, examined at day 0, day 10, and day 14 after wounding, and then digitally photographed. (b) Quantitative analysis of wound closure demonstrating a higher wound healing rate in the hAEC-treated group. Data was shown as means ± SD; $n = 6$; $^{***}P < 0.001$.

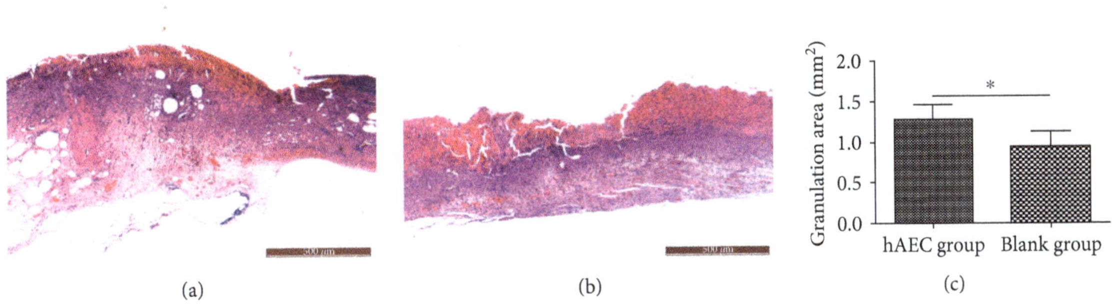

FIGURE 2: Histomorphometric analysis of diabetic wounds. Representative H&E staining of wound sections at day 10 from the hAEC group (a) and PBS group (b). Quantitative analysis of the granulation tissue area, showing the increased granulation tissue formation in the hAEC-treated group (c). Data was shown as means ± SD; $n = 6$; $^{*}P < 0.05$; scale bar = 500 μm.

incubating HUVECs for 6 hours, we took photographs with a microscope system (Leica, Germany) and then calculated the capillary-like structures. Complete medium was treated as a positive control medium, and serum-free high-glucose DMEM was used as a negative control medium.

2.8. HUVEC Migration Assay. We performed HUVEC migration assay by a transwell chamber with 8 μm pore size (BD Biosciences, USA). The upper chamber was plated with 1×10^5 HUVECs suspended in serum-free DMEM, and the bottom chamber was added with 600 μl hAEC-CM. After 24 hours, we fixed the filters with 10% formalin, stained them with 0.1% crystal violet (Sigma, USA), and then counted the migrated cells by Leica QWin image analysis software. Complete medium was treated as a positive control medium, and serum-free high-glucose DMEM was used as a negative control medium.

2.9. Western Blot Analysis. The macrophages were lysed in lysis buffer after washing with ice cold PBS buffer. Lysates were centrifuged, and the supernatants were collected for Western blot analysis. The protein concentration was determined by the BCA protein assay kit. Western blot analysis was performed with primary antibody against iNOS, CD206, and GAPDH as previously described [19].

2.10. Detection of Growth Factors and Inflammatory Cytokines in hAEC-CM. hAEC-CM was collected to detect the expression of growth factors and inflammatory cytokines by using human growth factor antibody array G1 and human inflammation antibody array G1 (RayBiotech Inc.), respectively, in accordance with the manufacturer's protocol.

2.11. Statistical Analysis. We expressed the results as mean ± SD and analyzed the data using two-tailed Student's t-test or one-way ANOVA by SPSS 16.0. $P < 0.05$ was considered as statistical significance.

3. Results

3.1. Topical Administration of hAECs Accelerated Diabetic Wound Healing. We treated diabetic wounds with hAECs or PBS and then examined at day 0, day 10, and day 14 after wounding (Figure 1(a)). At day 10, the wound healing rate was significantly higher in the hAEC-treated group (52.16 ± 6.80%) than that in the PBS-treated group (35.76 ± 6.19%, $P < 0.001$, Figure 1(b)). The gap of the wound healing rate between the two groups gradually increased along with time. Furthermore, we performed H&E staining (Figures 2(a) and 2(b)) and found that the granulation tissue area was

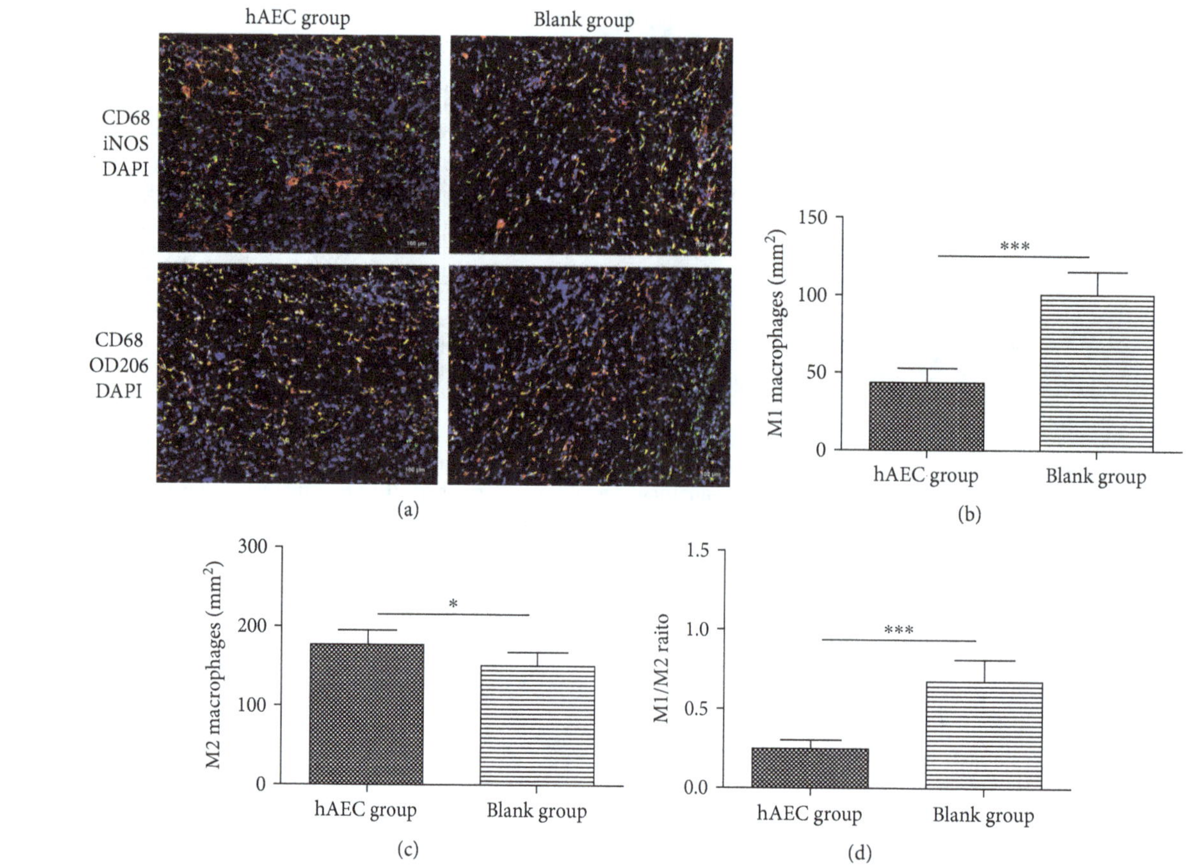

FIGURE 3: Macrophage phenotype was polarized toward M2 macrophage in the hAEC-treated group. (a) Representative immunofluorescent staining of M1 and M2 macrophages in day 10 wounds. M1 macrophages were shown in the upper panel to be yellow as $CD68^+iNOS^+DAPI^+$ triple-positive staining, and M2 macrophages were shown in the lower panel to be yellow as $CD68^+CD206^+DAPI^+$ triple-positive staining. (b, c, and d) The number of M1 macrophages was significantly reduced in the hAEC group (b), whereas the number of M2 macrophages was increased (c), resulting in a lower M1/M2 ratio (d). Data was shown as means ± SD; $n = 6$; $^*P < 0.05$; $^{***}P < 0.001$; scale bar = 100 μm.

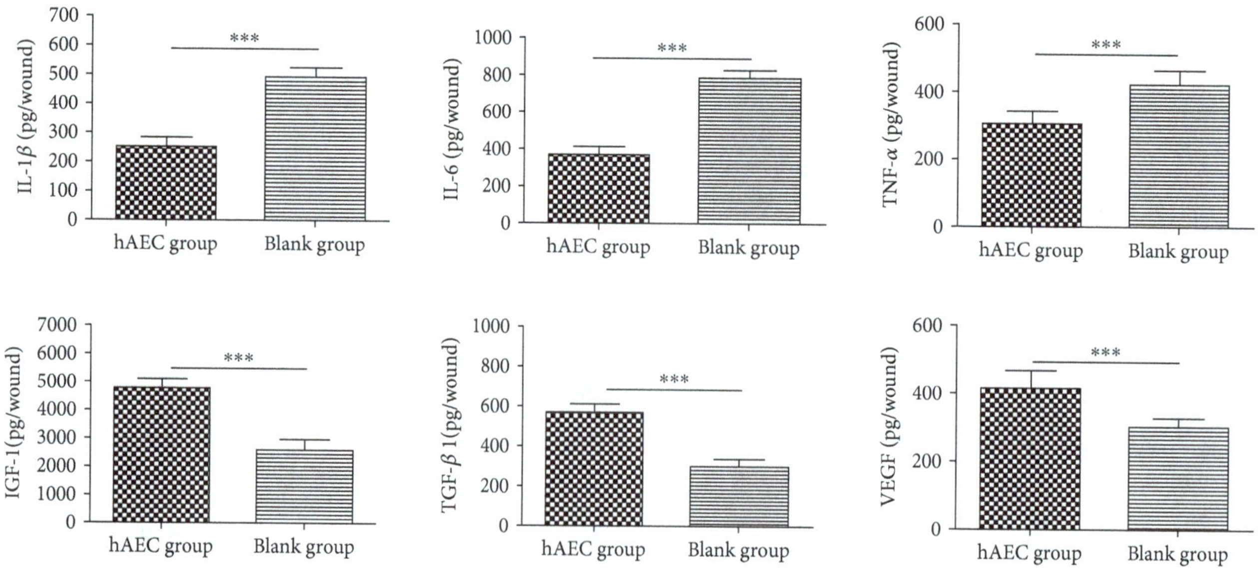

FIGURE 4: hAECs switched proinflammatory status into prohealing status of diabetic wounds. Expression levels of IL-6, IL-1β, TNF-α, VEGF, TGF-β1, and IGF-1 in day 10 diabetic wounds were detected by ELISA, showing reduced levels of proinflammatory cytokines and increased expression levels of prohealing cytokines in the hAEC group. Data was shown as means ± SD; $n = 6$; $^{***}P < 0.001$.

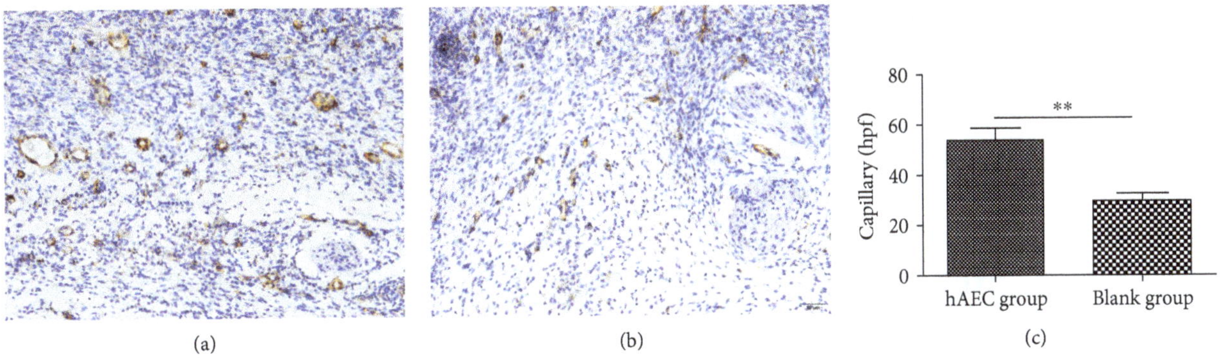

FIGURE 5: hAECs increased capillary density in diabetic wounds. Representative immunohistochemistry staining of CD31 at day 10 after wounding in the hAEC group (a) and PBS group (b). Statistical analysis of $CD31^+$ newly formed vessels showed that neovascularization was more obvious in hAEC-treated wounds (c). Data was shown as means ± SD; $n = 6$; $^{**}P < 0.01$; scale bars: 50 μm (a, b).

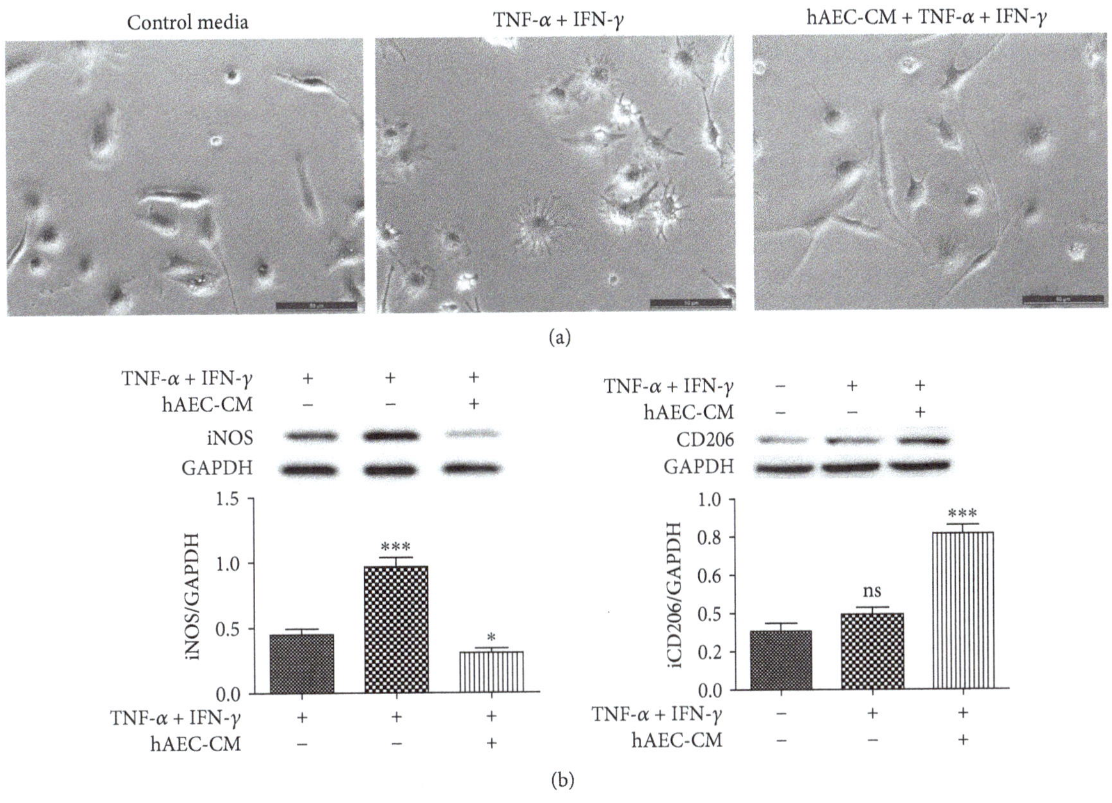

FIGURE 6: hAEC-CM promoted phenotype switch of macrophages toward M2-like in vitro. (a) Changes of macrophages in morphology when treated with IFN-γ and TNF-α with or without hAEC-CM. Complete medium without IFN-γ and TNF-α was treated as the control medium. (b) Protein expression levels of iNOS and CD206 when treated with the control medium, IFN-γ + TNF-α, or IFN-γ + TNF-α + hAEC-CM were measured by Western blot. Data was shown as means ± SD; $n = 3$; $^{*}P < 0.05$; $^{***}P < 0.001$; and ns: no significance; scale bars: 50 μm (a).

significantly higher in day 10 hAEC-treated wounds than that in PBS-treated wounds (Figure 2(c)).

3.2. hAECs Promoted Macrophage Phenotype Switch from M1 Macrophage to M2 Macrophage in Diabetic Wounds. The numbers of M1 and M2 macrophages in day 10 wounds were assessed by immunofluorescence (Figure 3(a)). Using iNOS as a marker of M1 macrophage and CD206 as a marker of M2 macrophage, we found that hAEC-treated wounds had fewer M1 macrophages (Figure 3(b)), more M2 macrophages (Figure 3(c)), and a significantly lower M1/M2 ratio (Figure 3(d)). We then measured the expression of inflammatory cytokines and prohealing cytokines in day 10 wounds using ELISA. The expression levels of proinflammatory cytokines IL-1β, IL-6, and TNF-α were significantly reduced in the hAEC group, and the levels of prohealing cytokines VEGF, TGF-β1, and IGF-1 were significantly increased in the hAEC group when compared with the PBS group

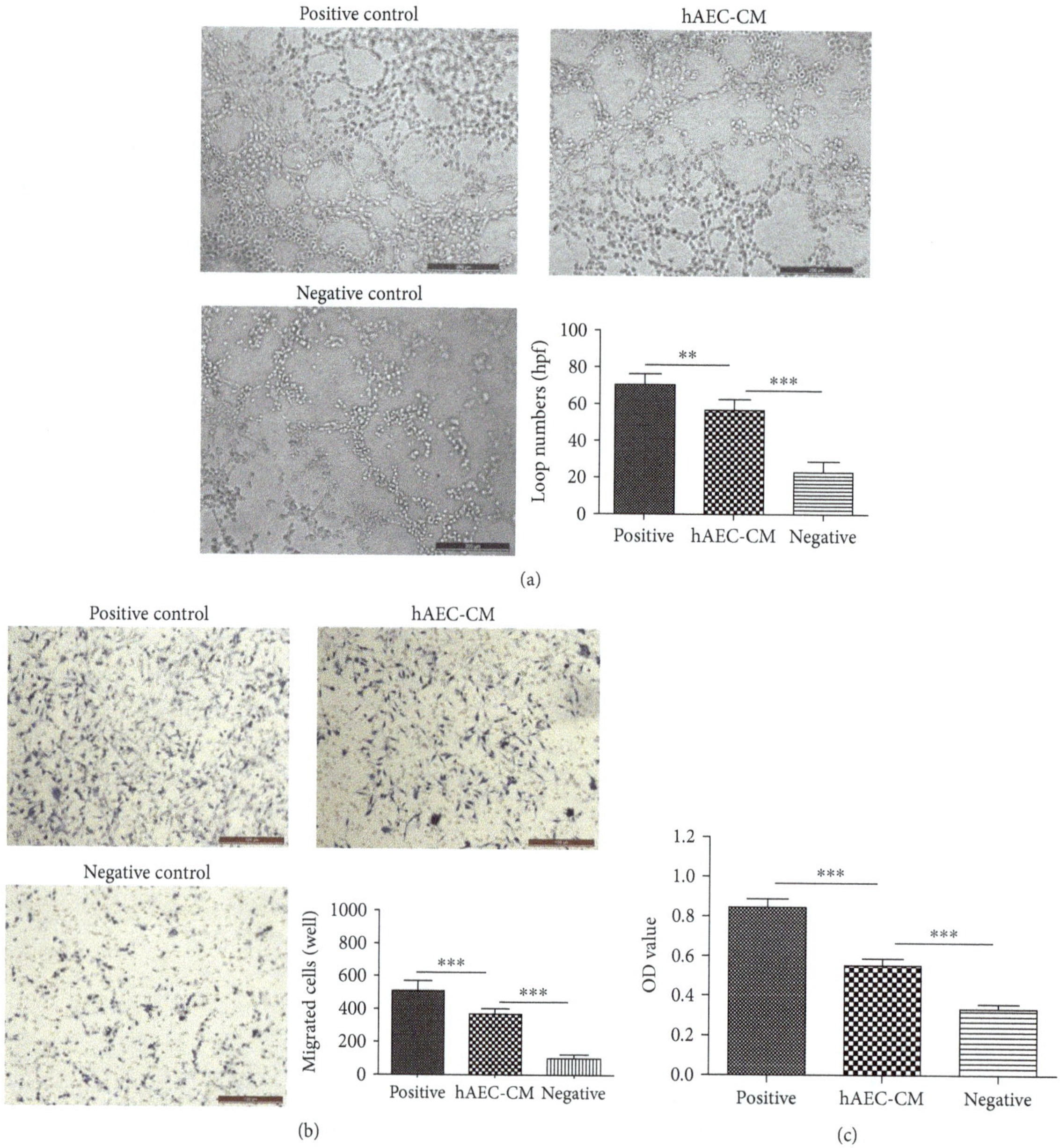

FIGURE 7: hAEC-CM exhibited chemoattractive, mitogenic, and angiogenic effects on HUVECs in vitro. (a) The tube formation assay was performed to investigate the effect of hAEC-CM on the angiogenic capacity of HUVECs. (b and c) Effect of hAEC-CM on the migration (b) and proliferation (c) of HUVECs was measured by transwell assay and CCK-8 assay, respectively. Complete medium was treated as positive control medium and serum-free DMEM as negative control medium, respectively. Data was shown as means ± SD; $n = 6$; $^{**}P < 0.01$; and $^{***}P < 0.001$. Scale bars: 200 μm (a); 100 μm (b).

(Figure 4), indicating that hAECs could switch proinflammatory status into prohealing status of diabetic wounds.

3.3. hAECs Increased Capillary Density in Diabetic Wounds. CD31 was a blood vessel endothelium cell marker, and immunohistochemistry staining of CD31 demonstrated that the newly formed vessels in the hAEC group were more obvious than that in the PBS group in day 10 wounds of db/db mice (Figures 5(a) and 5(b)). Capillary density in hAEC-treated wounds was 53.8 ± 11.8/hpf (high-power field), whereas the number was 29.7 ± 7.3/hpf in PBS-treated wounds ($P < 0.01$, Figure 5(c)).

3.4. hAEC-CM Promoted Phenotype Switch of Macrophages toward M2-Like In Vitro. The primary-cultured macrophages were small and round cultured in control media. When treated with IFN-γ + TNF-α, many macrophages processed multiple protrusions and showed dendritic morphology, whereas IFN-γ + TNF-α + hAEC-CM guided elongation of macrophages (Figure 6(a)). Moreover, hAEC-CM significantly increased the protein expression of CD206 and decreased the protein expression of iNOS measured by Western blot (Figure 6(b)). Taken together, these results enunciated that hAEC-CM could guide macrophage polarization toward M2-like in morphology and phenotype.

RayBio human inflammation antibody array G series

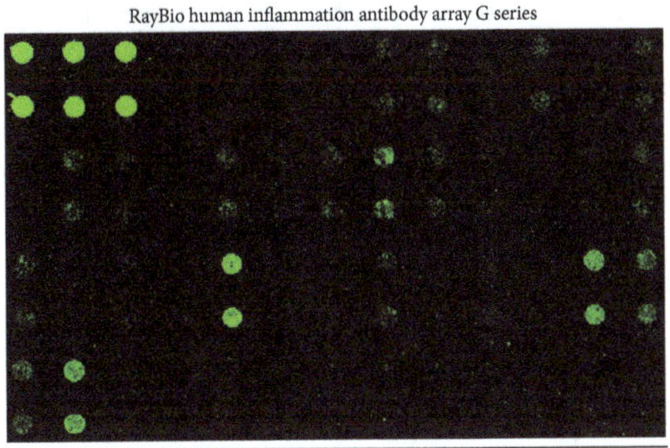

	A	B	C	D	E	F	G	H	I	J	K	L	M
1	POS1	POS2	POS3	NEG	NEG	EOTAXIN	EOTAXIN-2	GCSF	GM-CSF	ICAM-1	IFN-γ	I-309	IL-1α
2	POS1	POS2	POS3	NEG	NEG	EOTAXIN	EOTAXIN-2	GCSF	GM-CSF	ICAM-1	IFN-γ	I-309	IL-1α
3	IL-1b	IL-2	IL-3	IL-4	IL-6	IL-6sR	IL-7	IL-8	IL-10	IL-11	IL-12 p40	IL-12 p70	IL-13
4	IL-1b	IL-2	IL-3	IL-4	IL-6	IL-6sR	IL-7	IL-8	IL-10	IL-11	IL-12 p40	IL-12 p70	IL-13
5	IL-15	IL-16	IL-17	IP-10	MCP-1	MCP-2	M-CSF	MIG	MIP-1a	MIP-1b	MIP-1d	RANTES	TGF-β1
6	IL-15	IL-16	IL-17	IP-10	MCP-1	MCP-2	M-CSF	MIG	MIP-1a	MIP-1b	MIP-1d	RANTES	TGF-β1
7	TNF-α	TNF-β	s TNF RI	s TNF RII	PDGF-BB	TIMP-2	NEG	NEG	NEG	NEG	NEG	NEG	NEG
8	TNF-α	TNF-β	s TNF RI	s TNF RII	PDGF-BB	TIMP-2	NEG	NEG	NEG	NEG	NEG	NEG	NEG

RayBio human inflammation antibody array G series

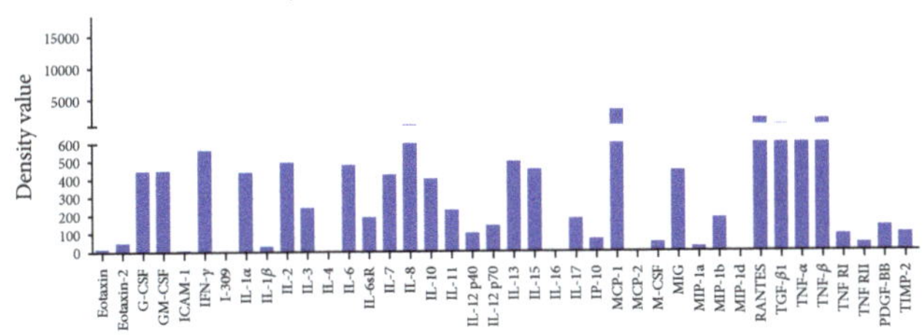

(a)

RayBio human growth factor antibody array G series

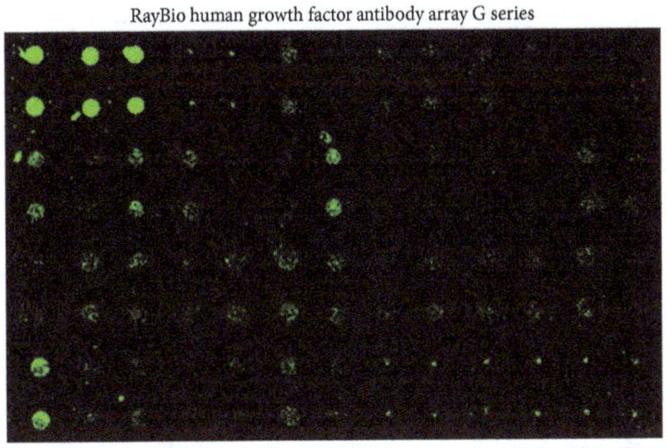

	A	B	C	D	E	F	G	H	I	J	K	L	M
1	POS1	POS2	POS3	NEG	NEG	AREG	bFGF	β-NGF	EGF	EGFR	FGF4	FGF6	FGF7
2	POS1	POS2	POS3	NEG	NEG	AREG	bFGF	β-NGF	EGF	EGFR	FGF4	FGF6	FGF7
3	CSF3	GDNF	CSF2	HB-EGF	HGF	IGFBP1	IGFBP2	IGFBP3	IGFBP4	IGFBP6	IGF1	IGF1R	IGF2
4	CSF3	GDNF	CSF2	HB-EGF	HGF	IGFBP1	IGFBP2	IGFBP3	IGFBP4	IGFBP6	IGF1	IGF1R	IGF2
5	CSF1	CSF1R	NT-3	NT-4	PDGF Rα	PDGF Rβ	PDGF-AA	PDGF-AB	PDGF-BB	PLGF	SCF	SCFR	TGF-α
6	CSF1	CSF1R	NT-3	NT-4	PDGF Rα	PDGF Rβ	PDGF-AA	PDGF-AB	PDGF-BB	PLGF	SCF	SCFR	TGF-α
7	TGF-β1	TGF-β2	TGF-β3	VEGF-A	VEGF R2	VEGF R3	VEGF-D	NEG	NEG	NEG	NEG	NEG	NEG
8	TGF-β1	TGF-β2	TGF-β3	VEGF-A	VEGF R2	VEGF R3	VEGF-D	NEG	NEG	NEG	NEG	NEG	NEG

RayBio human growth factor antibody array G series

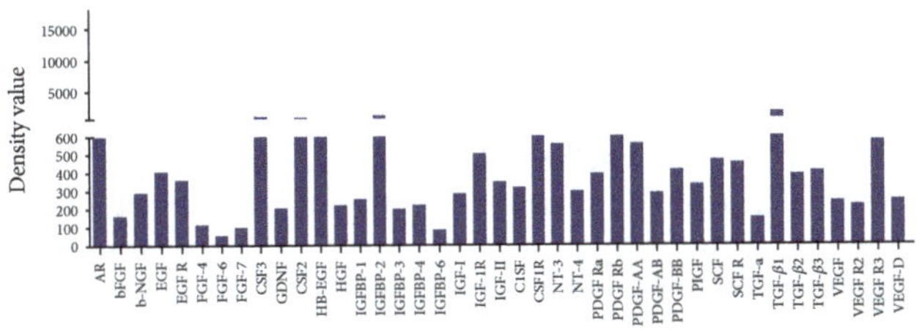

(b)

FIGURE 8: Inflammatory cytokines and growth factors in hAEC-CM. (a) RayBio human inflammatory cytokine antibody array was used to detect a panel of inflammatory cytokines in hAEC-CM. (b) RayBio human growth factor antibody array was used to detect a panel of growth factors in hAEC-CM.

3.5. hAEC-CM Promoted Migration, Proliferation, and Tube Formation of HUVECs In Vitro. The tube formation assay was performed to investigate the effect of hAEC-CM on the angiogenic capacity of HUVECs. We found that more networks formed when treated with hAEC-CM (Figure 7(a)). In addition, hAEC-CM significantly promoted the migration and proliferation of HUVECs performed by transwell assay and CCK-8 assay, respectively (Figures 7(b) and 7(c)).

3.6. Inflammatory Cytokines and Growth Factors in hAEC-CM. Of the 40 inflammatory cytokines showed in the human inflammation antibody array, IL-8, MCP-1, RANTES, MIP-1b, TGF-β1, TNF, and IL-13 in hAEC-CM represented the highest expression levels (Figure 8(a)). Of the 41 growth factors represented in the human growth factor antibody array, CSF2, CSF3, HB-EGF, IGFBP-2, CSF1R, PDGF, and TGF-β1 in hAEC-CM demonstrated the highest expression levels (Figure 8(b)). The results showed similar kinds of inflammatory cytokines and growth factors representing the higher expression levels with the previous study, which have performed a cytokine array containing 507 human cytokines on the hAEC-derived-conditioned medium [13].

4. Discussion

hAECs are nontumorigenic, highly abundant, and low immunogenic and possess multipotent differentiation ability, which make them become ideal alternative stem cell source for regenerative medicine. Previous studies have demonstrated the therapeutic potential of hAECs in various tissue repairs, including lung injury [10, 11, 14], brain injury [20], myocardial infarction [21], kidney injury [22], and liver fibrosis [23, 24]. Nonetheless, the therapeutic effect of hAECs on diabetic wound healing is still unknown. In this study, we first reported that hAECs significantly accelerated the diabetic wound healing rate and granulation tissue formation, at least partially, by regulating inflammation and promoting neovascularization.

Macrophage polarization plays an important part in normal wound healing progression. During the inflammatory phase, M1 macrophages initiate an urgent inflammatory response, whereas during the proliferative phase, M2 macrophages accelerate neovascularization and granulation tissue formation [25]. A poorly healing wound such as a diabetic wound is characterized by persevering inflammatory response with protracted aggregation of M1 macrophages along with high-level expression of inflammatory factors and low-level expression of prohealing cytokines [26, 27]. Previous studies have shown that promoting macrophage phenotype switch from the M1 macrophage to the M2 macrophage could accelerate diabetic wound healing effectively [28–30]. hAECs could reduce fibrosis and promote repair of damaged tissue by modulating inflammation and promoting macrophage polarization from M1 macrophage to M2 macrophage [14, 31], but the effect of hAECs on macrophage phenotype switch in diabetic wounds is at present unknown. In this study, we found that hAECs could promote macrophage phenotype switch from M1 macrophage to M2 macrophage and switch proinflammatory status into prohealing status of diabetic wounds. These results from our in vitro and in vivo experiments are consistent with the previously reported data. Using RayBio human inflammation antibody arrays, we found that hAECs secreted IL-13 and TGF-β1, which contributed to the polarization of macrophages [32, 33]. This finding may partly explain the promoting effect of hAECs on macrophage polarization in vitro and in vivo.

Another factor contributing to refractory diabetic wound healing is the inhibited neovascularization [27]. Previous studies have reported that hAECs could promote neovascularization in the damaged tissues, including chemotherapy-induced ovarian damage and hyperoxia-induced lung injury [13, 34]. However, whether hAECs could promote neovascularization in diabetic wounds is currently unaware. In this study, we found increased capillary density in hAEC-treated wounds. Two likely underlying reasons may lead to this result. First, we suspected that the prohealing local environment of the hAEC-treated diabetic wounds associated with increased number of M2 macrophages and elevated levels of various growth factors promoted neovascularization indirectly. Second, our results showed that hAEC-CM could promote proliferation, migration, and tube formation of endothelial cells, suggesting the paracrine effects of hAECs on neovascularization directly. Using RayBio human inflammation antibody arrays and growth factor antibody arrays, we found that a variety of active peptides (PDGF, IL-8, and TGF-β1) were secreted from hAECs and these peptides are strongly associated with neovascularization [35–37]. This finding may partly explain the direct promoting effect of hAECs on neovascularization.

The present study has its limitation. First, notwithstanding some potential active peptides screened by RayBio antibody arrays may explain the effects of hAECs on the function of macrophages and endothelial cells; further studies are still necessary to find out the key active peptides and illuminate related signaling passway. Second, although the potential mechanisms of hAECs in promoting tissue repairs are not yet well-understood, the main therapeutic mechanisms of stem cells have been explained by paracrine effects rather than transdifferentiation, considering that only a fraction of grafted hAECs could survive in the damaged tissues [13, 20, 38]. Furthermore, impaired diabetic wound healing is characterized by hypoxia, impaired neovascularization, and excessive inflammation, which are extremely detrimental to the survival of hAECs in the wounds. For all the above reasons, it suggests that hAECs are hard to survive in the diabetic wounds for a long period of time and paracrine effects rather than transdifferentiation may play a key role of hAECs in promoting diabetic wound healing. However, further researches are still necessary to provide the direct evidences to determine the fate of hAECs after transplantation onto diabetic wounds.

5. Conclusions

Taken together, the results of the present study first showed that hAECs significantly accelerated the diabetic wound healing rate and granulation tissue formation, at least partially, by regulating inflammation and promoting neovascularization. hAECs are nontumorigenic, highly abundant, and low immunogenic, suggesting that it might be a safe and effective therapeutic approach to treat diabetic ulcers and other chronic wounds in clinics.

Acknowledgments

This work was funded by the National Natural Science Foundation of China (81701905, 81772076, 81372058, 81571897, and 81501645), the Shanghai Pujiang Program (17PJD043), "Twelfth Five-Year" Scientific Program of China (AWS14C001, 201502028, and AWS11J008), Clinical Key Discipline Project of Shanghai and China, and Shanghai Health System Excellent Talent Training Program (2017BR037).

References

[1] A. J. M. Boulton, D. G. Armstrong, S. F. Albert et al., "Comprehensive foot examination and risk assessment. A report of the Task Force of the Foot Care Interest Group of the American Diabetes Association, with endorsement by the American Association of Clinical Endocrinologists," *Physical Therapy*, vol. 88, no. 11, pp. 1436–1443, 2008.

[2] G. Pelizzo, M. A. Avanzini, A. Icaro Cornaglia et al., "Mesenchymal stromal cells for cutaneous wound healing in a rabbit model: pre-clinical study applicable in the pediatric surgical setting," *Journal of Translational Medicine*, vol. 13, no. 1, p. 219, 2015.

[3] S. E. Hanson, K. R. Kleinbeck, D. Cantu et al., "Local delivery of allogeneic bone marrow and adipose tissue-derived mesenchymal stromal cells for cutaneous wound healing in a porcine model," *Journal of Tissue Engineering and Regenerative Medicine*, vol. 10, no. 2, pp. E90–E100, 2016.

[4] H. Doi, Y. Kitajima, L. Luo et al., "Potency of umbilical cord blood- and Wharton's jelly-derived mesenchymal stem cells for scarless wound healing," *Scientific Reports*, vol. 6, no. 1, p. 18844, 2016.

[5] C. Caliari-Oliveira, J. N. U. Yaochite, L. N. Z. Ramalho et al., "Xenogeneic mesenchymal stromal cells improve wound healing and modulate the immune response in an extensive burn model," *Cell Transplantation*, vol. 25, no. 2, pp. 201–215, 2016.

[6] S. Wolbank, A. Peterbauer, M. Fahrner et al., "Dose-dependent immunomodulatory effect of human stem cells from amniotic membrane: a comparison with human mesenchymal stem cells from adipose tissue," *Tissue Engineering*, vol. 13, no. 6, pp. 1173–1183, 2007.

[7] G. Pratama, V. Vaghjiani, J. Y. Tee et al., "Changes in culture expanded human amniotic epithelial cells: implications for potential therapeutic applications," *PLoS One*, vol. 6, no. 11, article e26136, 2011.

[8] A. Toda, M. Okabe, T. Yoshida, and T. Nikaido, "The potential of amniotic membrane/amnion-derived cells for regeneration of various tissues," *Journal of Pharmacological Sciences*, vol. 105, no. 3, pp. 215–228, 2007.

[9] S. Murphy, S. Rosli, R. Acharya et al., "Amnion epithelial cell isolation and characterization for clinical use," *Current Protocols in Stem Cell Biology*, vol. 13, no. 1, pp. 1E.6.1–1E.6.25, 2010.

[10] J. L. Tan, Y. Z. Tan, R. Muljadi et al., "Amnion epithelial cells promote lung repair via lipoxin A4," *Stem Cells Translational Medicine*, vol. 6, no. 4, pp. 1085–1095, 2017.

[11] S. Murphy, R. Lim, H. Dickinson et al., "Human amnion epithelial cells prevent bleomycin-induced lung injury and preserve lung function," *Cell Transplantation*, vol. 20, no. 6, pp. 909–924, 2011.

[12] Q. Yang, M. Luo, P. Li, and H. Jin, "Transplantation of human amniotic epithelial cells repairs brachial plexus injury: pathological and biomechanical analyses," *Neural Regeneration Research*, vol. 9, no. 24, pp. 2159–2163, 2014.

[13] Q. Zhang, S. Bu, J. Sun et al., "Paracrine effects of human amniotic epithelial cells protect against chemotherapy-induced ovarian damage," *Stem Cell Research & Therapy*, vol. 8, no. 1, p. 270, 2017.

[14] J. L. Tan, S. T. Chan, E. M. Wallace, and R. Lim, "Human amnion epithelial cells mediate lung repair by directly modulating macrophage recruitment and polarization," *Cell Transplantation*, vol. 23, no. 3, pp. 319–328, 2014.

[15] D. Baltzis, I. Eleftheriadou, and A. Veves, "Pathogenesis and treatment of impaired wound healing in diabetes mellitus: new insights," *Advances in Therapy*, vol. 31, no. 8, pp. 817–836, 2014.

[16] S. C. Bryer, G. Fantuzzi, N. Van Rooijen, and T. J. Koh, "Urokinase-type plasminogen activator plays essential roles in macrophage chemotaxis and skeletal muscle regeneration," *Journal of Immunology*, vol. 180, no. 2, pp. 1179–1188, 2008.

[17] Y. Zhang, X. Liang, S. Liao et al., "Potent paracrine effects of human induced pluripotent stem cell-derived mesenchymal stem cells attenuate doxorubicin-induced cardiomyopathy," *Scientific Reports*, vol. 5, no. 1, article 11235, 2015.

[18] N. S. Tan and W. Wahli, "Studying wound repair in the mouse," *Current Protocols in Mouse Biology*, vol. 3, no. 3, pp. 171–185, 2013.

[19] Y. Zheng, X. Wang, S. Ji et al., "Mepenzolate bromide promotes diabetic wound healing by modulating inflammation and oxidative stress," *American Journal of Translational Research*, vol. 8, no. 6, pp. 2738–2747, 2016.

[20] B. Leaw, D. Zhu, J. Tan et al., "Human amnion epithelial cells rescue cell death via immunomodulation of microglia in a mouse model of perinatal brain injury, *Stem Cell Research & Therapy*, vol. 8, no. 1, p. 46, 2017.

[21] Y. S. Song, H. W. Joo, I. H. Park et al., ""Transplanted human amniotic epithelial cells secrete paracrine proangiogenic cytokines in rat model of myocardial infarction," *Cell Transplantation*, vol. 24, no. 10, pp. 2055–2064, 2015.

[22] J. Liu, R. Hua, Z. Gong et al., "Human amniotic epithelial cells inhibit CD4+ T cell activation in acute kidney injury patients by influencing the miR-101-c-Rel-IL-2 pathway," *Molecular Immunology*, vol. 81, pp. 76–84, 2017.

[23] A. Hodge, D. Lourensz, V. Vaghjiani et al., "Soluble factors derived from human amniotic epithelial cells suppress collagen production in human hepatic stellate cells," *Cytotherapy*, vol. 16, no. 8, pp. 1132–1144, 2014.

[24] R. Lim, A. Hodge, G. Moore, E. M. Wallace, and W. Sievert, "A pilot study evaluating the safety of intravenously administered human amnion epithelial cells for the treatment of hepatic fibrosis," *Frontiers in Pharmacology*, vol. 8, p. 549, 2017.

[25] S. Gordon and F. O. Martinez, "Alternative activation of macrophages: mechanism and functions," *Immunity*, vol. 32, no. 5, pp. 593–604, 2010.

[26] R. Blakytny and E. Jude, "The molecular biology of chronic wounds and delayed healing in diabetes," *Diabetic Medicine*, vol. 23, no. 6, pp. 594–608, 2006.

[27] V. Falanga, "Wound healing and its impairment in the diabetic foot," *The Lancet*, vol. 366, no. 9498, pp. 1736–1743, 2005.

[28] R. E. Mirza, M. M. Fang, W. J. Ennis, and T. J. Koh, "Blocking interleukin-1β induces a healing-associated wound macrophage phenotype and improves healing in type 2 diabetes," *Diabetes*, vol. 62, no. 7, pp. 2579–2587, 2013.

[29] E. C. Leal, E. Carvalho, A. Tellechea et al., "Substance P promotes wound healing in diabetes by modulating inflammation and macrophage phenotype," *The American Journal of Pathology*, vol. 185, no. 6, pp. 1638–1648, 2015.

[30] A. Tellechea, E. C. Leal, A. Kafanas et al., "Mast cells regulate wound healing in diabetes," *Diabetes*, vol. 65, no. 7, pp. 2006–2019, 2016.

[31] U. Manuelpillai, D. Lourensz, V. Vaghjiani et al., "Human amniotic epithelial cell transplantation induces markers of alternative macrophage activation and reduces established hepatic fibrosis," *PLoS One*, vol. 7, no. 6, article e38631, 2012.

[32] J. R. Grunwell, S. M. Yeligar, S. Stephenson et al., "TGF-β1 suppresses the type I IFN response and induces mitochondrial dysfunction in alveolar macrophages," *The Journal of Immunology*, vol. 200, no. 6, pp. 2115–2128, 2018.

[33] S. Gordon, "Alternative activation of macrophages," *Nature Reviews Immunology*, vol. 3, no. 1, pp. 23–35, 2003.

[34] D. Zhu, R. Muljadi, S. T. Chan et al., "Evaluating the impact of human amnion epithelial cells on angiogenesis," *Stem Cells International*, vol. 2016, Article ID 4565612, 13 pages, 2016.

[35] K. T. Bauerle, R. E. Schweppe, G. Lund et al., "Nuclear factor κB-dependent regulation of angiogenesis, and metastasis in an in vivo model of thyroid cancer is associated with secreted interleukin-8," *The Journal of Clinical Endocrinology & Metabolism*, vol. 99, no. 8, pp. E1436–E1444, 2014.

[36] A. Dong, C. Seidel, D. Snell et al., "Antagonism of PDGF-BB suppresses subretinal neovascularization and enhances the effects of blocking VEGF-A," *Angiogenesis*, vol. 17, no. 3, pp. 553–562, 2014.

[37] A. K. Wara, S. Foo, K. Croce et al., "TGF-β1 signaling and

Krüppel-like factor 10 regulate bone marrow-derived proangiogenic cell differentiation, function, and neovascularization," *Blood*, vol. 118, no. 24, pp. 6450–6460, 2011.

[38] P. Kuchroo, V. Dave, A. Vijayan, C. Viswanathan, and D. Ghosh, "Paracrine factors secreted by umbilical cord-derived mesenchymal stem cells induce angiogenesis in vitro by a VEGF-independent pathway," *Stem Cells and Development*, vol. 24, no. 4, pp. 437–450, 2015.

12

New Strategies and In Vivo Monitoring Methods for Stem Cell-Based Anticancer Therapies

Ping Wang[1] **and Aitor Aguirre**[2,3]

[1]*Precision Health Program, Department of Radiology, College of Human Medicine, Michigan State University, East Lansing, MI 48823, USA*
[2]*Division of Developmental and Stem Cell Biology, Institute for Quantitative Health Science and Engineering, Michigan State University, East Lansing, MI 48823, USA*
[3]*Department of Biomedical Engineering, College of Engineering, Michigan State University, East Lansing, MI 48823, USA*

Correspondence should be addressed to Aitor Aguirre; aaguirre@msu.edu

Guest Editor: Tiago Fernandes

Cancer is a devastating disease and the second cause of death in the developed world. Despite significant advances in recent years, such as the introduction of targeted therapies such as receptor tyrosine kinase inhibitors and immunotherapy, current approaches are insufficient to stop the advance of the disease and many cancer types remain largely intractable. In this review, we describe the latest and most revolutionary stem cell-based approaches for the treatment of cancer. We also summarize the emerging imaging modalities being applied for monitoring anticancer stem cell therapy success and discuss the implications of these novel technologies for precision medicine.

1. Introduction

Cancer is the second cause of death of men and women in the United States and a major health problem worldwide [1]. Mortality data for 2018 predicts 1.7 million new cancer cases and 0.6 million cancer-related deaths only in the US [2]. There is however room for hope. Among the top 10 causes of death, cancer is the only one steadily declining (about 26% for men and women in the US in the last 25 years), reflecting continuous improvements in diagnosis, care, and treatment [2]. Therapeutic intervention has significantly advanced in the last two decades, particularly with the introduction of targeted therapeutics such as receptor tyrosine kinase inhibitors (e.g., erlotinib in 2003) [3, 4] and immunotherapy (e.g., pembrolizumab in 2014) [5, 6]. These compounds exhibit much higher selectivity for cancer cells over conventional treatments and minimize side effects. Unfortunately, despite the extensive efforts invested in clinical development of cancer therapeutics, many cancers remain difficult or impossible to treat by traditional approaches. Furthermore, tumors evolve under treatment, and cells become widely chemoresistant and highly invasive, reducing treatment options as the disease progresses [7, 8]. An innovative approach for cancer treatment in recent years is the use of stem cell-based therapies [9, 10]. In this context, rather than regenerating, repairing, or replenishing tissues, stem cells are carriers that infiltrate tumors to deliver lethal payloads and tell us about the mechanisms of cancer cell survival and immune evasion. Stem cells possess at least two unique biological characteristics that make them ideally suited to fight cancer. For starters, embryos and tumors share many characteristics, including surface antigens, production of growth factors, and the capacity to evade, at least partially, the immune system [9]. In 1838, these similarities led Muller to formulate what could be considered the first stem cell theory of cancer origin (still highly controversial) [11]. In 1906 Schone would show that vaccination of animals with fetal tissues could render them partially resistant to cancer, demonstrating the close connection existing between cancer cells and stem cells [11]. More recent efforts have established

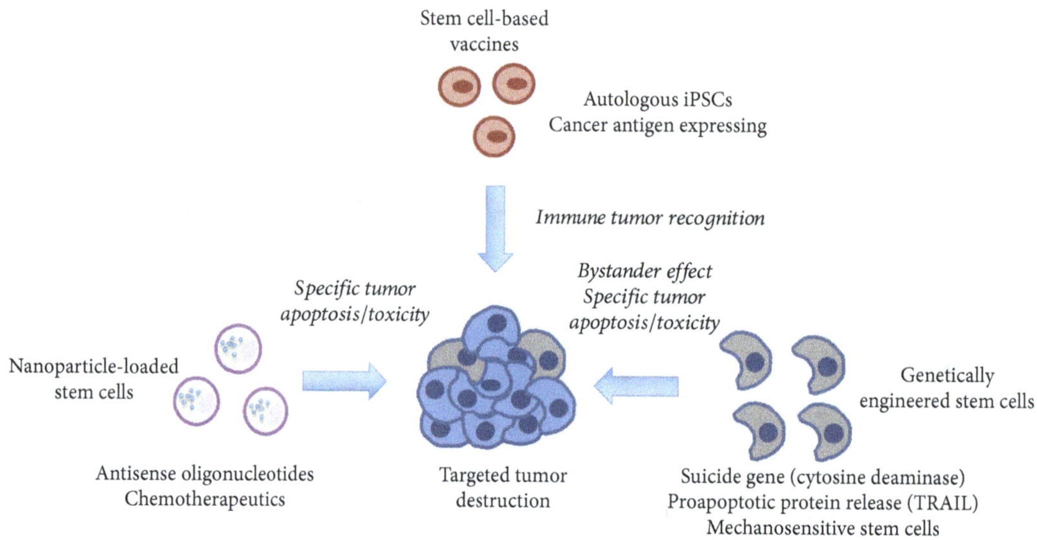

FIGURE 1: Stem cell-based strategies for anticancer therapy. Tumors can be specifically targeted with stem cells to make them vulnerable to therapy. Top: stem cell-based vaccines leverage the similarities between cancer cells and stem cells to promote immune tumor recognition; left: nanoparticle-loaded stem cells exhibit efficient homing to tumors, where they deliver their payload in the form of chemotherapies or apoptosis-inducing oligonucleotides; right: genetically engineered stem cells can express and release proapoptotic proteins or ligands in the tumor microenvironment or contain enzymes metabolizing prodrugs to their cytotoxic form (e.g., cytosine deaminase). Stem cells can also be engineered to recognize biophysical features of the tumor microenvironment before activating their engineered cytotoxic program.

beyond any doubt that stem cells and cancer cells share many common features at the molecular level, including the activation of developmental signaling pathways promoting cell survival, proliferation, self-renewal, and tissue invasion (e.g., Wnt, Notch, Hippo, and epithelial to mesenchymal transition) [12, 13]. It might be due to these similarities that stem cells also exhibit strong tropism towards tumors, which in turn makes them attractive candidates for targeted delivery of drugs or other compounds with minimal side effects. Strategies for fighting cancer with stem cell-based therapies fall into two broad categories: (1) stem cell vaccines, using the identity property, and (2) stem cell carriers, exploiting their tumor-tropic behavior. The different strategies and examples of their use can be found in Figure 1. Additionally, Table 1 includes a number of ongoing clinical trials in the US using stem cell-based therapies for anticancer treatment to highlight the relevance of this growing field for translational applications.

2. Stem Cell-Based Antitumor Vaccines

The idea of generating immunity against cancer cells (immunotherapy) is not new and has been pursued for many decades. In the 19th century, scientists noticed the similarity between embryonic cells and cancer cells. It was observed that when mice had been exposed to fetal tissue from another mouse, the recipient would reject transplanted tumors (for a detailed review on this topic, see [11]). These ideas were explored in-depth during the following decades, particularly during the 60s and 70s. Stem cells and cancer cells share significant cellular and molecular properties. Immunization with embryonal material was enough to prevent tumor growth and to suppress tumor formation by administration of carcinogens [11]. However, due to technical and ethical limitations at the time (inoculation of human fetal tissue would not be feasible in humans), these approaches were progressively abandoned. This changed at the turn of the century, with the enormous expansion in the stem cell biology in the last two decades, the establishment of numerous human embryonic stem cell lines and the introduction of induced pluripotent stem cells [14, 15]. These advances render the previous ethical and social concerns associated with fetal immunization obsolete, leading to a resurging interest in human anticancer stem cell-based vaccines.

In a breakthrough study published very recently, Kooreman et al. reported using irradiated induced pluripotent stem cells in conjunction with adjuvant therapy to vaccinate mice against a wide number of cancer types, including breast cancer, mesothelioma, and melanoma with great success [16]. Using RNA-seq, the authors found that iPSCs and cancer cells possessed a similar signature in several potential cancer antigens, suggesting that iPSCs could be used to prime the host's immune system. This approach has several advantages, including use of autologous cells minimizing host rejection and exposure to known and unknown cancer-associated antigens simultaneously to promote a more solid immune response against the tumor. As a proof of concept, the authors injected mouse iPSCs in mice and then transplanted cancer cells (breast, melanoma) in subcutaneous and orthotopic models. In all cases, a spectacular regression of the tumors was observed when compared with nonvaccinated control mice [16]. It was possible to determine that B and T lymphocytes were primarily responsible for this activity. Although iPSC vaccination was successful in preventing or reducing tumor growth, it was insufficient as a therapy to prevent the growth of established tumors, suggesting tumor immunosuppressive mechanisms

Table 1: Current clinical trials using stem cell-based therapies for anticancer treatment in the US.

Title	NCT number	Status	Sponsors	Enrollment	Funding	Start	Location
Generation of Cancer Antigen-Specific T-cells From Human Induced Pluripotent Stem Cells (iPSC) for Research and Potential Future Therapy	NCT03407040	Enrolling by invitation	National Cancer Institute (NCI), National Institutes of Health Clinical Center (CC)	7000	NIH	30 Jan. 18	National Institutes of Health Clinical Center, Bethesda
Stem Cells in NF1 Patients with Tumors of the Central Nervous System	NCT03332030	Recruiting	Children's Research Institute	20	Other	27 Nov. 15	Children's National Medical Center, Washington
Neural Stem Cell Based Virotherapy of Newly Diagnosed Malignant Glioma	NCT03072134	Recruiting	Northwestern University	36	Other	24 Apr. 17	Northwestern Memorial Hospital, Chicago
Umbilical & Cord Blood (CB) Derived CAR-Engineered NK Cells for B Lymphoid Malignancies	NCT03056339	Recruiting	MD Anderson Cancer Center	36	Other	21 Jun. 17	University of Texas MD Anderson Cancer Center, Houston
Mesenchymal Stem Cells (MSC) for Ovarian Cancer	NCT02530047	Active, not recruiting	MD Anderson Cancer Center	5	Other	16 May 16	University of Texas MD Anderson Cancer Center, Houston
MV-NIS Infected Mesenchymal Stem Cells in Treating Patients with Recurrent Ovarian Cancer	NCT02068794	Recruiting	Mayo Clinic, National Cancer Institute (NCI)	54	Other, NIH	Mar. 14	Mayo Clinic, Rochester
Genetically Modified Neural Stem Cells, Flucytosine, and Leucovorin for Treating Patients with Recurrent High-Grade Gliomas	NCT02015819	Active, not recruiting	City of Hope Medical Center, National Cancer Institute (NCI)	18	Other, NIH	7 Oct. 14	City of Hope Medical Center, Duarte
Allogeneic Human Bone Marrow Derived Mesenchymal Stem Cells in Localized Prostate Cancer	NCT01983709	Terminated	Sidney Kimmel Comprehensive Cancer Center at Johns Hopkins	7	Other	Oct. 13	Johns Hopkins Hospital, Baltimore
Stem Cell Transplantation as Immunotherapy for Hematologic Malignancies	NCT00143559	Completed	St. Jude Children's Research Hospital	17	Other	Aug. 05	St. Jude Children's Research Hospital, Memphis

Data was obtained from NIH clinicaltrials.gov by performing searches for cancer-related clinical trials using the following terms: stem cell-based anticancer vaccine, engineered stem cells, targeted stem cell therapy, stem cell virus carrier, stem cell nanoparticle carrier, and stem cell immunotherapy.

might be still too strong [16]. Combination of iPSC-based vaccines with targeted immunotherapy might be an interesting avenue for treatment in the future. Of note, the authors did not detect any negative effects derived from iPSC vaccination, such as autoimmunity or teratoma formation, making this approach more attractive for translation into the clinic.

An alternative approach at stem cell-based anticancer vaccination is the use of iPSCs to derive dendritic cells (DCs), which play an essential role in T cell activation, engineered to express tumor-specific antigens. Kitadani et al. applied this concept to the treatment of gastrointestinal cancer [17]. After generating iPSC-derived DCs (iPSDCs) with typical DC markers and cytokine secretion, iPSDCs were engineered to express carcinoembryonic antigen (CEA) employing adenoviral transduction. T cells from healthy human donors were exposed to the CEA-iPSDCs in vitro and then c-cultured with a panel of gastrointestinal cancer cell lines. Human T cells responded with strong cytotoxic activity to cancer cells expressing CEA, but not others [17]. Transplantation of mouse iPSDCs into a mouse subcutaneous model of gastrointestinal cancer resulted in remarkable cytotoxicity and tumor growth inhibition (~4-fold smaller tumor volume compared to controls) [17]. More studies will be necessary to determine the safety and efficacy of stem cell-based vaccines for controlling or eradicating human tumors; however, present advances support their feasibility and guarantee further research.

3. Targeted Suicide Stem Cells to Destroy Tumors

Stem cells have a significant capacity to home to tumors due to shared chemotactic and signaling pathways with cancer cells [9]. This property can be exploited for targeted therapies by placing specific stem cell types into the tumor mass. Protocols for growing and maintaining many different types of tissue-specific stem cells are now available and have significantly improved over the last decade [18, 19]. Introducing genetic modifications in stem cells is now easier than ever before since the implementation of CRISPR technologies [20]. These technical advances facilitate the making of engineered stem cell types for targeting tumors based on their origin and characteristics with minimal side effects in other tissues or organs. Successful attempts following this strategy can be found for the treatment of aggressive brain tumors, which are among the most deadly and challenging cancers to treat. Survival for patients with glioblastoma multiforme (GBM) ranges from 12 to 15 months, and treatment options are very limited and consist on aggressive chemo and radiotherapy [21]. Attempts to efficiently target glioblastoma have traditionally been insufficient for sustained therapeutic benefit [21]. Using a transdifferentiation approach, Bagó et al. generated autologous neural stem cells from skin fibroblasts for theranostic applications (iNSCs) [22]. The authors determined that iNSCs exhibited strong tumor-homing activity towards GBM cell lines due to CXCR4 chemotaxis [22]. The authors decided to genetically engineer iNSCs to express a secreted variant of the proapoptotic molecule TRAIL (TNF-related apoptosis-inducing ligand) and transplanted cells intravenously into mice carrying human glioblastoma xenografts. Over a period of 3 weeks, iNSCs lead to a 250-fold tumor mass reduction and a median increase in survival from 22 to 49 days. Other genetic modifications of iNSCs, such as ganciclovir prodrug therapy, were also successful. To mimic the postoperative setting in humans, mice with xenografted GBM were subjected to surgical resection and iNSC therapy. The treatment delayed the regrowth of GBMs 3-fold and extended survival from 46 to 60 days [22]. Taken together, these results suggest that tumor-homing stem cells are a powerful option for therapy, particularly in inaccessible tumors. Locally residing stem cells are present in almost every tissue in the body, potentially making this approach applicable to other tumor types.

4. Targeting the Metastatic Niche with Mechanosensitive Stem Cells

Another aspect of cancer that can be tackled with stem cell therapy is metastasis. Cancer metastases are responsible for 90% of cancer deaths [23, 24]. Treatments to directly target metastatic tumors are sorely lacking, and surgical resection is not always a feasible option, particularly when multiple metastatic sites are present. Interestingly, metastases frequently differ from their tissues of origin by possessing largely altered extracellular microenvironments, which leads to altered matrix stiffness, particularly in tumors with strong lysyl oxidase (LOX) expression (e.g., breast cancer metastases have 15-fold increased stiffness versus normal breast tissue) [25, 26]. Taking these properties into consideration, Liu et al. hypothesized that a mechanosensitive mesenchymal stem cell-based system, named mechanoresponsive cell system (MRCS), could be created to target cancer metastases [27]. Systemically infused MSCs target tumor sites due to naturally occurring combinations of tumor tropic molecules (growth factors, cytokines), and matrix stiffness is an important contributor to their behavior, including chemotaxis and differentiation, indicating that a fine-tuned mechanoresponsive machinery is already present in this cell type [27, 28]. Autologous MSCs can be easily obtained from a patient's adipose tissue or differentiated from iPSCs and expanded *in vitro* [29]. MSCs sense and transduce extracellular mechanical cues through the Hippo pathway effector YAP. In soft substrates, YAP remains in the cytoplasm in its inactive form, while hard substrates promote YAP nuclear translocation and associated transcriptional programs [30]. Taking advantage of this property, the authors genetically engineered MSCs to express the suicide gene cytosine deaminase (CD) under the control of the YAP promoter (referred to as CD-MCRS) [27]. In this system conditions, systemically infused CD-MCRS cells are attracted to metastatic sites and, once exposed to the matrix stiffness present at those locations, start expressing CD. Administration of 5-fluorocytosine at this point specifically kills metastatic cells by the bystander effect. To provide proof of concept on this approach, Liu et al. used mice transplanted with MDA-MB-231 breast cancer cells into the lung to mimic metastatic spread [27]. As expected, infused CD-MCRS homed to the lungs and activated CD expression. When administered in conjunction with 5-fluorocytosine, metastatic tumors shrank 2- to 3-fold and treated animals experienced significantly improved survival [27]. Overall, these results show great promise for the treatment of metastatic cancer and highlight the importance of using the biophysical properties of the tumor environment for targeted therapies.

5. Stem Cells as a Nanoparticle Delivery System

The tumor homing characteristics of stem cells can be leveraged to specifically deliver particles to tumor sites [31]. In a similar approach to the one described before for metastatic mechanosensing, MSCs can be induced to take up drug-loaded nanoparticles. Zhao et al. attempted this approach by loading MSCs with doxorubicin-containing poly-lactic-coglycolic acid nanoparticles (PLGA-DOX) [32]. MSCs readily took up PLGA-DOX and, due to low bioavailability of the drug in this composition, received low cytotoxicity. When transplanted into mice bearing lung metastases, MSCs homed to the tumor sites and locally released DOX, resulting in a significantly reduced number of tumor nodules (~3-fold reduction) [32]. An interesting recent variation of this approach involves the use of a physical phenomenon known as magnetic hyperthermia. Magnetic hyperthermia consists on the heating of tissues by means of magnetic nanoparticles and alternating magnetic fields (AMF). MSCs can be loaded with superparamagnetic iron oxide nanoparticles (SPIONs), which have minimal toxicity [33]. Once MSCs have homed into the tumor, SPIONs are delivered to the surrounding cells by exosome delivery. At this point, application of a high-frequency AMF will produce a localized hyperthermic effect reaching temperatures of 42–45 Celsius at intervals of 20 minutes. This localized effect exerts extensive damage to tumor cells in vitro, with up to 80% growth inhibition [33]. Although very promising, stem cell-mediated-magnetic hyperthermia therapeutic effects have not been explored *in vivo* in enough detail yet.

6. Stem Cells as Oncolytic Virus Carriers

Oncolytic viruses are an emerging class of cancer therapeutics. In 2017, the FDA approved the first immunogenic oncolytic virus (OV) for therapy in advanced melanoma [34]. However, the systemic administration of OV can lead to serious side effects. To circumvent this problem, Du et al. designed a strategy in which MSCs could act as oncolytic herpes simplex virus (oHSV) carriers into the tumor mass [34]. Using a mouse model that closely recapitulates melanoma progression, the authors demonstrated the therapeutic efficacy of oHSV-loaded MSCs. The cells, which were delivered via carotid artery, efficiently homed to the tumor metastases and reduced tumor size and foci number by ~2- to 4-fold [34]. Furthermore, treatment also extended survival by approximately 20 days. The authors have also demonstrated the efficacy of this approach in other tumor types before [35]. Overall, oncolytic virus therapies remain a strong option for therapy in the close future and this study demonstrates that further refinement using stem cells as carriers can improve therapeutic outcomes and minimize side effects.

7. Stem Cell Reprogramming Technologies for Cancer Immunotherapy

The field of cancer immunotherapy has seen important advances in recent years, including several clinical trials and approval of pembrolizumab. Transfer of T cell receptor (TCR) genes into patients' peripheral T cells has achieved good clinical outcomes [36], indicating that targeting a single antigen can be effective for some types of cancer. In addition, T cell expressing chimeric antigen receptor (CAR), an engineered receptor molecule, which combines an antibody recognition domain and cytoplasmic signaling domains, has demonstrated therapeutic effect in a certain type of leukemia [37]. In both TCR and CAR engineering, peripheral T cells are transduced by a retrovirus, bringing about the risk of tumorigenicity due to the random integration of a transfected gene into the genome. Moreover, in the autologous setting, it would be costly to produce T cells. To address this issue, a strategy has been proposed to regenerate T cells utilizing iPSC technology. Themeli et al. reported that CAR-expressing T cells were regenerated from iPSCs transduced with a CAR gene. iPSCs were generated by retrovirus reprogramming T cells isolated from peripheral blood of healthy donors. The CAR sequence specific for CD19 was inserted into iPSCs using CRISPR/Cas9. iPSC-derived CAR specific-T cells were phenotypically similar to innate T$\gamma\delta$ cells and showed ability to inhibit tumor growth in a xenograft animal model [38–40]. This strategy brings hope that CAR-T therapy may also work for other types of cancer beside hematologic malignancies. Certain obstacles associated with CAR-T including further customization of the technology to recognize specific/other tumor types and predicting and limiting cross-reactivity need to be resolved. CRISPR/Cas9 technologies will be useful to target CAR-T gene constructs to genomic safe harbor sites, reducing the risk of undesired effects. However, challenges related to the use of this cutting-edge technology for human therapy remain. Two recently published studies reported that stem cells whose genomes were successfully edited by CRISPR-Cas9 had the potential to be tumorigenic themselves due to p53 mutations. These results indicated that p53 and related genes should be monitored when developing stem cell-based therapies utilizing CRISPR-Cas9 [41, 42].

8. New Imaging Modalities for Stem Cell Theranostics in Cancer

Stem cell-based therapies have enormous potential for cancer treatment. For maximal efficacy, these promising therapies require targeted cell delivery to specific sites followed by successful cell engraftment. Various imaging methods have been applied for in vivo tracing of stem cells, including optimal imaging, nuclear imaging, and magnetic resonance imaging. Each imaging modality has its advantages and limitations in terms of sensitivity, tissue penetration, spatial

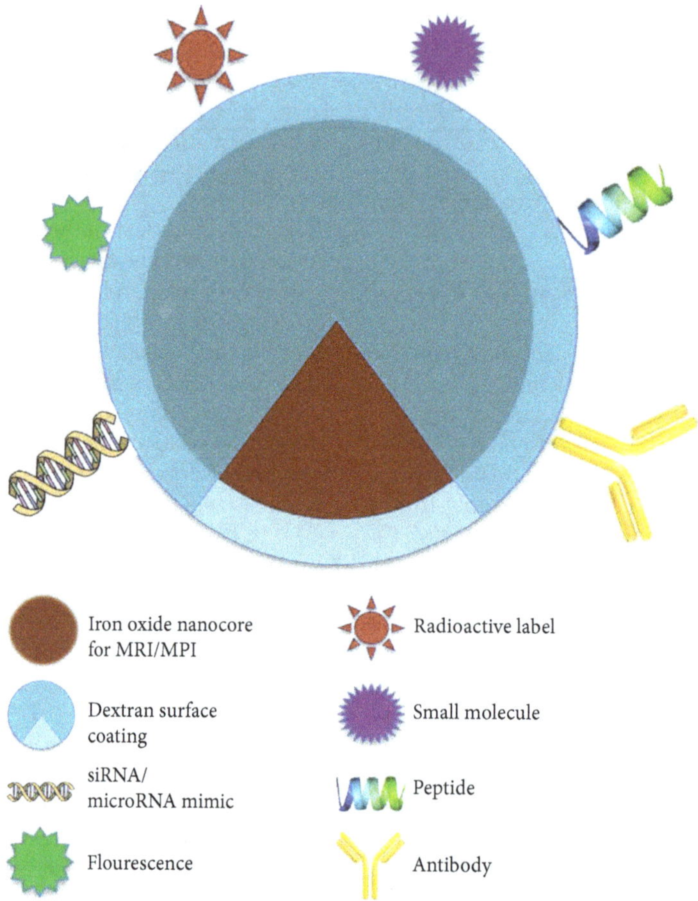

FIGURE 2: Theranostic magnetic nanoparticles for stem cell anticancer therapy. Iron oxide nanoparticles can be functionalized by applying a dextran coating. Different biologically active substances (antibodies, RNA/DNA, and drugs) intended to target or damage the tumor, or labeling probes for tracing and diagnostics, can be then tethered to the nanoparticle for theranostic applications.

resolution, and clinical potential [43, 44]. Optical imaging is a group of technologies that produce the image formed by the light rays from a self-luminous or an illuminated object that traverse an optical system. So far, this method is mainly restricted in tracking transplanted cells in animal models. In addition, low spatial resolution and limited tissue penetration are some disadvantages related to this method [45]. Nuclear imaging is based on the use of radiolabeled ligands targeting cell-specific antigens, receptors, metabolites, or pharmacologic agents. Many isotopes and labeling strategies have been investigated for stem cell labeling for nuclear imaging [46]. Lack of available isotopes, low spatial resolution, poor cellular uptake, and potential negative affect in cellular proliferation are some weaknesses of this modality. Magnetic resonance imaging (MRI) has some advantages over other modalities used for in vivo cellular imaging. It is clinically applicable and does not use radiation; it has high spatial resolution and unlimited tissue penetration, which can provide anatomical information of localizing transplanted cells. For MRI detection, stem cells usually need to be labeled with imaging contrast agents before transplantation. Superparamagnetic iron oxide (SPIO) nanoparticles, which result in signal-intensity voids or hypointense regions in T2-weighted or T2*-weighted MR images [43], are the most common imaging probes used for tracking transplanted stem cells using MRI. However, signal voids in MR images produced by iron-labeled cells/cell clusters were difficult to distinguish from other low MR signals produced by tissue including intestine and blood vessel structures or artifacts [47]. Magnetic particle imaging (MPI) is an emerging imaging technique introduced in 2005 that directly identifies the intense magnetization of SPIOs rather than indirectly detecting SPIOs via signal dropouts, which could potentially overcome the disadvantages of cell tracking with MRI. MPI unambiguously detects superparamagnetic iron oxide nanoparticles with high specificity and sensitivity and other advantages over previous methods, such as the absence of background signal, linear quantitative ability, and high potential for clinic translation. MPI's great specificity results from its high image contrast, since magnetic particles serve as the only source for signal [48]. MPI's high sensitivity derives from the direct detection of the electronic magnetization of SPIO nanoparticles, which is 10^8 times larger than the nuclear magnetization of protons seen in MRI [49], translating to a sensitivity to detect hundreds of magnetic nanoparticle-labeled cells with current hardware. MPI's safety is driven using clinically approved iron oxide nanoparticles, which have been proven safe for patients with compromised renal function. This new imaging modality has been tested for in vivo monitoring of transplanted stem cells. Zheng et al. firstly utilized MPI to monitor SPIO-labeled human embryonic stem cell- (hESC-) derived neural progenitor cells (NPCs) in vivo in a rat model. The results showed a 200-cell detection limit in vitro and in vivo, allowing them to monitor graft clearance over 87 days in the animal's brain using MPI [50]. In a more recent study, Zheng and colleagues imaged intravenously transplanted mesenchymal stem cells (MSCs) using MPI. Their studies demonstrated that labeled MSCs immediately entrapped in the lung tissue posttransplantation and then relocated to the liver within one day. Longitudinal MPI demonstrated a clearance half-life of MSC iron- oxide labels in the liver at 4.6 days [51]. These first in vivo MPI results indicate that MPI offers strong utility for quantitating transplanted stem cells labeled using SPIO. These results demonstrate that MPI's quantitative capacity arises from the linear signal change with nanoparticle concentration, which occurs independent of tissue depth. For clinical translation, a whole-body human MPI system for high-speed imaging is currently being developed and the first one has already delivered initial images. In terms of SPIO probe availability for MPI, there are several FDA-approved iron oxide nanoparticles under several brand names including ferucarbotran (Resovist®, Schering AG, Germany), ferumoxtran-10 (Sinerem®, Guerbet, France; Combidex® Advanced Magnetics Inc., MA, USA), and ferumoxytol (Feraheme®, AMAG Pharmaceuticals, Cambridge, MA) [52]. In addition, VivoTrax™ is provided for preclinical use by Magnetic Insight, CA, USA. Iron oxide nanoparticles used for cell labeling in MRI/MPI serve not only as imaging probes but also as nanocarriers for therapies. Various functional moieties could be attached to the coating of nanoparticle that serve as targeting macromolecules, therapeutic payloads, or additional imaging tags for multimodality in vivo imaging [53, 54]. These multifunctional nanodrugs could be carried by stem cells towards cancer cells for theranostic cancer treatment (Figure 2).

9. Perspectives and Conclusions

In conclusion, stem cell-based anticancer therapies offer great promise for the treatment of cancer. Although stem cells might be useful as cancer therapies of their own, they might also serve as powerful adjuvants in combination with traditional chemoradiotherapy treatment, or after surgery. Furthermore, cancer patient-derived iPSCs can be used to draw association between genotype and treatment responses and to identify biomarkers to inform patient selection for precision oncology [55, 56]. Emerging technologies such as CRISPR/Cas9 genome engineering and novel theranostic tools will be important factors in the successful implementation and continued improvement of stem cell-based anticancer therapies [57]. Many challenges remain, particularly regarding safety of stem cell transplants and CRISPR/Cas9 genomic manipulations. These issues are the focus of intense research and will be progressively clarified in the near future.

Acknowledgments

The work in the Aguirre Laboratory is supported by the National Heart, Lung, and Blood Institute of the National Institutes of Health under award number K01HL135464.

References

[1] R. L. Siegel, K. D. Miller, and A. Jemal, "Cancer statistics, 2017," *CA: a Cancer Journal for Clinicians*, vol. 67, no. 1, pp. 7–30, 2017.

[2] R. L. Siegel, K. D. Miller, and A. Jemal, "Cancer statistics, 2015," *CA: a Cancer Journal for Clinicians*, vol. 65, no. 1, pp. 5–29, 2015.

[3] F. A. Shepherd, J. Rodrigues Pereira, T. Ciuleanu et al., "Erlotinib in previously treated non-small-cell lung cancer," *The New England Journal of Medicine*, vol. 353, no. 2, pp. 123–132, 2005.

[4] M. Hojjat-Farsangi, "Small-molecule inhibitors of the receptor tyrosine kinases: promising tools for targeted cancer therapies," *International Journal of Molecular Sciences*, vol. 15, no. 8, pp. 13768–13801, 2014.

[5] N. L. Syn, M. W. L. Teng, T. S. K. Mok, and R. A. Soo, "De-novo and acquired resistance to immune checkpoint targeting," *The Lancet Oncology*, vol. 18, no. 12, pp. e731–e741, 2017.

[6] R. H. Vonderheide and K. L. Nathanson, "Immunotherapy at large: the road to personalized cancer vaccines," *Nature Medicine*, vol. 19, no. 9, pp. 1098–1100, 2013.

[7] L. N. Abdullah and E. K.-H. Chow, "Mechanisms of chemoresistance in cancer stem cells," *Clinical and Translational Medicine*, vol. 2, no. 1, p. 3, 2013.

[8] H. C. Zheng, "The molecular mechanisms of chemoresistance in cancers," *Oncotarget*, vol. 8, no. 35, pp. 59950–59964, 2017.

[9] D. W. Stuckey and K. Shah, "Stem cell-based therapies for cancer treatment: separating hope from hype," *Nature Reviews. Cancer*, vol. 14, no. 10, pp. 683–691, 2014.

[10] C. L. Zhang, T. Huang, B. L. Wu, W. X. He, and D. Liu, "Stem cells in cancer therapy: opportunities and challenges," *Oncotarget*, vol. 8, no. 43, pp. 75756–75766, 2017.

[11] B. G. Brewer, R. A. Mitchell, A. Harandi, and J. W. Eaton, "Embryonic vaccines against cancer: an early history," *Experimental and Molecular Pathology*, vol. 86, no. 3, pp. 192–197, 2009.

[12] E. Batlle and H. Clevers, "Cancer stem cells revisited," *Nature Medicine*, vol. 23, no. 10, pp. 1124–1134, 2017.

[13] D. Nassar and C. Blanpain, "Cancer stem cells: basic concepts and therapeutic implications," *Annual Review of Pathology*, vol. 11, no. 1, pp. 47–76, 2016.

[14] K. Takahashi, K. Tanabe, M. Ohnuki et al., "Induction of pluripotent stem cells from adult human fibroblasts by defined factors," *Cell*, vol. 131, no. 5, pp. 861–872, 2007.

[15] J. A. Thomson, J. Itskovitz-Eldor, S. S. Shapiro et al., "Embryonic stem cell lines derived from human blastocysts," *Science*, vol. 282, no. 5391, pp. 1145–1147, 1998.

[16] N. G. Kooreman, Y. Kim, P. E. de Almeida et al., "Autologous iPSC-based vaccines elicit anti-tumor responses *in vivo*," *Cell Stem Cell*, vol. 22, no. 4, pp. 501–513.e7, 2018.

[17] J. Kitadani, T. Ojima, H. Iwamoto et al., "Cancer vaccine therapy using carcinoembryonic antigen - expressing dendritic cells generated from induced pluripotent stem cells," *Scientific Reports*, vol. 8, no. 1, p. 4569, 2018.

[18] J. Wu and J. C. Izpisua Belmonte, "Stem cells: a renaissance in human biology research," *Cell*, vol. 165, no. 7, pp. 1572–1585, 2016.

[19] C. E. Murry and G. Keller, "Differentiation of embryonic stem cells to clinically relevant populations: lessons from embryonic development," *Cell*, vol. 132, no. 4, pp. 661–680, 2008.

[20] W. T. Hendriks, C. R. Warren, and C. A. Cowan, "Genome editing in human pluripotent stem cells: approaches, pitfalls, and solutions," *Cell Stem Cell*, vol. 18, no. 1, pp. 53–65, 2016.

[21] M. Davis, "Glioblastoma: overview of disease and treatment," *Clinical Journal of Oncology Nursing*, vol. 20, no. 5, pp. S2–S8, 2016.

[22] J. R. Bagó, O. Okolie, R. Dumitru et al., "Tumor-homing cytotoxic human induced neural stem cells for cancer therapy," *Science Translational Medicine*, vol. 9, no. 375, article eaah6510, 2017.

[23] A. W. Lambert, D. R. Pattabiraman, and R. A. Weinberg, "Emerging biological principles of metastasis," *Cell*, vol. 168, no. 4, pp. 670–691, 2017.

[24] S. Valastyan and R. A. Weinberg, "Tumor metastasis: molecular insights and evolving paradigms," *Cell*, vol. 147, no. 2, pp. 275–292, 2011.

[25] D. A. Kirschmann, E. A. Seftor, S. F. Fong et al., "A molecular role for lysyl oxidase in breast cancer invasion," *Cancer Research*, vol. 62, no. 15, pp. 4478–4483, 2002.

[26] T. H. Wang, S. M. Hsia, and T. M. Shieh, "Lysyl oxidase and the tumor microenvironment," *International Journal of Molecular Sciences*, vol. 18, no. 1, 2017.

[27] L. Liu, S. X. Zhang, W. Liao et al., "Mechanoresponsive stem cells to target cancer metastases through biophysical cues," *Science Translational Medicine*, vol. 9, no. 400, article eaan2966, 2017.

[28] A. J. Engler, S. Sen, H. L. Sweeney, and D. E. Discher, "Matrix elasticity directs stem cell lineage specification," *Cell*, vol. 126, no. 4, pp. 677–689, 2006.

[29] P. A. Zuk, M. Zhu, P. Ashjian et al., "Human adipose tissue is a source of multipotent stem cells," *Molecular Biology of the Cell*, vol. 13, no. 12, pp. 4279–4295, 2002.

[30] F. X. Yu and K. L. Guan, "The hippo pathway: regulators and regulations," *Genes & Development*, vol. 27, no. 4, pp. 355–371, 2013.

[31] M. R. Reagan and D. L. Kaplan, "Concise review: mesenchymal stem cell tumor-homing: detection methods in disease model systems," *Stem Cells*, vol. 29, no. 6, pp. 920–927, 2011.

[32] Y. Zhao, S. Tang, J. Guo et al., "Targeted delivery of doxorubicin by nano-loaded mesenchymal stem cells for lung melanoma metastases therapy," *Scientific Reports*, vol. 7, no. 1, 2017.

[33] U. Altanerova, M. Babincova, P. Babinec et al., "Human mesenchymal stem cell-derived iron oxide exosomes allow targeted ablation of tumor cells via magnetic hyperthermia," *International Journal of Nanomedicine*, vol. 12, pp. 7923–7936, 2017.

[34] W. du, I. Seah, O. Bougazzoul et al., "Stem cell-released oncolytic herpes simplex virus has therapeutic efficacy in brain metastatic melanomas," *Proceedings of the National Academy of Sciences of the United States of America*, vol. 114, no. 30, pp. E6157–E6165, 2017.

[35] M. Duebgen, J. Martinez-Quintanilla, K. Tamura et al., "Stem cells loaded with multimechanistic oncolytic herpes simplex virus variants for brain tumor therapy," *JNCI: Journal of the National Cancer Institute*, vol. 106, no. 6, article dju090, 2014.

[36] P. F. Robbins, R. A. Morgan, S. A. Feldman et al., "Tumor regression in patients with metastatic synovial cell sarcoma and melanoma using genetically engineered lymphocytes reactive with NY-ESO-1," *Journal of Clinical Oncology*, vol. 29, no. 7, pp. 917–924, 2011.

[37] S. S. Neelapu, S. Tummala, P. Kebriaei et al., "Chimeric antigen receptor T-cell therapy - assessment and management of toxicities," *Nature Reviews. Clinical Oncology*, vol. 15, no. 1, pp. 47–62, 2018.

[38] M. Themeli, C. C. Kloss, G. Ciriello et al., "Generation of tumor-targeted human T lymphocytes from induced pluripotent stem cells for cancer therapy," *Nature Biotechnology*, vol. 31, no. 10, pp. 928–933, 2013.

[39] H. Kawamoto, K. Masuda, S. Nagano, and T. Maeda, "Cloning and expansion of antigen-specific T cells using iPS cell technology: development of "off-the-shelf" T cells for the use in allogeneic transfusion settings," *International Journal of Hematology*, vol. 107, no. 3, pp. 271–277, 2018.

[40] F. Rami, H. Mollainezhad, and M. Salehi, "Induced pluripotent stem cell as a new source for cancer immunotherapy," *Genetics Research International*, vol. 2016, Article ID 3451807, 9 pages, 2016.

[41] R. J. Ihry, K. A. Worringer, M. R. Salick et al., "p53 inhibits CRISPR-Cas9 engineering in human pluripotent stem cells," *Nature Medicine*, vol. 24, no. 7, pp. 939–946, 2018.

[42] E. Haapaniemi, S. Botla, J. Persson, B. Schmierer, and J. Taipale, "CRISPR-Cas9 genome editing induces a p53-mediated DNA damage response," *Nature Medicine*, vol. 24, no. 7, pp. 927–930, 2018.

[43] P. Wang and A. Moore, "Molecular imaging of stem cell transplantation for neurodegenerative diseases," *Current Pharmaceutical Design*, vol. 18, no. 28, pp. 4426–4440, 2012.

[44] P. Wang, F. Petrella, L. Nicosia, M. Bellomi, and S. Rizzo, "Molecular imaging of stem cell transplantation for liver diseases: monitoring, clinical translation, and theranostics," *Stem Cells International*, vol. 2016, Article ID 4058656, 8 pages, 2016.

[45] M. Mangoni, L. Livi, G. Biti et al., "Stem cell tracking: toward clinical application in oncology?," *Tumori*, vol. 98, no. 5, pp. 535–542, 2012.

[46] C. Wu, G. Ma, J. Li et al., "In vivo cell tracking via ^{18}F-fluorodeoxyglucose labeling: a review of the preclinical and clinical applications in cell-based diagnosis and therapy," *Clinical Imaging*, vol. 37, no. 1, pp. 28–36, 2013.

[47] P. Wang, Z. Medarova, and A. Moore, "Molecular imaging: a promising tool to monitor islet transplantation," *Journal of Transplantation*, vol. 2011, Article ID 202915, 14 pages, 2011.

[48] N. Panagiotopoulos, R. L. Duschka, M. Ahlborg et al., "Magnetic particle imaging: current developments and future directions," *International Journal of Nanomedicine*, vol. 10, pp. 3097–3114, 2015.

[49] P. Wang, P. W. Goodwill, P. Pandit et al., "Magnetic particle imaging of islet transplantation in the liver and under the kidney capsule in mouse models," *Quantitative Imaging in*

Medicine and Surgery, vol. 8, no. 2, pp. 114–122, 2018.

[50] B. Zheng, T. Vazin, P. W. Goodwill et al., "Magnetic particle imaging tracks the long-term fate of *in vivo* neural cell implants with high image contrast," *Scientific Reports*, vol. 5, article 14055, 2015.

[51] B. Zheng, M. P. von See, E. Yu et al., "Quantitative magnetic particle imaging monitors the transplantation, biodistribution, and clearance of stem cells *in vivo*," *Theranostics*, vol. 6, no. 3, pp. 291–301, 2016.

[52] Y. X. J. Wáng and J.-M. Idée, "A comprehensive literatures update of clinical researches of superparamagnetic resonance iron oxide nanoparticles for magnetic resonance imaging," *Quantitative Imaging in Medicine and Surgery*, vol. 7, no. 1, pp. 88–122, 2017.

[53] A. Allegra, G. Penna, A. Alonci, V. Rizzo, S. Russo, and C. Musolino, "Nanoparticles in oncology: the new theragnostic molecules," *Anti-Cancer Agents in Medicinal Chemistry*, vol. 11, no. 7, pp. 669–686, 2011.

[54] Z. Fan, P. P. Fu, H. Yu, and P. C. Ray, "Theranostic nanomedicine for cancer detection and treatment," *Journal of Food and Drug Analysis*, vol. 22, no. 1, pp. 3–17, 2014.

[55] E. P. Papapetrou, "Patient-derived induced pluripotent stem cells in cancer research and precision oncology," *Nature Medicine*, vol. 22, no. 12, pp. 1392–1401, 2016.

[56] D. Zhu, C. S. L. Kong, J. A. Gingold, R. Zhao, and D. F. Lee, "Induced pluripotent stem cells and induced pluripotent cancer cells in cancer disease modeling," in *Advances in Experimental Medicine and Biology*, Springer, New York, NY, 2018.

[57] C. Reinshagen, D. Bhere, S. H. Choi et al., "CRISPR-enhanced engineering of therapy-sensitive cancer cells for self-targeting of primary and metastatic tumors," *Science Translational Medicine*, vol. 10, no. 449, article eaao3240, 2018.

13

The Mechanobiology of the Actin Cytoskeleton in Stem Cells during Differentiation and Interaction with Biomaterials

X. Ambriz,[1] P. de Lanerolle,[2] and J. R. Ambrosio[1]

[1]*Departamento de Microbiologia y Parasitologia, Facultad de Medicina, UNAM, 04510 Ciudad de México, Mexico*
[2]*Department of Physiology and Biophysics, College of Medicine, University of Illinois at Chicago, 60612 Chicago, Illinois, USA*

Correspondence should be addressed to J. R. Ambrosio; jrah@unam.mx

Academic Editor: Xingbin Hu

An understanding of the cytoskeleton's importance in stem cells is essential for their manipulation and further clinical application. The cytoskeleton is crucial in stem cell biology and depends on physical and chemicals signals to define its structure. Additionally, cell culture conditions will be important in the proper maintenance of stemness, lineage commitment, and differentiation. This review focuses on the following areas: the role of the actin cytoskeleton of stem cells during differentiation, the significance of cellular morphology, signaling pathways involved in cytoskeletal rearrangement in stem cells, and the mechanobiology and mechanotransduction processes implicated in the interactions of stem cells with different surfaces of biomaterials, such as nanotopography, which is a physical cue influencing the differentiation of stem cells. Also, cancer stem cells are included since it is necessary to understand the role of their mechanical properties to develop new strategies to treat cancer. In this context, to study the stem cells requires integrated disciplines, including molecular and cellular biology, chemistry, physics, and immunology, as well as mechanobiology. Finally, since one of the purposes of studying stem cells is for their application in regenerative medicine, the deepest understanding is necessary in order to establish safety protocols and effective cell-based therapies.

1. Introduction

Stem cells are undifferentiated cells with the potential to generate diverse lineages, but they are also capable of maintaining their own population, a process well known as self-renewal. Stem cells can be obtained from various tissues, with diverse potential properties, being able to generate from one to all kinds of cells (Figure 1).

Embryonic stem cells (ESCs) are isolated from the blastocyst and have the potential to generate any kind of cells from the three germ lines: ectoderm, mesoderm, and endoderm [1]. Mouse ESCs have been intensely studied for their capability of self-renewal, totipotency, and genome stability in comparison to human ESCs [2]. The interest in these kinds of cells is not solely for totipotency and regenerative use, but also for immunotherapy as well as a vehicle for drug delivery. At the moment, the use of ESCs in cellular therapy is controversial, due to ethical issues requiring human oocytes in obtaining these cells. Despite their legal use in some countries, most other countries prohibit the use of this tissue.

Inducible pluripotent stem cells (iPS or iPSCs) are generated by viral transfection of fibroblasts from adult humans, with these key transcriptional factors: Oct4/3 (octamer-binding transcription factor 4/3), Sox2 (sex determining region Y), Klf4 (kruppel-like factor 4), and c-Myc (avian myelocytomatosis virus oncogene cellular homologue) [3]. This strategy generates "stem cell-like" cells similar to the ESCs. They both share ethical controversy, but in this case, because iPSs are generated by viral transfection and because the stability of the incorporated genes is still unknown, this issue has to be solved before using iPS in humans.

Adult stem cells or somatic stem cells, also referred to as tissue-specific stem cells, are cells that can be obtained from already born animals and humans, not necessarily adults, because infants also have adult stem cells. These stem cells

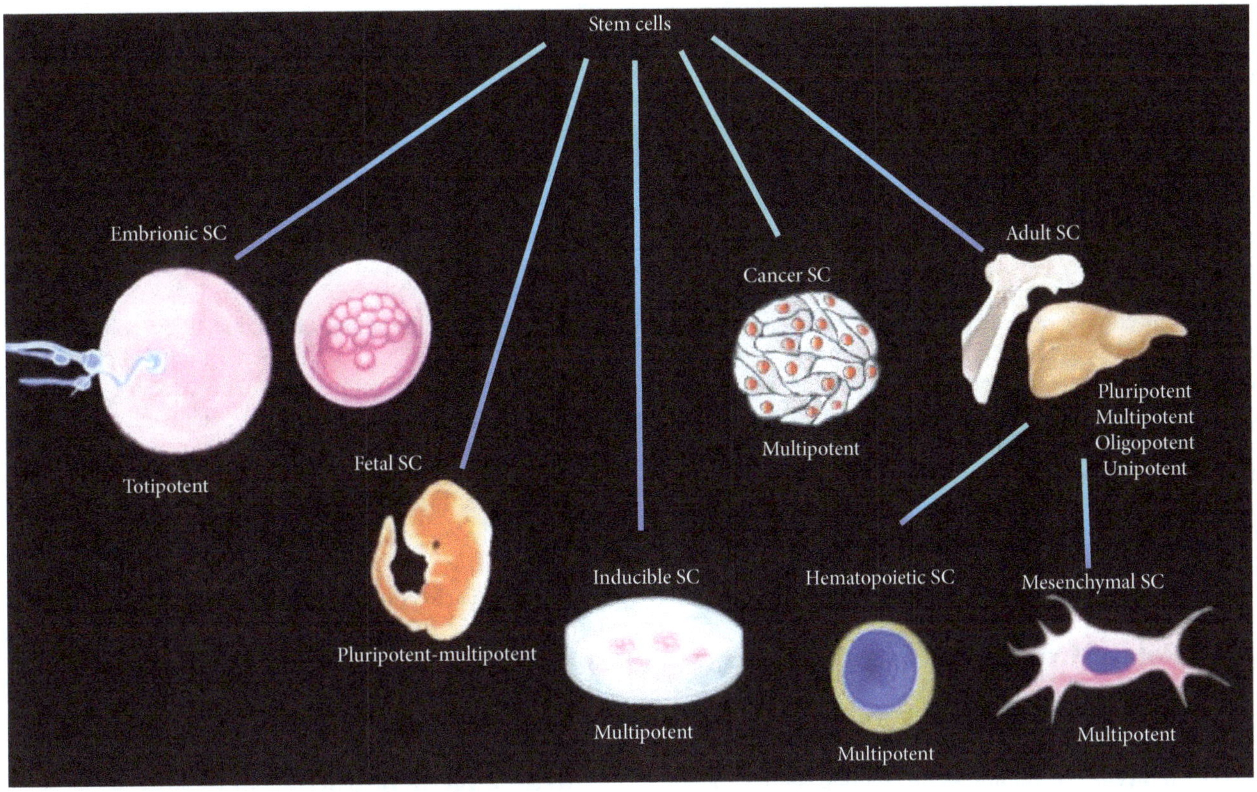

FIGURE 1: Kinds of stem cells and their differentiation potencies. Stem cells can be obtained from various tissues, with different potential properties (by Dr. Ambriz, 2018).

are necessary to maintain the body during its lifetime, with a self-renewing capability but without the potency to generate cells from the three germ lines.

Mesenchymal stem cells (MSCs) are a type of adult stem cell that is self-renewing and pluripotent. MSCs have the capacity to differentiate into several lineages, mainly adipocytes, chondrocytes, and osteocytes. On the other hand, hematopoietic stem cells (HSCs), another kind of adult stem cells, have the potential to generate blood cells like lymphocytes, dendritic cells, natural killer cells, monocytes, and others, while neural stem cells (NSCs) can generate lineages from the nervous system, neurons, and glia (astrocytes and oligodendrocytes).

Cancer stem cells (CSCs), also known as "cancer stem-like cells" or "tumor-initiating cells" (TICs) are a kind of stem cells which may express surface markers present on human ESCs and/or adult stem cells [4]. These cancer cells share the same properties of self-renewal and differentiation with stem cells, and for that reason are included into this category. CSCs are defined as cells capable of generating many cancer types and the failure of chemotherapy, which will be discussed later.

In order to regulate the recovery and characterization of stem cells, the International Society for Cellular Therapy (ISCT) established the minimum criteria to define them as stem cells [5], including specific recommendations that need to be followed in order to identify and avoid "unproven cellular therapies," any manufacturing of products, and loss of trust in the field. Furthermore, the ISCT strongly encourages the sharing of efforts and the contributions of involved professionals, as well as establishing the identification of key features of unproven cellular interventions. In this context, in order to have standard culture conditions for the maintenance of stem cells and the possibility of testing the effect of any kind of biomaterial on these cells, it is mandatory to elucidate intracellular events produced by the involvement of the cytoskeleton and mechanotransduction, which is the transduction of mechanical stimulus into intracellular signaling, both chemical and biophysical. Moreover, a higher scope of knowledge of these events and description of the involved mechanism will result in an increasing confidence for new cellular therapy protocols.

Steady-state conditions and differentiation processes are key aspects for the establishment of stem cell culture. However, the limitations involved in the access to organs or prostheses narrow the study of the implantation of stem cells, pushing more attention into the development of cell therapies [6].

Additionally, other important challenges that require examination are phenotype stability and maintenance in culture conditions, self-renewal and control of lineage commitment to ensure the identity of stem cells introduced to a body and, finally, the stability of a specific phenotype inside the body, avoiding aberrant differentiation, like that of cancer-like cells.

Biophysical aspects, such as the role of the actin cytoskeleton-mediated mechanobiology of stem cells, are important to consider. The conjunction and comprehension of these aspects present a better way for establishing all the possible interactions between biomaterials, cells, and organisms in order to be used for medical purposes.

The ability to design biomaterials to mimic natural scaffolds is a novel perspective for improving or developing more efficient stem cell-based therapies in regenerative medicine, requiring a deep understanding of stem cell biology.

Considering that regenerative medicine is a promising field for developing and applying new medical therapies, based on stem cell use, there is a continuous necessity to explain how these cell types are controlling self-renewal and differentiation. In this context, we could be close to developing "living implants" for humans, with their high capability of integration to a body without rejection, as well as the induction of a cellular replacement in situations of tissue damage, using the extracellular components of the host.

2. The Role of Cytoskeletal Proteins in Stem Cells

The cytoskeleton is a highly dynamic web composed of different molecules including actin, tubulin, and vimentin, whose role is dependent on the context and structures generated in each condition, but it also relies on the cell type. In this way, the cells have a specialized manner to respond to the environment, always trying to survive and adapt. The response of adherent or nonadherent cells involves different mechanisms, including surface molecules, like integrins and selectins that help with adhesion, and generate a link between the physical microenvironment from outside and within the cell. Thus, the cytoskeleton provides the support for stem cells in culture conditions or homing and establishment inside the body. Considering that, in both cases, the mechanisms are not completely understood, this section focuses solely on the physical signals the cells receive, excluding soluble factors, which are also relevant, as most of the literature already addresses them.

Cytoskeletal rearrangement is induced by several stimuli like chemokines, growth factors, differences in the stiffness of a substrate, and others. As mentioned above, the extracellular environment is connected to the inner cell, including the nucleus [7, 8]. In that case, the characteristics of the substrate may generate a reaction inside the cells, and the reaction is led by a reorganization of the F-actin structuring and the modulation of actin dynamics, like polymerization/depolymerization cycles.

In this context, actin reorganization is required during stem cell differentiation, as well as adhesion, cellular spreading, force distribution, stress fiber formation, and others, all of which are completely dependent on the cytoskeleton, a complex scaffold constituted of different kinds of filaments distributed throughout the cytoplasm. Thus, rigidity, structure, and support are not the only functions, but also subcellular organization, inner transport of molecules, motility and migration, cellular division, and mechanotransduction [9–11].

3. Cytoskeletal Structures Implied in Cellular Morphology and Lineage Commitment

Stem cells have a fibroblastic shape, which is considered as one of its morphological characteristics. There are specific structures that may serve in the stem cell progression of differentiation. These include the cytoskeleton and specific structures generated to make possible to establish stem cells in culture, as well as in stem cells during differentiation to specific lineages [12–17].

Osteogenic differentiation, induced by soluble factors, showed modification of the actin cytoskeleton. This morphology modification is a consequence of parallel arrangement and orientation of the actin filaments, to the rearrangement of F-actin in well-defined stress fibers as well as a change in its pattern. FA distribution and cellular density are altered by physical characteristics of the substrate and/or its matrix. Therefore, the analysis of cell spreading and F-actin arrangement helps identify the kind of response induced in each context and subsequently the manipulation of specific physical cues to deliberately induce a stem cell's fate [15].

4. Mechanotransduction and Cytoskeletal Rearrangement during Stem Cell Differentiation

Considering that actin filaments are assembled by noncovalent interactions, this provides a higher potential of exchange between the monomeric and the filamentous states. In motile cells, actin dynamics are activated by extracellular stimuli, which in turn trigger intracellular signaling, including Rho-family small GTPases, focal adhesion kinases, cofilin, LIM kinases, capping proteins, polymerization complexes, and other actin binding proteins (ABPs) [18, 19]. Generally, the shift between F-actin and G-actin elicits the acquisition of specific structures and in turn, the change of shape. For example, from spherical to spread shape (or in the opposite direction), the ratio between F-actin and G-actin changes, while in spreading, F-actin helps to generate contact adhesions and stress fibers, as well as membrane protrusions. In both "steady-state" or stimulated conditions, the turnover between filamentous and monomeric actin is continuous [20–22]. G-actin is bound to profilin or thymosin beta 4 (Tβ4). These proteins maintain the stock of G-actin and, along with other ABPs, prevent spontaneous actin polymerization. Profilin can release the G-actin easier than Tβ4 when the polymerization is required [18].

Tβ4 plays a role in human bone marrow-derived MSC differentiation. Tβ4 is known to suppress osteogenic differentiation by sequestering G-actin and preventing its polymerization [23]. It has shown a biophysical effect using exogenous Tβ4, without altering gene expression, measured by monitoring Runt-related transcription factor 2 (Runx2) and peroxisome proliferator-activated receptor gamma (PPARγ) genes during early osteogenic differentiation. Despite a lack of change in gene expression, one cannot rule out the possibility of alteration in other genes not included in this study, since alteration in the actin cytoskeleton may modify gene expression via mechanotransduction. On the other hand, this study has shown that in these conditions, the adipogenic differentiation was promoted, but chondrogenic differentiation was not altered, pointing out the difference in requirements and importance of F-actin during these processes [23].

The cytoskeleton is linked to the extracellular matrix (ECM) by adhesion molecules like integrins, selectins, laminin receptors, and syndecans, and it participates during homing inside an organism or in culture conditions. This contact adhesion also generates a direct link from ECM to the nucleus and confers mechanical properties in a dynamic fashion. In this context, integrins play a crucial role during stem cell maintenance and differentiation. ECM interacts with integrins, and this activates outside-in signaling, while intracellular signaling also induces the conformational change of integrins, as well as modulating its avidity by clustering [24].

Integrins may mediate focal adhesions, considered as mechanosensors that link the substrate to the cytoskeleton. From outside of the cell, these structures are integrin clusters, but in the cytoplasm many molecules are recruited to generate a complex structure (Figure 2), with different proteins like focal adhesion kinase (FAK), talin, vinculin, and paxilin, which link receptors with the cytoskeleton [25, 26].

Because stem cells require the activity of integrins, it is important to understand how focal adhesions are regulated and how they can be modulated by biomaterials, inducing more or less adhesion and then altering the differentiation potential of stem cells.

For example, focal adhesion size and intracellular tension induced by ECM proteins regulate stem cell differentiation, as well as self-renewal [27]. Initial contacts and early adhesion generate tension that plays a crucial role in the internalization of signals, including activation of molecules like FAK and mitogen-activated protein kinases (MAPKs).

Myosins are molecular motors that provide mechanical properties and contribute to the tension generated in response to a substrate (adhesion). Myosin II, along with F-actin, generate the actomyosin complex that is largely responsible for establishing the mechanical properties of a cell. Myosin II in smooth muscle and nonmuscle cells is regulated by phosphorylation of myosin light chains (MLC) by myosin light chain kinase [28]. MLC phosphorylation enables the interaction of myosin II with actin filaments and tension generation. Myosin II is also regulated downstream of the Rho family of small GTPases.

The Rho family of GTPases (guanosine triphosphatases) are small molecules involved in regulating actin polymerization. These molecules orchestrate coordinated cytoskeletal reorganizations by generating different structures, like filopodium, lamellipodium, or uropod, depending on the type of GTPase activated, that is, Cdc42, Rac, or RhoA, respectively [29]. In HSCs, the GTPase family also takes part during self-renewal, proliferation, apoptosis, migration, and adhesion. Rac1 and Cdc42 mediate proliferation; Rac2 and Cdc42 mediate apoptosis; and Cdc42, Rac1, and RhoA mediate self-renewal [30]. However, we have to consider that GTPase functions are more complex. In general, these molecules have an activation/inactivation cycle mediated by the exchange of GTP/GDP, respectively. GEFs and GAPs regulate Rho GTPase activity in a stimulus-dependent fashion [31].

As shown in studies with MSCs, RhoA, ROCKII, and the tension that might be generated are important in cell fate, since high activity of RhoA is associated with osteogenic differentiation, while adipogenic differentiation requires a minor activity of the GTPase [32]. In this study they use C3H10T1/2 progenitor cells as a model of primary bone marrow- (BM-) MSCs with a stable population. Expression of Runx2, PPARγ, and Sox9 were analyzed to determine regulation of osteogenic, adipogenic, and chondrogenic differentiation, respectively. By oscillatory fluid flow, the possibility to activate RhoA and then to modulate cellular fate have been measured. This model has shown that RhoA activated by flow may upregulate the expression of Runx2 [32].

Specifically, RhoA/ROCK is involved in the tension induced by fibrous substrates. In this context, RhoA/ROCK signaling generates myosin contractility and this results in increased osteogenic differentiation. In addition, the substrate influences focal adhesion (FA) formation and maturation [33]. Furthermore, by modulating the activity of RhoA it is possible to change the lineage commitment. For instance, the expression of the dominant-negative of RhoA leads hMSCs to differentiate into adipocytes, while the constitutively active RhoA results in osteogenesis [13].

RhoA effectors, ROCK I/II, regulate the actomyosin complex by inhibiting MLC dephosphorylation. Phosphorylation by ROCK inactivates a myosin phosphatase, retaining myosin II in the phosphorylated or active state [34, 35]. ROCK and downstream molecules lead to the interaction of myosin motor molecules with actin filaments [36]. These motor molecules, in association with actin polymerization, contribute to the FAs' assembly, while along with force generation, FAs become more stable and that is known as FA maturation [26].

LIM domain-containing protein kinase (LIMK) regulates actin dynamics by phosphorylating cofilin at Serine3. Cofilin is a member of the actin depolymerizing factors (ADF)/cofilin family of molecules. It was shown that pharmacological inhibition of LIMK1 increased adipocyte differentiation of BM-hMSCs [37], while the opposite result was obtained after siRNA-mediated knockdown of CFL1 and DSTN in human BM-derived primary MSCs, which resulted in osteoblast differentiation [12]. In the same study, the authors analyzed the effect of Cyto-D and phalloidin in human and murine BM-MSCs, confirming that actin polymerization is essential for osteoblast differentiation.

Cofilin is activated by serine/threonine phosphatases like PP1/PP2A [38], calcineurin PP2B [39], Slingshot (SSH1L, -2L, and -3L) [40, 41], and chronophin [42]. Also, membrane phosphoinositides PIP and PIP2 regulate cofilin activity by sequestration. PP2A also regulates phosphoinositide 3-kinase (PI3K), AKT (PKB), mitogen-activated protein kinase (MEK)/ERK, and GSK-3b pathways, which participate in proliferation and apoptosis. In hESCs, PP2A promotes

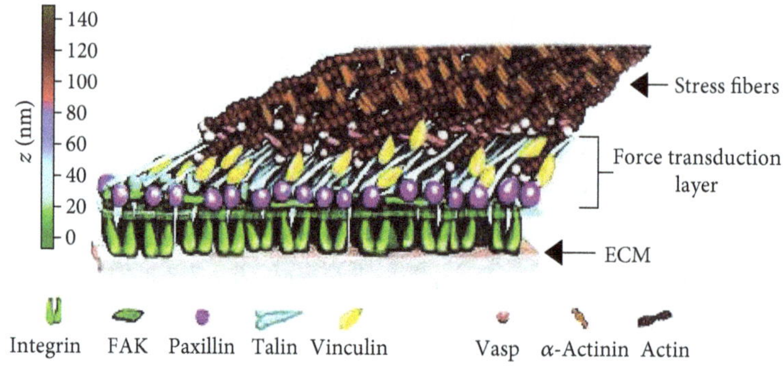

FIGURE 2: Molecular structure of contact adhesion. Different proteins are involved and are necessary for focal adhesion, like focal adhesion kinase (FAK), talin, vinculin, and paxilin, linking receptors with the cytoskeleton. Outside the membrane, adhesion receptors, like integrins and selectines link the membrane with the substrate.

differentiation [43]. This study found incremental activity of PP2A during differentiation of hESCs. Also, inducing the overexpression of this phosphatase or the addition of C2-ceramide (activator of PP2A) promoted differentiation. Hence, by inactivating PP2A with okadaic acid and plurypotency markers, the expression and telomerase activity with normal karyotypes were maintained. This indicated the regulatory role of PP2A in the differentiation/self-renewal of hESCs.

5. Mechanobiology: Propagation of Forces through the Cytoskeleton in Linear and Nonlinear Fashions

Since the cell is not a homogenous gel, we have to understand how the forces are distributed and generated by spreading and adhesion. It is necessary to review Newton's Second Law for a better comprehension of this topic. A force is an interaction between two objects, such as stem cells and biomaterials, which may cause acceleration of mass, like gravity, as well as compression (push) or tension (pull) that changes its momentum.

Cells are not static, homogenous entities; on the contrary they are highly dynamic and heterogeneous gels. Analyzing cellular response to a biomaterial is possible, while fixing a point in time as well as a single subcellular compartment. This utilizes Young's modulus, or tensile elasticity, helping measure the extension of cells as a result of biomaterial interaction. In other words, how much a material will deform in response to a stress placed on it can be measured. Materials with a higher Young's modulus are stiffer and do not deform easily. Before differentiation, hMSCs have a Young's modulus value of 3.2 kPa [44].

The disruption of actin filaments causes a decrease in the average elastic modulus of the cellular membrane. Using atomic force microscopy (AFM), Titushkin and Cho [45] reported that osteoblasts have a Young's modulus value of 1.7 kPa. This study also found that hMSCs exposed to an osteogenic medium for 10 days exhibited a significant decrease in the elastic modulus from 3.2 kPa to 2 kPa. Moreover, adipocytes have a lower stiffness than hMSCs and osteoblasts [46]. Darling et al. reported an elastic modulus of 0.61 kPa for adipocytes; this relatively low modulus implies that adipocytes do not have a denser cytoskeleton network in comparison to hMSCs and osteoblasts. The same author reported that chondrocytes have a stiffness of 1.2 kPa, which is a value between that of MSCs and adipocytes (3.2 kPa and 0.61 kPa, respectively) [46].

Tension or compression might be caused by biomaterials or any substrate in which cells will be seeded. As described by Ingber, tensegrity or tensional integrity is the mechanical stability produced by the cellular network and its control of shape and structure [47]. In this regard, the cytoskeletal filament is a network in an isomeric tension state, but it is resilient with a high capability to respond to external forces generating mechanical stress.

Models of tensed elastic strings and interconnected straws can predict actomyosin complex behavior, and the forms created with these models resemble structures observed in living cells [47]. According to Ingber's model, actin networks of hMSCs visualized with a confocal microscope (Figure 3) mirrored the model's pattern, changing the orientation of actin filaments, depending on its localization, whether cortical or closer to the nucleus.

Applied stress by Newtonian fluids can be measured as viscosity. Biopolymers have mechanical properties, ranging from pure fluid to elastic solid, which are considered viscoelastic [48]. Cells also respond to the intrinsic properties of biomaterials by restructuring F-actin networks, complicating the measurement of force distribution along the cytoplasm or cellular membrane [49]. Moreover, ABPs provide a dynamic way to rearrange actin filaments, linking or severing F-actin, as well as by conferring greater elasticity to the filament. Cofilin association to F-actin changes the filament twist in ~4 to 5° per subunit [50]. Therefore, the cytoskeleton network displays a nonlinear elastic response [46], since stiffness or softening are regulated by F-actin and myosin II, not just actin. This was first suggested by Eliot Elson in the 1990s. Subsequently, Cai et al. showed that myosin light chain kinase plays a crucial role in regulating cell stiffness by phosphorylating myosin II [51]. These cellular characteristics and properties have to be included in the design of biomaterials and scaffolds, as well as stem cell therapies, since they can transduce signals provided by nanotopography and stiffness of biomaterials.

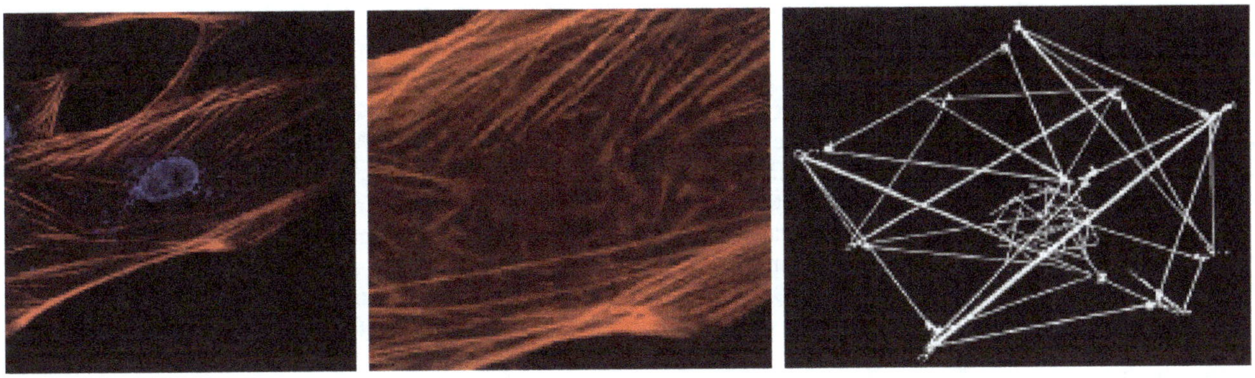

FIGURE 3: Actin networks of MSCs visualized by a confocal microscope. hMSCs transfected with β-actin-RFP (red) and stained with DAPI (blue) (by Dr. Ambriz, 2016). Actin networks resemble the same pattern from Ingber's model [47] in which tensed elastic strings and straws that are interconnected can predict the actomyosin complex behaviour. Actin filament orientation changes depending on its distance to the nucleus.

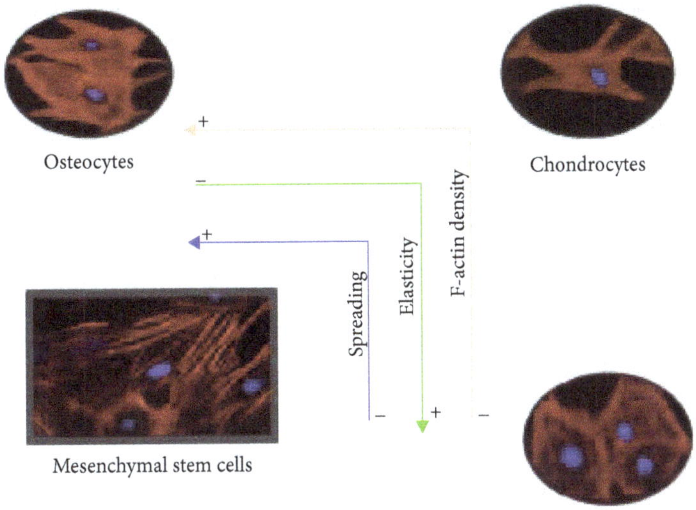

FIGURE 4: Actin cytoskeleton in stem cell differentiation. Cellular spreading (blue line), elasticity (green line), and F-actin density (orange line) are some of the properties that change during stem cell differentiation and can predict the cell's fate. Substrates with different mechanical characteristics influence the rearrangement of the F-actin cytoskeleton in the differentiation process modulating cellular spreading, elasticity, and F-actin. In the case of adipocytes, they have less F-actin and spreading but are more elastic compared to chondrocytes and osteocytes. On the other hand, osteocytes have the opposite context than adipocytes. They are less elastic but with higher F-actin and spreading. Chondrocytes display intermediate properties of adipocytes and osteocytes considering these three properties (by Dr. Ambriz, 2018).

6. Nanotopography of Biomaterials and the Role of the Cytoskeleton during Stem Cell Interaction

Actin and tubulin, in contrast to vimentin, are cytoskeletal molecules generating, in a highly dynamic fashion, specialized structures in just a few seconds after a signal is initiated. This property provides a cell the capability of adapting if the microenvironment changes, or if it is required in other processes, like cell migration.

Stem cells share an exceptional plasticity and adaptation to microenvironmental conditions. According to the plasticity potential, cells respond and adhere easily, acquiring a spherical or spread shape. Stem cells are unspecialized with a remarkable potential to renew themselves, as well as the potential to differentiate into mature specialized tissue; both functions are maintained in balance. With *in vitro* models, these properties can be manipulated by employing different strategies, like cocktails of growth factors. Another approach is to use scaffolds, like mechanical cues [16, 17], which can be manipulated to generate specific changes in cellular shape, spreading, rearrangement of F-actin, stress fiber formation, and inducing adhesion patterns and differentiation [52, 53] (Figure 4).

In the human body, stem cells interact with ECM, which vary in composition depending on the site. ECM is mainly composed of collagen, fibronectin, and laminin [54], as well as proteins like glycosaminoglycans and proteoglycans. Niche compositions rely on the abundance of these molecules and contribute to the differentiation process in which stem cells generate specific adhesion arrangements, maintaining or modifying its cellular shape and migration capability to other sites.

When stem cells are maintained in culture, it is crucial to avoid any possible stimulus that can trigger the differentiation process. For example, fibronectin binds to integrins like α5β1, α4β1, and αvβ3. This interaction results in an intracellular actin reorganization and induces a specific change of shape and the activation of intracellular signaling pathways, which results in chondrocyte differentiation. On the other hand, in vitro self-renewal of ES cells has been shown to be dependent on the interaction with type I or type IV collagen substrates [55].

Induction of morphological changes of hMSCs have been studied by the generation of specific micropatterns [25, 56] causing topography-mediated differentiation [56]. ECM proteins have been used to "print" patterns, lines or dots, with different spacing between each one, resulting in the induction of tension or compression, as the cells attempt to generate different distributions of FAs.

To illustrate the influence of nanotopography, consider nanoislands of fibronectin. With spacing below 60 nm, it is possible to generate FAs, while longer spacing results in impairment of FA formation and cellular spreading. Moreover, the organization of patterns seems to be significant since disordered nanopatterns do not cause cellular spreading. Furthermore, FA maturation and cell adhesion strength were constant at 60 nm of spacing, in comparison to 70 and 120 nm of micropatterned substrates [25]. These results are highly significant if it is considered that biomaterials, with specific micro- or nanopatterned designs can modulate the maturation of FAs, which in turn has consequences in stem cell proliferation, self-renewal, and differentiation, as described above.

Adhesion structures are required sites for binding to the substrate. These molecular structures function as links between the substrate and the actin cytoskeleton. Furthermore, motor molecules like myosins, FAKs activated by integrins, and the activation of the molecular machinery responsible for actin polymerization generate mature or immature contact adhesions. These contacts in turn modify the affinity and valency of integrins and are the main features during the adaptation of stem cells to a surface. The molecular machinery involved and adhesion structures' organization that was generated rely on the mechanical properties of the substrate.

For example, the stiffness of the substrate influences adhesion structuring as well as stress fibers, establishing the actomyosin complex. If the substrate is soft, the shape of the cell will be more rounded with a low density of stress fibers. If substrate stiffness is increased, the density of stress fibers and the spreading of the cell will also increase [54–56]. The stiffness of the substrate can be manipulated, allowing the design of specific conditions and the induction of stem cell differentiation.

Other techniques exist, measuring the physical forces and mechanical properties of cells, making possible the analysis of conformational changes by AFM and Förster resonance energy transfer (FRET). Single cell analysis of mechanobiology is also possible by microelectromechanical systems (MEMS), AFM, optical stretchers, and micropipette aspirations [56]. These techniques create standards required to control stem cell differentiation.

Mechanical forces produced during the interaction between substrate or biomaterials and stem cells cause mechanical stimulus, and this may be translated in intracellular signaling, both chemical and biophysical [57, 58]. In this context, the actin cytoskeleton plays an active role in the interpretation of the microenvironmental conditions that drive and link directly to the cytoplasm and nucleus, having the consequence of molecular activation and/or gene transcription [59–62].

7. Cancer Stem Cells: Targeting Their Biomechanics

The complexity within stem cell niches elicits the interaction of CSCs with other cells. All of them could be involved in some kind of regulation but these aspects need to be defined specifically, as they are all related with those molecules involved in biophysical interactions of CSCs. Inside of cancer cell niches, several types of cells exist, such as tumor, stromal, and vascular cells where as part of them, CSCs are maintained in a quiescent stage until adequate conditions, including cellular and molecular events, induce them to proliferate, invade, and metastasize [63].

The expression "awakening the beast" has been used to describe the activation of CSCs following chemotherapeutic treatment [64]. CSCs have clear properties of self-renewal, clonal tumor initiation capacity, clonal long-term repopulation potential, transitions from a nonstem cell state to stem cell state, evasion of cell death, metastasis, and dormancy for long periods of time [65]. CSCs can also be activated by direct or indirect interactions with different cell types present inside of niches [65, 66] and by biophysical interactions within cancer cell niches surrounding ECM or ECM molecules [67, 68]. In those niches, the local cells produce factors capable of stimulating CSCs, inducing angiogenesis, and recruiting immune and other stromal cells that secrete additional factors while promoting tumor cell metastasis and invasion. CSCs can also produce exosomes, which facilitate ingress of RNA molecules that facilitate the ingress of multidrug resistance in tumor cells [65].

In tumor niches or tissues, there is a production and concentration of several molecules that could activate CSCs. Biochemical and biophysical signals come from growth factors, cytokines, and matrix-remodeling proteins [63]. Potentially, all of them are capable of activating and/or inducing growth and differentiation of quiescent CSCs that develop into more aggressive stages. Part of those molecules are noncellular components derived from degradation of ECM due to the action of matrix metalloproteinases coming from activated cells inside of niches; the importance of the produced ECM is due to its constitution remaining as a physical barrier, as well as the integrity of CSCs blocking any possible harmful condition such as the action of chemotherapeutic agents found in solid tumors. Therefore, the release of cytokines, growth factors, and other molecules enable the degradation of the ECM because of the action of metalloproteinases which are factors facilitating angiogenesis, tumor cell metastasis, and invasion associated with therapeutic resistance. Cross talk between CSCs and their niches have the basis of activation of these types of cells [65].

It is clear that those factors present in the microenvironment of cells have an important influence on different stem cell phenotypes. Such factors are composed of materials surrounding the cells that can compete with biochemical supplements. They influence or induce the activation and/or the differentiation of stem cells by inducing or activating signaling pathways through mechanotransduction because of its mechanosensing [68]. Therefore, those conditions involving cancer therapy, where there is a manipulation of the components of the microenvironment of cancer niches or tissues, could produce an effective strategy for cancer treatment or the induction of resistance to cancer therapy and the prevention or the maintaining of malignancy and metastasis of CSCs [65].

Materials in cellular environments are capable of being inductors/activators of stem cells which is a crucial consideration for CSC niches. If these molecules are part of the surrounding niches, their surfaces could become inductors of CSC activation that can be involved in mechanotransduction and mechanosensing events (as those described in the present revision for stem cells). These conditions could trigger growth, expansion, and drug resistance as shown by these types of cancer cells. It is mandatory to consider whether their engineering and utilization could be the reason why some quiescent CSCs become capable of expanding and developing resistance to anticancer drugs [69]. There are several properties of synthetic materials which can induce changes in cellular activity, and these include stiffness, molecular flexibility, nanotopography, cell adhesiveness, binding affinity, chemical functionality, degradability, and/or degradation by-products. Materials could produce specific stem cell behavior which need to be always considered during the design and use of materials [68], and CSC biology and niche factors have to be involved during the use of materials for regenerative medicine purposes.

The significance of cell fate and mechanotransduction has been discussed above, but to understand how they are involved in CSCs' progression to metastasis requires describing the signaling pathways activated when a mechanical disruption occurs and cell-cell contact is lost. There is a tensional homeostasis within cells when there is a disruption, and it may play a role in oncogenic transformation. Considering that stiffness is measured by mechanosensors in cancer stem cells and solid tumors have high mechanical stress, this may impede drug delivery driving tumor progression. Biomechanic forces can drive tumor aggression in the case of a mesenchymal-like switch, developing tumor-initiating or stem-like cell properties, as well as elevated tissue mechanics promoting aggression. These events open the possibility of manipulating mechanical properties of CSCs to break drug resistance by its stem cell phenotype [70].

8. Signaling Molecules Involved in Biomechanics and Drug Resistance in Cancer Stem Cells

In most solid tumors, recent studies show the relevance of the oncogenes Yes-associated protein (YAP) and transcriptional coactivator with PDZ-binding motif (TAZ) transcriptional regulators. YAP/TAZ activation provides not only stem cell properties in cells, but also chemoresistance. Considering these molecules as mechanosensors, it is highly relevant to understand its function in normal or pathological conditions and how its activation potentially is a key factor for cancer treatment and designing anticancer drugs [71, 72].

YAP/TAZ proteins are mechanosensors and mechanotransducers that respond to physical stimulus in which the actin cytoskeleton is involved, such as the rigidity of extracellular matrix, cell geometry, cell density, and cell polarity [73]. For this purpose, it is important to maintain that molecules in ECM are polymers such as collagen or fibrin, which also self-ensemble into gels. For example, increasing the amount of collagen in a tissue enhances its stiffness. Moreover, cytoskeletal stress causes protein stabilisation to maintain cell integrity, and one good example is the nuclear structure protein lamin A, whose protein and transcript levels increase with collagen-I and tissue stiffness. Then, mechanogenomic processes are pivotal inducers in mutations and cause cancer related to tissue stiffness [74]. Approaches to reduce tumor aggression include reducing or inhibiting TGFβ, LOXL2, or collagen deposition and cross-linking [70].

YAP/TAZ have been shown to play positive as well as negative roles in the Wnt signaling pathway. This pathway is important to measure cell-cell contact, among other functions. YAP/TAZ are integral components of the β-catenin destruction complex, which they may translocate to the nucleus after Wnt pathway activation [75]. Other hypotheses support the notion that ECM stiffness is the extracellular activator of YAP/TAZ downstream G protein coupled receptor (GPCR)/lipid rafts/Rho/ROCK signaling pathway, leading to CSC survival [76, 77].

On the other hand, integrin and FAK activation result in focal adhesion formation, which in turn activates Rho-GTPases and elicits the formation of stress fibers. This leads to the activation of other kinases such as LATS1/2 and inhibition of YAP/TAZ transcription factors causing a negative effect in CSCs [76, 77]. In this context, actin polymerization is required in focal adhesions. After cellular spreading, myosin II increases tension on the actin network while depolymerization of F-actin decreases the tension, and this maintains the tension in equilibrium.

Mechanical properties of CSCs will be essential in the design of personalised medicine in order to develop more efficient treatments. Then, it is necessary to consider the disruption of tumor microenvironment barriers, such as stromal cells, vasculature, and collagen cross-linking, which restrict drug entry and then affect the chemotherapeutic efficiency. If there are well-designed nanomaterials [78] and nanoparticles [79], such as nanocarriers used to reach the target cell, it will improve drug delivery and provide access for drugs to cancer cells, including CSCs. Also, biomaterials which may modulate and reduce the chances of wrong activation of the CSCs should be designed.

9. Conclusions and Perspectives

Mechanotransduction helps comprehend the mechanism by which the nanotopography of biomaterials can direct the differentiation of stem cells. Intracellular tension generated by the adhesion to a biomaterial is transduced like a chemical signal with the possibility of gene expression. In this manner, interactions with physical cues provided by nanotopography, nanopatterns, stiffness of the substrate, and other physical properties of biomaterials, can modulate stem cell fate and must be considered in the study of these cells and the use of stem cells in regenerative medicine and cellular therapy.

Understanding cytoskeleton arrangement and its implication during stem cell interactions with biomaterials, as well as the importance of nanotopography, creates new aspects of integration with other fields of knowledge, in order to improve cell-based therapies and regenerative medicine.

Along with the considerations of the present work, clearly it is mandatory to have new ways of focusing the design and engineering of new biomaterials with intentions of using it for therapeutic purposes. Not taking into account these considerations could be a determinant for inducing abnormal activation or differentiation of stem cells.

It is a big risk to design and build a biomaterial without evaluating their physical aspects, such as the stiffness, porosity, nanotopography, chemical composition, and interaction with other types of surfaces. Moreover, the aberrant growth of cells or the wrong differentiation of the stem cells can be triggered by alterations in their physical microenvironment. As indicated, under these considerations, activated cells could be redirected to produce pathological situations or in the case of CSCs to develop resistance to anticancer drugs due to epigenetic changes. It is important to carry out the characterization of the new biomaterials, in order to establish if they are adequate for the terms of any potential use in regenerative medicine and, more importantly, if they do not have the capability to "awake the beast."

In conclusion, the mechanobiology of stem cell differentiation and cytoskeletal dynamics provide the knowledge to develop cellular therapies with higher efficiency, as well as the possibility of understanding its involvement in pathological conditions and its effect on cellular biology.

Acknowledgments

The authors gratefully acknowledge the assistance of Dr. Rocio Tirado in revising and preparing the manuscript. The authors are also grateful to Javier Carmona, MFA, for style correction and manuscript editing. Financial support was provided by PAPIIT-UNAM IN224316, PAPIME-UNAM PE211115, and FM-UNAM. Dr. Xochitl Ambriz Peña was supported by a postdoctoral scholarship of DGAPA, UNAM (2016–2018) and the School of Medicine (UNAM).

References

[1] J. A. Thomson, J. Itskovitz-Eldor, S. S. Shapiro et al., "Embryonic stem cell lines derived from human blastocysts," *Science*, vol. 282, no. 5391, pp. 1145–1147, 1998.

[2] I. Ullah, R. B. Subbarao, and G. J. Rho, "Human mesenchymal stem cells—current trends and future prospective," *Bioscience Reports*, vol. 35, no. 2, pp. 1–18, 2015.

[3] K. Takahashi and S. Yamanaka, "Induction of pluripotent stem cells from mouse embryonic and adult fibroblast cultures by defined factors," *Cell*, vol. 126, no. 4, pp. 663–676, 2006.

[4] W.-T. Kim and C. J. Ryu, "Cancer stem cell surface markers on normal stem cells," *BMB Reports*, vol. 50, no. 6, pp. 285–298, 2017.

[5] M. Dominici, K. Le Blanc, I. Mueller et al., "Minimal criteria for defining multipotent mesenchymal stromal cells. The International Society for Cellular Therapy position statement," *Cytotherapy*, vol. 8, no. 4, pp. 315–317, 2006.

[6] N. S. Hwang, S. Varghese, and J. Elisseeff, "Controlled differentiation of stem cells," *Advanced Drug Delivery Reviews*, vol. 60, no. 2, pp. 199–214, 2008.

[7] B. Sen, Z. Xie, G. Uzer et al., "Intranuclear actin regulates osteogenesis," *Stem Cells*, vol. 33, no. 10, pp. 3065–3076, 2015.

[8] B. Sen, G. Uzer, R. M. Samsonraj et al., "Intranuclear actin structure modulates mesenchymal stem cell differentiation," *Stem Cells*, vol. 35, no. 6, pp. 1624–1635, 2017.

[9] P. A. Janmey, "The cytoskeleton and cell signaling: component localization and mechanical coupling," *Physiological Reviews*, vol. 78, no. 3, pp. 763–781, 1998.

[10] A. Pullikuth and A. Catling, "Scaffold mediated regulation of MAPK signaling and cytoskeletal dynamics: a perspective," *Cellular Signalling*, vol. 19, no. 8, pp. 1621–1632, 2007.

[11] D. A. Fletcher and R. D. Mullins, "Cell mechanics and the cytoskeleton," *Nature*, vol. 463, no. 7280, pp. 485–492, 2010.

[12] L. Chen, K. Shi, C. E. Frary et al., "Inhibiting actin depolymerization enhances osteoblast differentiation and bone formation in human stromal stem cells," *Stem Cell Research*, vol. 15, no. 2, pp. 281–289, 2015.

[13] R. McBeath, D. M. Pirone, C. M. Nelson, K. Bhadriraju, and C. S. Chen, "Cell shape, cytoskeletal tension, and RhoA regulate stem cell lineage commitment," *Developmental Cell*, vol. 6, no. 4, pp. 483–495, 2004.

[14] P. Müller, A. Langenbach, A. Kaminski, and J. Rychly, "Modulating the actin cytoskeleton affects mechanically induced signal transduction and differentiation in mesenchymal stem cells," *PLoS One*, vol. 8, no. 7, article e71283, 2013.

[15] C. Huang, J. Dai, and X. A. Zhang, "Environmental physical cues determine the lineage specification of mesenchymal stem cells," *Biochimica et Biophysica Acta (BBA) - General Subjects*, vol. 1850, no. 6, pp. 1261–1266, 2015.

[16] P. Angele, J. U. Yoo, C. Smith et al., "Cyclic hydrostatic pressure enhances the chondrogenic phenotype of human mesenchymal progenitor cells differentiated in vitro," *Journal of Orthopaedic Research*, vol. 21, no. 3, pp. 451–457, 2003.

[17] P. Angele, D. Schumann, M. Angele et al., "Cyclic, mechanical compression enhances chondrogenesis of mesenchymal

progenitor cells in tissue engineering scaffolds," *Biorheology*, vol. 41, no. 3-4, pp. 335–346, 2004.

[18] T. D. Pollard, L. Blanchoin, and R. D. Mullins, "Molecular mechanisms controlling actin filament dynamics in nonmuscle cells," *Annual Review of Biophysics and Biomolecular Structure*, vol. 29, no. 1, pp. 545–576, 2000.

[19] T. D. Pollard, L. Blanchoin, and R. D. Mullins, "Actin dynamics," *Journal of Cell Science*, vol. 114, no. 1, pp. 3-4, 2001.

[20] E. S. Chhabra and H. N. Higgs, "The many faces of actin: matching assembly factors with cellular structures," *Nature Cell Biology*, vol. 9, no. 10, pp. 1110–1121, 2007.

[21] A. E. Carlsson, "Actin dynamics: from nanoscale to microscale," *Annual Review of Biophysics*, vol. 39, no. 1, pp. 91–110, 2010.

[22] A. Nurnberg, T. Kitzing, and R. Grosse, "Nucleating actin for invasion," *Nature Reviews Cancer*, vol. 11, no. 3, pp. 177–187, 2011.

[23] J. H. Ho, W. H. Ma, Y. Su, K. C. Tseng, T. K. Kuo, and O. K. Lee, "Thymosin beta-4 directs cell fate determination of human mesenchymal stem cells through biophysical effects," *Journal of Orthopaedic Research*, vol. 28, no. 1, pp. 131–138, 2010.

[24] T. Kinashi, "Intracellular signalling controlling integrin activation in lymphocytes," *Nature Reviews. Immunology*, vol. 5, no. 7, pp. 546–559, 2005.

[25] S. Di Cio and J. E. Gautrot, "Cell sensing of physical properties at the nanoscale: mechanisms and control of cell adhesion and phenotype," *Acta Biomaterialia*, vol. 30, pp. 26–48, 2016.

[26] P. Kanchanawong, G. Shtengel, A. M. Pasapera et al., "Nanoscale architecture of integrin-based cell adhesions," *Nature*, vol. 468, no. 7323, pp. 580–584, 2010.

[27] R. J. McMurray, M. J. Dalby, and P. M. Tsimbouri, "Using biomaterials to study stem cell mechanotransduction, growth and differentiation," *Journal of Tissue Engineering and Regenerative Medicine*, vol. 9, no. 5, pp. 528–539, 2015.

[28] P. de Lanerolle and R. J. Paul, "Myosin phosphorylation/dephosphorylation and regulation of airway smooth muscle contractility," *American Journal of Physiology-Lung Cellular and Molecular Physiology*, vol. 261, no. 2, pp. L1–14, 1991.

[29] V. L. J. Tybulewicz and R. B. Henderson, "Rho family GTPases and their regulators in lymphocytes," *Nature Reviews Immunology*, vol. 9, no. 9, pp. 630–644, 2009.

[30] R. C. Nayak, K.-H. Chang, N.-S. Vaitinadin, and J. A. Cancelas, "Rho GTPases control specific cytoskeleton-dependent functions of hematopoietic stem cells," *Immunological Reviews*, vol. 256, no. 1, pp. 255–268, 2013.

[31] M. S. Samuel and M. F. Olson, "Rho-GTPases in embryonic stem cells," in *Embryonic Stem Cells - Basic Biology to Bioengineering*, M. Kallos, Ed., InTech, 2011.

[32] E. J. Arnsdorf, P. Tummala, R. Y. Kwon, and C. R. Jacobs, "Mechanically induced osteogenic differentiation—the role of RhoA, ROCKII and cytoskeletal dynamics," *Journal of Cell Science*, vol. 122, no. 4, pp. 546–553, 2009.

[33] R. K. Das, O. F. Zouani, C. Labrugère, R. Oda, and M. C. Durrieu, "Influence of nanohelical shape and periodicity on stem cell fate," *ACS Nano*, vol. 7, no. 4, pp. 3351–3361, 2013.

[34] T. Kaneko-Kawano, F. Takasu, H. Naoki et al., "Dynamic regulation of myosin light chain phosphorylation by rho-kinase," *PLoS One*, vol. 7, no. 6, article e39269, 2012.

[35] S. J. Heasman and A. J. Ridley, "Multiple roles for RhoA during T cell transendothelial migration," *Small GTPases*, vol. 1, no. 3, pp. 174–179, 2014.

[36] G. Bardi, V. Niggli, and P. Loetscher, "Rho kinase is required for CCR7-mediated polarization and chemotaxis of T lymphocytes," *FEBS Letters*, vol. 542, no. 1-3, pp. 79–83, 2003.

[37] L. Chen, H. Hu, W. Qiu, K. Shi, and M. Kassem, "Actin depolymerization enhances adipogenic differentiation in human stromal stem cells," *Stem Cell Research*, vol. 29, pp. 76–83, 2018.

[38] Y. Samstag and G. Nebl, "Interaction of cofilin with the serine phosphatases PP1 and PP2A in normal and neoplastic human T lymphocytes," *Advances in Enzyme Regulation*, vol. 43, no. 1, pp. 197–211, 2003.

[39] Y. Wang, F. Shibasaki, and K. Mizuno, "Calcium signal-induced cofilin dephosphorylation is mediated by Slingshot via calcineurin," *The Journal of Biological Chemistry*, vol. 280, no. 13, pp. 12683–12689, 2005.

[40] M. Nishita, C. Tomizawa, M. Yamamoto, Y. Horita, K. Ohashi, and K. Mizuno, "Spatial and temporal regulation of cofilin activity by LIM kinase and Slingshot is critical for directional cell migration," *The Journal of Cell Biology*, vol. 171, no. 2, pp. 349–359, 2005.

[41] S. Kurita, Y. Watanabe, E. Gunji, K. Ohashi, and K. Mizuno, "Molecular dissection of the mechanisms of substrate recognition and F-actin-mediated activation of cofilin-phosphatase Slingshot-1," *The Journal of Biological Chemistry*, vol. 283, no. 47, pp. 32542–32552, 2008.

[42] A. Gohla, J. Birkenfeld, and G. M. Bokoch, "Chronophin, a novel HAD-type serine protein phosphatase, regulates cofilin-dependent actin dynamics," *Nature Cell Biology*, vol. 7, no. 1, pp. 21–29, 2005.

[43] B. S. Yoon, E. K. Jun, G. Park et al., "Optimal suppression of protein phosphatase 2A activity is critical for maintenance of human embryonic stem cell self-renewal," *Stem Cells*, vol. 28, no. 5, pp. 874–884, 2010.

[44] P. S. Mathieu and E. G. Loboa, "Cytoskeletal and focal adhesion influences on mesenchymal stem cell shape, mechanical properties, and differentiation down osteogenic, adipogenic, and chondrogenic pathways," *Tissue Engineering. Part B, Reviews*, vol. 18, no. 6, pp. 436–444, 2012.

[45] I. A. Titushkin and M. R. Cho, "Controlling cellular biomechanics of human mesenchymal stem cells," in *2009 Annual International Conference of the IEEE Engineering in Medicine and Biology Society*, Minneapolis, MN, USA, September 2009.

[46] E. M. Darling, M. Topel, S. Zauscher, T. P. Vail, and F. Guilak, "Viscoelastic properties of human mesenchymally-derived stem cells and primary osteoblasts, chondrocytes, and adipocytes," *Journal of Biomechanics*, vol. 41, no. 2, pp. 454–464, 2008.

[47] D. E. Ingber, "Tensegrity-based mechanosensing from macro to micro," *Progress in Biophysics and Molecular Biology*, vol. 97, no. 2-3, pp. 163–179, 2008.

[48] M. L. Gardel, K. E. Kasza, C. P. Brangwynne, J. Liu, and D. A. Weitz, "Chapter 19. Mechanical response of cytoskeletal networks," *Methods in Cell Biology*, vol. 89, pp. 487–519, 2008.

[49] J. Stricker, T. Falzone, and M. L. Gardel, "Mechanics of the F-actin cytoskeleton," *Journal of Biomechanics*, vol. 43, no. 1, pp. 9–14, 2010.

[50] A. McGough, B. Pope, W. Chiu, and A. Weeds, "Cofilin changes the twist of F-actin: implications for actin filament dynamics and cellular function," *The Journal of Cell Biology*, vol. 138, no. 4, pp. 771–781, 1997.

[51] S. Cai, L. Pestic-Dragovich, M. E. O'Donnell et al., "Regulation of cytoskeletal mechanics and cell growth by myosin light chain phosphorylation," *American Journal of Physiology-Cell Physiology*, vol. 275, no. 5, pp. C1349–C1356, 1998.

[52] N. Rodríguez-Fuentes, A. G. Rodríguez-Hernández, J. Enríquez-Jiménez et al., "Nukbone® promotes proliferation and osteoblastic differentiation of mesenchymal stem cells from human amniotic membrane," *Biochemical and Biophysical Research Communications*, vol. 434, no. 3, pp. 676–680, 2013.

[53] N. Rodríguez-Fuentes, O. Reynoso-Ducoing, A. Rodríguez-Hernández et al., "Isolation of human mesenchymal stem cells and their cultivation on the porous bone matrix," *Journal of Visualized Experiments*, no. 96, article e51999, 2015.

[54] G. C. Reilly and A. J. Engler, "Intrinsic extracellular matrix properties regulate stem cell differentiation," *Journal of Biomechanics*, vol. 43, no. 1, pp. 55–62, 2010.

[55] J. Hao, Y. Zhang, D. Jing et al., "Mechanobiology of mesenchymal stem cells: perspective into mechanical induction of MSC fate," *Acta Biomaterialia*, vol. 20, pp. 1–9, 2015.

[56] E. K. F. Yim and M. P. Sheetz, "Force-dependent cell signaling in stem cell differentiation," *Stem Cell Research & Therapy*, vol. 3, no. 5, p. 41, 2012.

[57] E. K. Paluch, C. M. Nelson, N. Biais et al., "Mechanotransduction: use the force(s)," *BMC Biology*, vol. 13, no. 1, p. 47, 2015.

[58] N. Wang, J. D. Tytell, and D. E. Ingber, "Mechanotransduction at a distance: mechanically coupling the extracellular matrix with the nucleus," *Nature Reviews Molecular Cell Biology*, vol. 10, no. 1, pp. 75–82, 2009.

[59] Y. Chou, W. Huang, J. Dunn, T. Miller, and B. Wu, "The effect of biomimetic apatite structure on osteoblast viability, proliferation, and gene expression," *Biomaterials*, vol. 26, no. 3, pp. 285–295, 2005.

[60] J. W. Shin, J. Swift, I. Ivanovska, K. R. Spinler, A. Buxboim, and D. E. Discher, "Mechanobiology of bone marrow stem cells: from myosin-II forces to compliance of matrix and nucleus in cell forms and fates," *Differentiation*, vol. 86, no. 3, pp. 77–86, 2013.

[61] J. Du, Y. Zu, J. Li et al., "Extracellular matrix stiffness dictates Wnt expression through integrin pathway," *Scientific Reports*, vol. 6, no. 1, article 20395, 2016.

[62] G. Kanellos, J. Zhou, H. Patel et al., "ADF and Cofilin1 control actin stress fibers, nuclear integrity, and cell survival," *Cell Reports*, vol. 13, no. 9, pp. 1949–1964, 2015.

[63] F. Broders-Bondon, T. H. Nguyen Ho-Bouldoires, M. E. Fernandez-Sanchez, and E. Farge, "Mechanotransduction in tumor progression: the dark side of the force," *The Journal of Cell Biology*, vol. 217, no. 5, pp. 1571–1587, 2018.

[64] J. D. Lathia, "Awakening the beast: chemotherapeutic activation of cancer stem cells," *Science Translational Medicine*, vol. 7, no. 269, article 269ec3, 2015.

[65] V. Plaks, N. Kong, and Z. Werb, "The cancer stem cell niche: how essential is the niche in regulating stemness of tumor cells?," *Cell Stem Cell*, vol. 16, no. 3, pp. 225–238, 2015.

[66] Y. Kfoury and D. T. Scadden, "Mesenchymal cell contributions to the stem cell niche," *Cell Stem Cell*, vol. 16, no. 3, pp. 239–253, 2015.

[67] L. Liu, S. X. Zhang, W. Liao et al., "Mechanoresponsive stem cells to target cancer metastases through biophysical cues," *Science Translational Medicine*, vol. 9, no. 400, article eaan2966, 2017.

[68] W. L. Murphy, T. C. McDevitt, and A. J. Engler, "Materials as stem cell regulators," *Nature Materials*, vol. 13, no. 6, pp. 547–557, 2014.

[69] R. X. Wu, X. Y. Xu, J. Wang, X. T. He, H. H. Sun, and F. M. Chen, "Biomaterials for endogenous regenerative medicine: coaxing stem cell homing and beyond," *Applied Materials Today*, vol. 11, pp. 144–165, 2018.

[70] J. J. Northey, L. Przybyla, and V. M. Weaver, "Tissue force programs cell fate and tumor aggression," *Cancer Discovery*, vol. 7, no. 11, pp. 1224–1237, 2017.

[71] F. Zanconato, M. Cordenonsi, and S. Piccolo, "YAP/TAZ at the roots of cancer," *Cancer Cell*, vol. 29, no. 6, pp. 783–803, 2016.

[72] F. Zanconato, G. Battilana, M. Cordenonsi, and S. Piccolo, "YAP/TAZ as therapeutic targets in cancer," *Current Opinion in Pharmacology*, vol. 29, pp. 26–33, 2016.

[73] B. C. Low, C. Q. Pan, G. V. Shivashankar, A. Bershadsky, M. Sudol, and M. Sheetz, "YAP/TAZ as mechanosensors and mechanotransducers in regulating organ size and tumor growth," *FEBS Letters*, vol. 588, no. 16, pp. 2663–2670, 2014.

[74] D. E. Discher, L. Smith, S. Cho, M. Colasurdo, A. J. García, and S. Safran, "Matrix mechanosensing: from scaling concepts in 'omics data to mechanisms in the nucleus, regeneration, and cancer," *Annual Review of Biophysics*, vol. 46, no. 1, pp. 295–315, 2017.

[75] L. Azzolin, T. Panciera, S. Soligo et al., "YAP/TAZ incorporation in the β-catenin destruction complex orchestrates the Wnt response," *Cell*, vol. 158, no. 1, pp. 157–170, 2014.

[76] E. Jabbari, S. K. Sarvestani, L. Daneshian, and S. Moeinzadeh, "Optimum 3D matrix stiffness for maintenance of cancer stem cells is dependent on tissue origin of cancer cells," *PLoS One*, vol. 10, no. 7, article e0132377, 2015.

[77] L. Daneshian and E. Jabbari, "Determination of optimum matrix stiffness for maintenance of human colon cancer stem cells," *Tissue Engineering Part A*, vol. 21, article S222, 2015.

[78] A. Orza, D. Casciano, and A. Biris, "Nanomaterials for targeted drug delivery to cancer stem cells," *Drug Metabolism Reviews*, vol. 46, no. 2, pp. 191–206, 2014.

[79] B. Li, Q. Li, J. Mo, and H. Dai, "Drug-loaded polymeric nanoparticles for cancer stem cell targeting," *Frontiers in Pharmacology*, vol. 8, p. 51, 2017.

14

A Comparison of the Preservation of Mouse Adipose Tissue-Derived Mesenchymal Stem Cells using the University of Wisconsin Solution and Hank's Balanced Salt Solution

Saifun Nahar,[1] Yoshiki Nakashima,[2] Chika Miyagi-Shiohira,[2] Takao Kinjo,[3] Naoya Kobayashi,[4] Issei Saitoh,[5] Masami Watanabe,[6] Hirofumi Noguchi,[2] and Jiro Fujita[1]

[1]*Department of Infectious, Respiratory, and Digestive Medicine, Graduate School of Medicine, University of the Ryukyus, Okinawa 903-0215, Japan*
[2]*Department of Regenerative Medicine, Graduate School of Medicine, University of the Ryukyus, Okinawa 903-0215, Japan*
[3]*Department of Basic Laboratory Sciences, School of Health Sciences in the Faculty of Medicine, University of the Ryukyus, Okinawa 903-0215, Japan*
[4]*Okayama Saidaiji Hospital, Okayama 704-8192, Japan*
[5]*Division of Pediatric Dentistry, Graduate School of Medical and Dental Science, Niigata University, Niigata 951-8514, Japan*
[6]*Department of Urology, Okayama University Graduate School of Medicine, Dentistry and Pharmaceutical Sciences, Okayama 700-8558, Japan*

Correspondence should be addressed to Yoshiki Nakashima; nakasima@med.u-ryukyu.ac.jp and Hirofumi Noguchi; noguchih@med.u-ryukyu.ac.jp

Academic Editor: Sangho Roh

Preservation of adipose tissue before the isolation of cells is one of the most important steps in maintaining the cell viability of adipose tissue-derived mesenchymal stem cells (ADSCs) for clinical use. Hank's balanced salt solution (HBSS) is one of the main ADSC preservation solutions used clinically. However, this step is known to lead to decreased cell viability. The University of Wisconsin (UW) solution is recognized by transplant physicians as an excellent organ preservation solution. We aimed to investigate the effectiveness of UW solution in preservation of the viability of ADSCs. We collected adipose tissue from the inguinal fat pad of mice and compared preservation in UW solution and HBSS overnight by measuring cell viability after isolation. We found that the number of viable cells harvested per gram of adipose tissue mass was higher in UW solution- than HBSS-preserved tissue.

1. Introduction

Mesenchymal stem cells (MSCs) [1] are a source of cell therapy in regenerative medicine. MSCs have the ability to undergo self-renewal and to form differentiated cells, including adipocytes, chondrocytes, neuronal cells, and osteocytes [2]. MSCs also regulate biological functions such as growth factor release [3] and have immunosuppressive effects. Among several sources of MSCs, adipose tissue-derived mesenchymal stem cells (ADSCs) [4, 5] have become a renowned therapeutic tool in clinical use [6–8].

Most clinical researchers using ADSCs follow their own particular protocol for isolating ADSCs, and there is no optimal storage medium for preserving adipose tissue after collection. There are several reasons why facilities that perform cell therapy with ADSCs use a preserving solution. First, it can take from several hours to as long as a day to transport the tissue from the operating room to the cell processing center. Second, some clinical researchers believe that overnight preservation using a mixture of storage medium and penicillin/streptomycin is necessary to prevent bacterial infection. The selection of a storage solution is therefore critically important for maintaining the function of ADSCs for clinical use. Nevertheless, cell survival rates decrease when ADSCs are stored in preservation solution for 12–24 hours [9].

Hank's balanced salt solution (HBSS) [10, 11] and phosphate-buffered saline (PBS) solution are the most common solutions used for preserving certain types of cells. The essential function of HBSS is to maintain the pH and osmotic balance as well as provide the cells with water and inorganic ions. HBSS also contains glucose, which provides the cells with energy. Meanwhile, some studies have reported that the University of Wisconsin (UW) solution [12–14] has a better tissue preservation ability than other types of preservation solutions for certain types of cells [15].

Here, we compared the cell viability of ADSCs preserved in UW solution and HBSS.

2. Materials and Methods

2.1. Reagents. UW solution (Viaspan) was obtained from Astellas Pharma Inc. (Tokyo, Japan). HBSS and collagenase type IV solution were obtained from Thermo Fisher Scientific (Tokyo, Japan). All other materials used were of the highest commercial grade.

2.2. Animal Care. All experimental protocols were in accordance with the guidelines for the care and use of laboratory animals set by the Research Laboratory Center, Faculty of Medicine, and the Institute for Animal Experiments, Faculty of Medicine, University of the Ryukyus (Okinawa, Japan). The experimental protocol was approved by the Committee on Animal Experiments of the University of the Ryukyus (permit number: A2017101).

C57BL/6 male mice (8 weeks old; Japan SLC, Shizuoka, Japan) were maintained under controlled temperature (23 ± 2°C) and light conditions (lights on from 08:30–20:30). Animals were fed standard rodent chow pellets and had ad libitum access to water. All efforts were made to minimize the suffering of the animals.

2.3. Isolation of ADSCs from Adipose Tissue. Adipose tissue was extracted from the inguinal fat pad of 8-week-old mice (male, $n = 3$). The tissues were divided into three groups: nonpreserved control, HBSS-preserved, and UW solution-preserved groups. In the control group, ADSCs were isolated without preserving adipose tissue overnight. In the preservation groups, adipose tissue was submerged in HBSS or UW solution at 4°C for 16 h until the isolation procedure. Isolation of ADSCs from adipose tissue was conducted as previously described [16]. Briefly, the adipose tissue was stored in HBSS at 4°C temperature and washed vigorously three times using HBSS before tissue digestion. The adipose tissue was cut into small fragments using a scalpel and digested enzymatically (2 mg collagenase type IV/ml; HBSS) in 50 ml tubes with shaking (rotation speed 20 speeds/min at 37°C for 120 min; BioShaker BR-42FM, TAITEC, Saitama, Japan). The tubes were subsequently centrifuged (800 × g) for 5 minutes. The cell pellet containing ADSCs was collected and washed with fresh Dulbecco's Modified Eagle Medium (DMEM) containing 10% fetal bovine serum (FBS; Gibco-Invitrogen, Carlsbad, CA, USA) to remove residual enzyme after the digestion, and the digested cells were incubated in a T25 flask (illustration of the procedure is shown in Figure 1). All mouse studies were approved by the Institutional Animal Care and Use Committee of University of the Ryukyus.

2.4. Assessment of the Cellular Viability. The viability of ADSCs after isolation was assessed using 0.4% *w/v* Trypan blue solution (Wako Pure Chemical Corporation, Osaka, Japan) and C-Chip™ hemocytometers (NanoEnTek Inc., MA, USA).

2.5. Flow Cytometry. Cell flow cytometry was performed using a NovoCyte® Flow Cytometer (ACEA Biosciences Inc., San Diego, CA, USA) according to the manufacturer's instructions. Briefly, ADSCs (1×10^5 cells) were mixed into 0.5 ml of Perfusion Solution (CORNING, Manassas, VA, USA). Each antibody (1/100 of the volume) was added to the cell mixture and incubated on ice for 30 minutes. After washing the cells with Brilliant Stain Buffer (BD Biosciences, Franklin Lakes, NJ, USA), fluorescence-activated cell sorting (FACS) measurements were conducted. The following primary antibodies were used: Brilliant Violet 421™ Rat Anti-Mouse CD44 (BD Biosciences), Fluorescein Isothiocyanate (FITC) Rat Anti-Mouse CD90.2 (BD Biosciences), PerCP/Cy5.5 Anti-Mouse CD34 (BioLegend, San Diego, CA, USA), and PE/Cy7 Rat Anti-Mouse CD45 (BD Biosciences). Isotype-identical antibodies were used as controls.

2.6. Real-Time PCR and RT-PCR. RNA was prepared for a qPCR using a RNeasy® Mini kit and QuantiTect® Reverse Transcription kit according to the manufacturer's instructions (Qiagen, Hilden, Germany). AmpliTaq Gold® 360 Master mix was used according to the manufacturer's instructions (Thermo Fisher Scientific, Tokyo, Japan). Real-time PCR analyses were performed using a LightCycler 96 Real-Time PCR system (Roche, Basel, Switzerland). The Taqman® Universal Master Mix II, no UNG (Applied Biosystems, USA) was used according to the manufacturer's instructions. An RT-PCR was performed using a GeneAtlas 482 thermal cycler (Astec Co. Ltd., Fukuoka, Japan). Images were recorded using an Aplegen® Omega Lum C (Gel Company, San Francisco, CA, USA).

The primers used for the RT-PCR included the following:

(i) Mouse HGF forward, ACTCTTACCAAGGAAG ACCCATTAC

(ii) Mouse HGF reverse, ATACCAGTAGCATCGT TTTCTTGAC

(iii) Mouse EGF forward, TATCCATCGGTAATAA GGGTGAAC

(iv) Mouse EGF reverse, CCAGCACACACTCATC TATATCAGA

(v) Mouse VEGF forward, TGTCTTCACTGGATAT GTTTGACTG

(vi) Mouse VEGF reverse, TTCTCTGTCATCATCT GTCTCTCTG

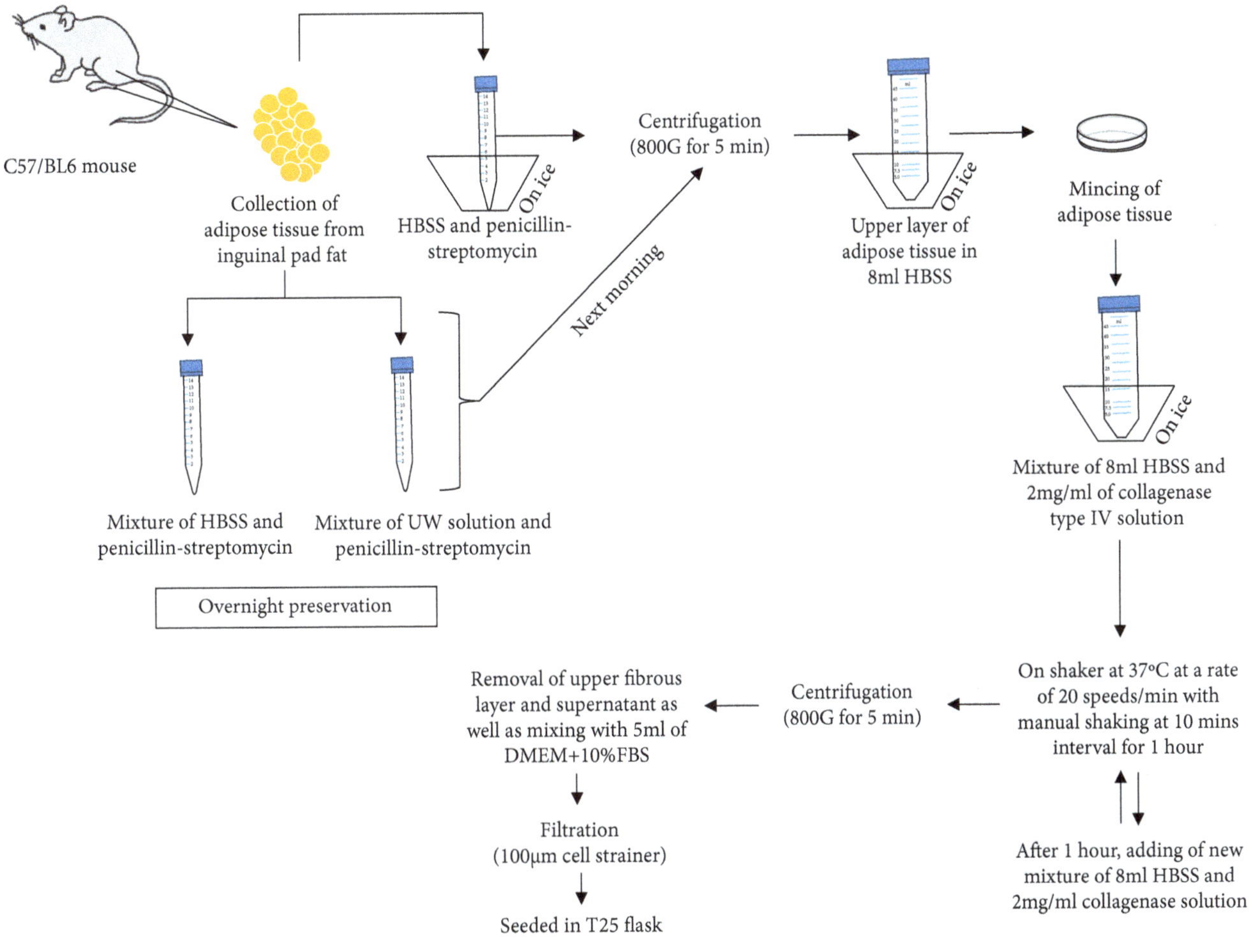

FIGURE 1: Illustration of the collection and preservation of adipose tissue-derived mesenchymal stem cells (ADSCs). ADSCs were isolated after storage of adipose tissue overnight in preservation solution (HBSS or UW solution). In the control group, ADSCs were isolated without preserving adipose tissue overnight.

(vii) Mouse SCAI forward, GGTTGTTTTCAGTACC TCTTTCCTG

(viii) Mouse SCAI reverse, CATGCTCATTACTAGA AAAGCCAGG

(ix) Mouse GAPDH forward, AACTCACTCAAGAT TGTCAGCAATG

(x) Mouse GAPDH reverse, GCTGTAGCCGTATT CATTGTCATAC

2.7. Cell Proliferation. The cells were seeded onto 24-well plates at a density of 1.0×10^4 cells/well. The slides were photographed with a microscope (×40) and the number of cells in the image was counted. The relative cell proliferation rate was calculated by converting the number of cells on the day of cell seeding to 100%.

2.8. Cell Differentiation. Adipogenic differentiation was examined using OriCell™ Mesenchymal Stem Cell Adipogenic Differentiation Medium (GUXMX-90031, Cyagen Biosciences) and the Lipid Assay Kit (AK09F, Cosmo Bio Co. Ltd, Tokyo, Japan) according to the manufacturer's instructions. Osteogenic differentiation was examined using OriCell™ Mesenchymal Stem Cell Osteogenic Differentiation Medium (GUXMX-90021, Cyagen Biosciences) and the Calcified Nodule Staining Kit (AK21, Cosmo Bio Co. Ltd, Tokyo, Japan) according to the manufacturer's instructions.

2.9. Statistical Analyses. The data are presented as the mean ± standard error (SE). The differences among three groups were analyzed using two-way ANOVA. *P* values of <0.05 were considered statistically significant.

3. Results and Discussion

3.1. Characteristics of ADSCs Isolated without Preservation. ADSCs isolated without preservation served as the control group. They were cultured to 80% confluence in DMEM containing 10% FBS. Microscopy was performed to confirm the absence of abnormalities with regard to cell size and shape and culture state (Figure 2(a)). Flow cytometry was performed using markers of mouse MSCs (CD44 and CD90.2), hematopoietic stem cells (CD34), and leukocytes (CD45). We observed the expression of CD44 and CD90.2 but not CD34 and CD45 (Figure 2(a)), confirming that the isolated

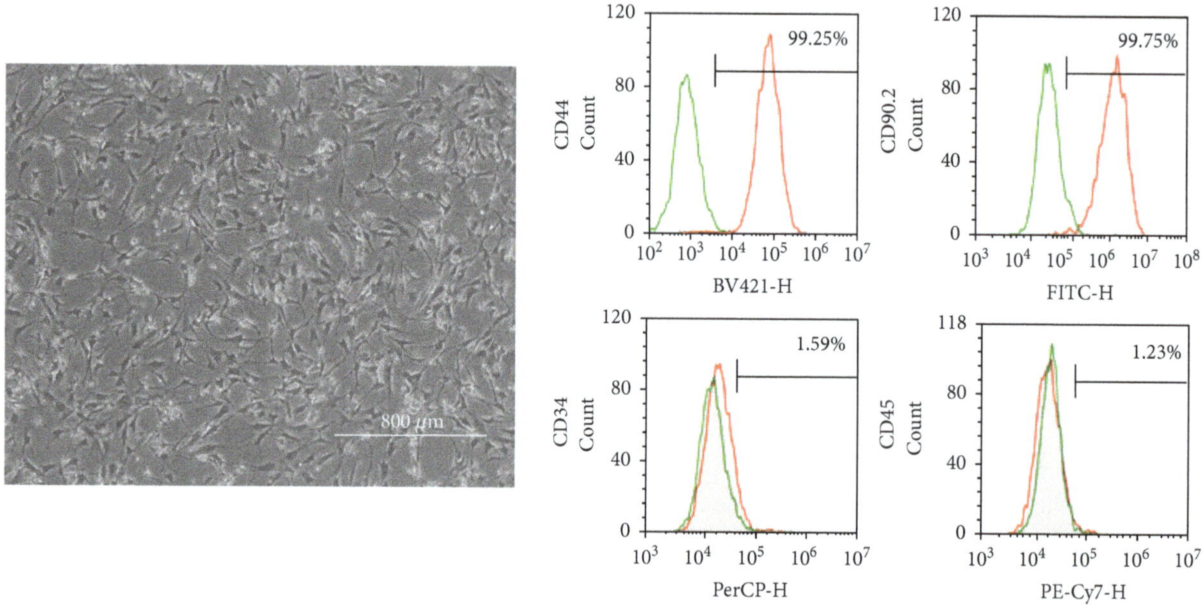

(a)

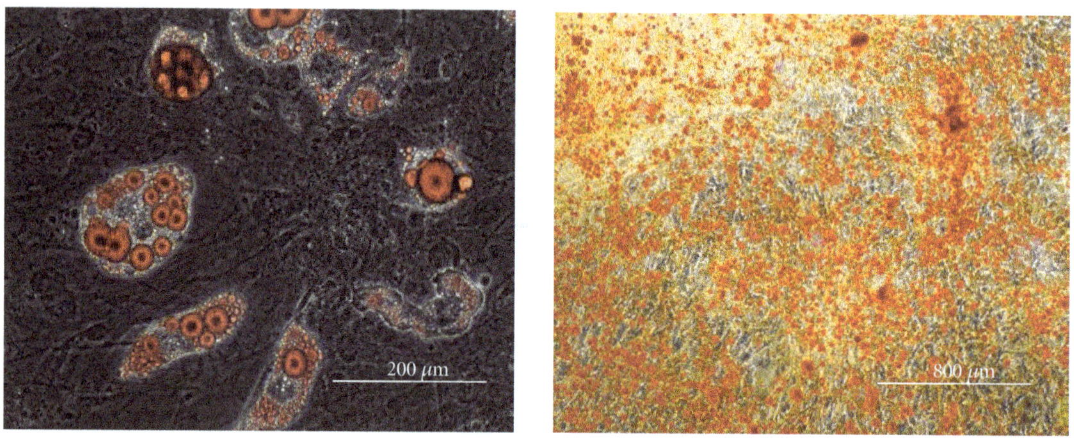

(b)

Figure 2: Phenotype and differentiation potential of ADSCs isolated without preservation, which served as control group. Morphological appearance of ADSCs (passage 2) (a, left panel) and cell surface markers of ADSCs by flow cytometry (passage 2) (a, right panel). Representative images of adipocyte (b, left panel) and osteocyte differentiation (b, right panel) from mouse ADSCs (passage 2) cultured in differentiation medium.

cells were MSCs. We induced differentiation of the ADSCs into adipocytes (Figure 2(b)) and osteoblasts (Figure 2(b)). Mature adipocytes were stained with Oil Red O, and mature osteoblasts were stained with Alizarin Red S.

3.2. Cell Viability of ADSCs after Preservation in HBSS or UW Solution. To assess the cell viability in each group, we measured the total cell number/tissue weight (mg) and live cell number/tissue weight (mg). There were no significant differences in the total cell number between the control group ($1.37 \pm 0.43 \times 10^7$/g) and two preservation groups (HBSS group, $1.43 \pm 0.16 \times 10^7$/g; UW solution group, $1.52 \pm 0.33 \times 10^7$/g) ($n = 3$) (Figure 3(a)). These data suggest that the isolation of ADSCs in the control and two preservation groups were of similar processing efficiency. We also calculated the live cell number/total cell number ratio. There was a significant difference in cell viability between the control and HBSS-preserved group but not the UW-preserved group (control group: 0.83 ± 0.03, HBSS group: 0.74 ± 0.03, UW solution group: 0.82 ± 0.01) ($n = 3$) (Figure 3(b)). These data suggest that the cell viability of ADSCs after preservation in HBSS was significantly decreased compared to both the control and UW solution-preserved groups. ADSCs in each group were seeded at a concentration of 1×10^4 cells/24 well and the number of cells on days 3 and 5 was then counted (Figure 3(c)). The cell proliferation rate on days 3 and 5 of the UW group was equivalent to that of the control group. However, the cell proliferation rate on days 3 and 5 of the HBSS group was significantly lower than that of the control group. ADSC preserved in UW solution maintained a cell proliferation ability equivalent to that of the control group.

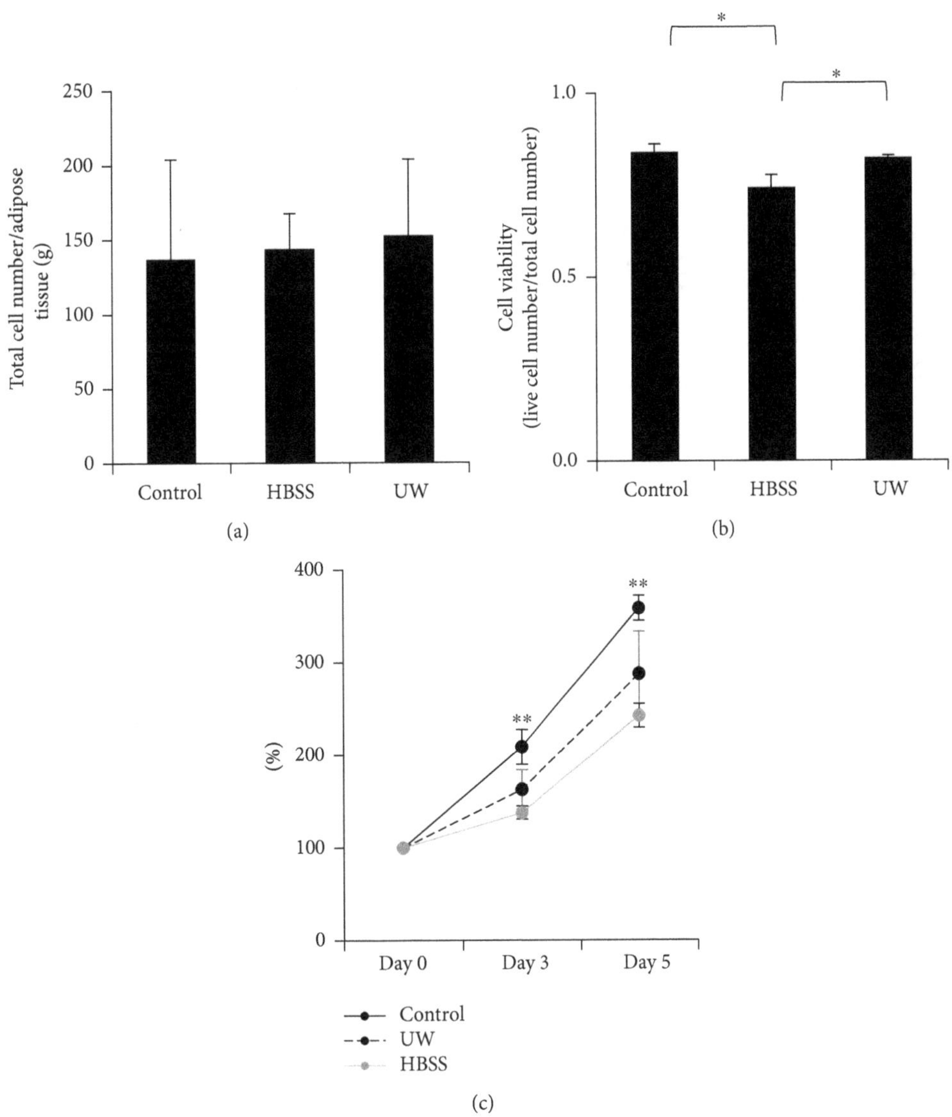

FIGURE 3: Total cell number and cell viability of ADSCs after preservation for 16 h in Hank's balanced salt solution (HBSS) or University of Wisconsin (UW) solution. Graphical representation of the total number of cells yielded from 1 gram of mouse adipose tissue after overnight preservation in UW and HBSS. ADSCs isolated without preservation served as control group (a). Cellular viability was determined by counting the number of live cells (not stained with 0.4% *w/v* Trypan blue solution) under a microscope. The decrease in cell viability of the HBSS group compared with both the control and UW groups was significant. Data are expressed as the mean ± SE (control group: 0.83 ± 0.03, HBSS group: 0.74 ± 0.03; $^*P < 0.05$. UW solution group: 0.82 ± 0.01; $^*P < 0.05$, $n = 3$) (b). Cell proliferation rate in the HBSS group on days 3 and 5 was significantly lower than that of the control group. Data are mean ± SE. The relative value is shown with the number of cells on day 0 as 100%. Day 0 (control group: 100.0 ± 0.0, UW group: 100.0 ± 0.0, HBSS group: 100.0 ± 0.0, $n = 5$). Day 3 (control group: 208.5 ± 18.9, UW group: 162.5 ± 21.2, HBSS group: 137.5 ± 7.1; $^{**}P < 0.01$, $n = 5$). Day 5 (control group: 358.0 ± 13.7, UW group: 287.0 ± 45.4, HBSS group: 242.3 ± 12.9; $^{**}P < 0.01$, $n = 5$) (c).

3.3. Characteristics of the Isolated ADSCs after Preservation Using HBSS or UW Solution. The characteristics of mouse ADSCs after preservation are shown in Figure 4. ADSCs were cultured to 80% confluence in DMEM medium containing 10% FBS. Microscopy was performed to confirm the absence of abnormalities with regard to cell size and shape and the culture state in the HBSS- (Figure 4(a)) and UW solution-preserved groups (Figure 4(c)). Flow cytometry was performed using markers of mouse MSCs (CD44, CD90.2), hematopoietic stem cells (CD34), and leukocytes (CD45). We observed the expression of CD44 and CD90.2 but not CD34 or CD45 in cells that were preserved in HBSS (Figure 4(a)) and UW solution (Figure 4(c)), indicating the presence of MSCs. We confirmed the expression level of ADSC surface markers (CD34, CD44, and CD45) of the control, HBSS and UW groups using the PCR measurement method. Results were similar to those of flow cytometer analysis (data not shown). PCR was used to examine the mRNA expression levels of hepatocyte growth factor (HGF), epidermal growth factor (EGF), vascular endothelial growth factor (VEGFA), and a suppressor of cancer cell invasion (SCAI) expressed in ADSC. As a result, cell functions of the

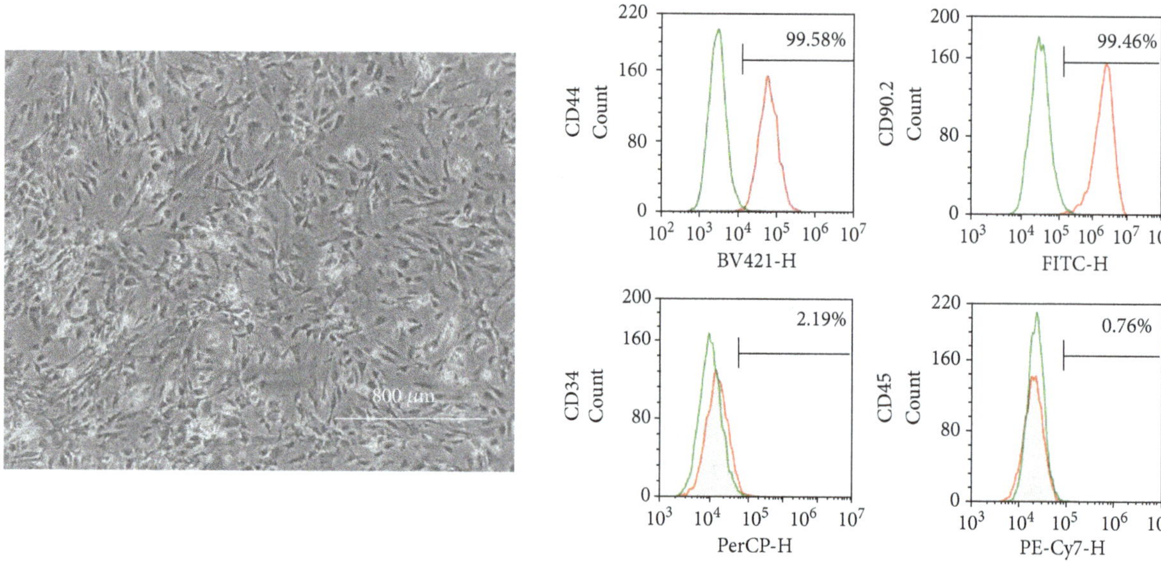

(a)

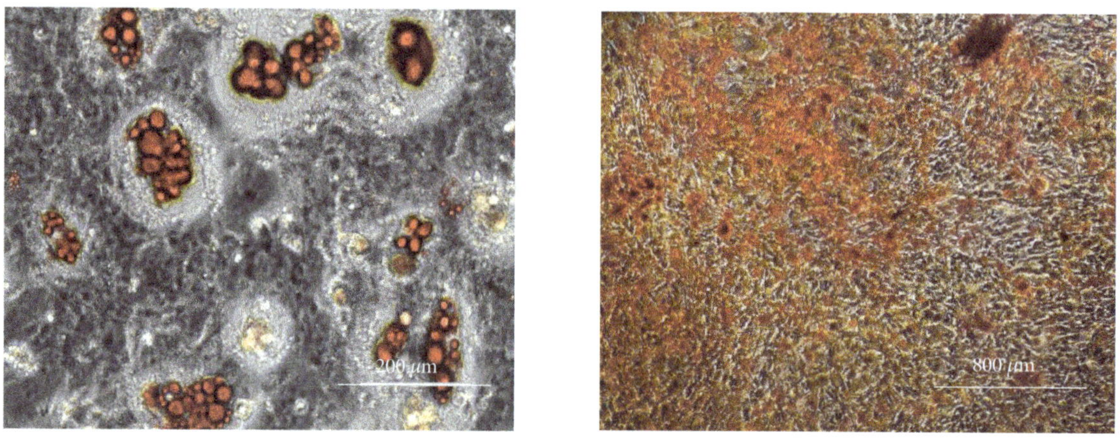

(b)

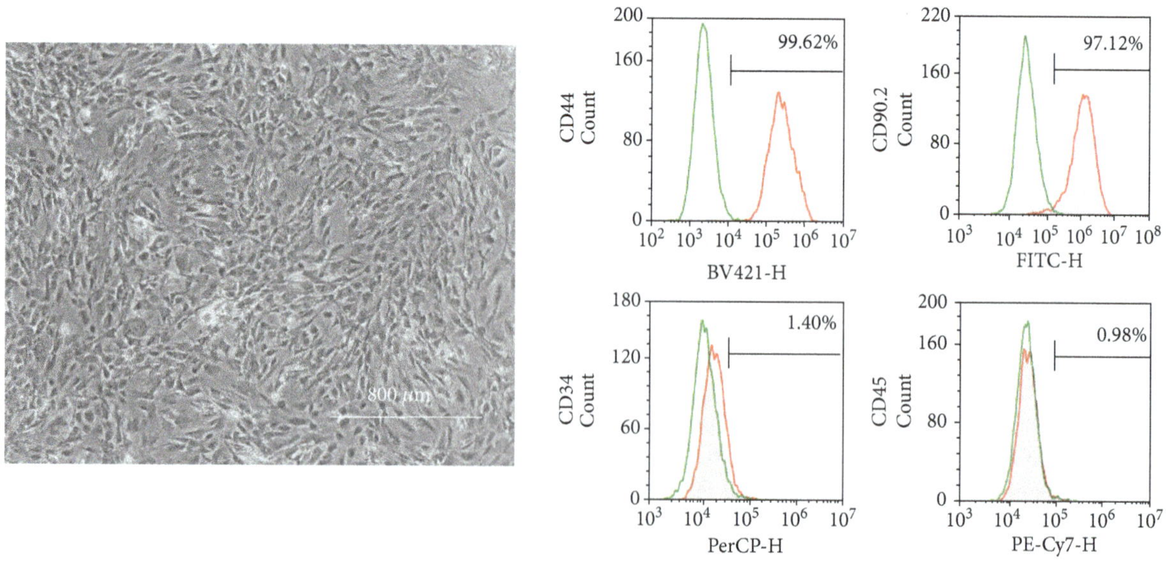

(c)

FIGURE 4: Continued.

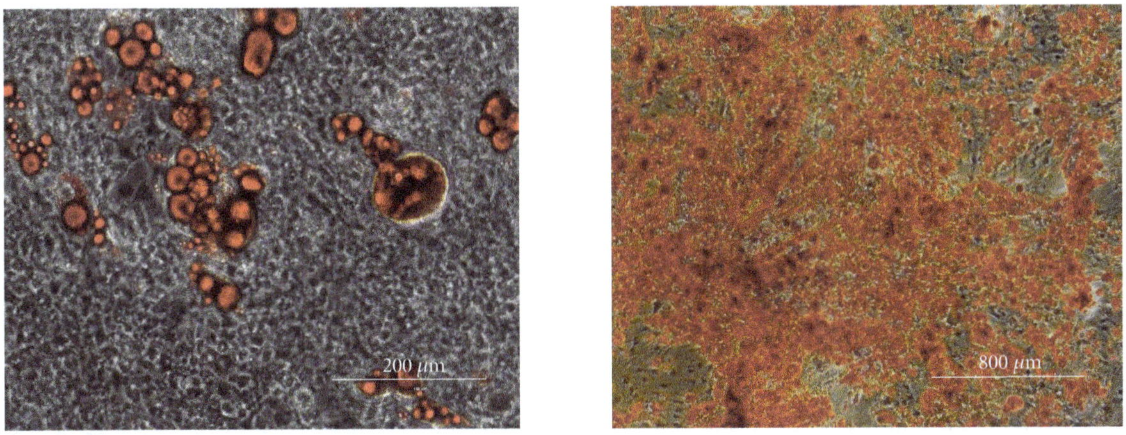

(d)

FIGURE 4: Phenotype and differentiation potential of ADSCs after preservation for 16 h in HBSS or UW solution. Morphological appearance of ADSCs (passage 2) in the HBSS- (a, left panel) and UW solution-preserved groups (c, left panel). Cell surface markers of ADSCs (passage 2) preserved in HBSS (a, right panels) or UW solution (c, right panels) by flow cytometry. Representative images of differentiated adipocytes from ADSCs preserved in HBSS (b, left panel) and UW solution (d, left panel), and differentiated osteocytes from ADSCs preserved in HBSS (b, right panel) and UW solution (d, right panel).

control, HBSS and UW groups were evaluated as equivalent (Supplemental Figure 1A). We induced differentiation of ADSCs in the HBSS (Figure 4(b)) and UW solution-preserved groups (Figure 4(d)) into adipocytes. We also induced differentiation of the ADSCs in the HBSS (Figure 4(b)) and UW solution-preserved groups (Figure 4(d)) into osteoblasts. The presence of mature adipocytes and osteoblasts was confirmed by staining with Oil Red O and Alizarin Red S, respectively. Maintenance of differentiation potential was demonstrated as osteogenic and adipogenic differentiation.

Adipose tissue is considered a reliable and abundant source of adult stem cells for regenerative therapy. To yield good quality ADSCs, adipose tissue must be preserved in an appropriate solution before isolation. We investigated the effectiveness of two storage solutions (HBSS and UW solution) for preserving adipose tissue overnight before isolation of ADSCs by examining subsequent cell viability. We found that cell viability was higher in the UW solution group (82%) than the HBSS group (74%). However, UW solution has an inhibitory effect on collagenase digestion. That tissue digestion is the most important step in the isolation of ADSCs from adipose tissue makes this a major disadvantage. To overcome this, we washed the adipose tissue with HBSS or Dulbecco's phosphate-buffered saline (DPBS). Table 1 shows the compositions of UW solution and HBSS. The UW solution contains higher potassium (120 mmol/l), magnesium (5 mmol/l), and phosphorus (25 mmol/l) than HBSS. It also contains many additional components such as lactobionate (100 mmol/l), raffinose (30 mmol/l), adenosine (5 mmol/l), allopurinol (1 mmol/l), and glutathione (3 mmol/l). These components might have contributed to maintaining the survival rate of ADSCs. However, the UW solution is ten times more expensive than the HBSS solution. Meanwhile, the composition of HBSS is similar to that of PBS and is characterized by its containing glucose (5.6 mmol/l) and low price. Interestingly, however, our results suggest that there is almost no influence of glucose on adipose tissue preservation for 16 h. This is in agreement with previous reports that revealed that glucose concentration does not affect the cell proliferation of human MSCs [17]. In other reports, however, bone marrow-derived MSCs were observed to have fewer mitochondria in the glycolysis system and lower glucose metabolism [18]. In addition, there are reports that high glucose promotes bone differentiation of MSCs [19]. Therefore, glucose containing preservation solution may not be necessary to maintain quality of ADSCs.

TABLE 1: The specific composition of UW solution and HBSS.

	University of Wisconsin (UW) solution	Hank's balanced salt solution (HBSS)
Natrium [Na^+] (mmol/l)	30	142.8
Kalium [K^+] (mmol/l)	120	5.8
Magnesium [Mg^{2+}] (mmol/l)	5	0.9
Calcium [Ca^{2+}] (mmol/l)	—	1.3
Carbonate [$CO3^{2-}$] (mmol/l)	—	4.2
Chlorine [Cl^-] (mmol/l)	—	146.8
Phosphate [$PO4^{3-}$] (mmol/l)	25	0.8
Sulfate [$SO4^{2-}$] (mmol/l)	5	0.4
Lactobionate (mmol/l)	100	—
Raffinose (mmol/l)	30	—
Adenosine (mmol/l)	5	—
Allopurinol (mmol/l)	1	—
Glutathione (mmol/l)	3	—
Glucose (mmol/l)	—	5.6
HES (g/l)	50	—
pH	7.4	7.2

4. Conclusions

UW solution has been confirmed to significantly enhance cell survival and cell proliferation ability as a preservation solution of ADSCs. However, considering that UW solution is substantially more expensive than HBSS, our findings also suggest that HBSS possess sufficient function as a preservative solution.

Authors' Contributions

SN, YN, CS, and HN designed the study. SN, YN, CS, and HN conducted the study. SN, YN, CS, TK, and HN collected the data. SN, YN, CS, TK, and HN analyzed the data. SN, YN, CS, TK, and HN interpreted the data. TM, NK, IS, MW, and JF provided the materials. SN, YN, and HN provided the manuscript. SN, YN, and HN drafted the manuscript. SN, YN, and HN revised the content of the manuscript. SN, YN, CS, TK, NK, IS, MW, JF, and HN approved the final version of the manuscript. SN takes responsibility for the integrity of all of the data analyses.

Acknowledgments

We thank Naomi Kakazu (University of the Ryukyus) for clerical assistance and Saki Uema, Yuka Onishi, Maki Higa, Yuki Kawahira, and Saori Adaniya (University of the Ryukyus) for providing technical support. This work was supported by the Research Laboratory Center, Faculty of Medicine, and the Institute for Animal Experiments, Faculty of Medicine, University of the Ryukyus. This work was supported in part by the Japan Society for the Promotion of Science (JSPS; KAKENHI Grant number 16H07094), Japan Agency for Medical Research and Development, Naito Foundation, and Okinawa Science and Technology Promotion Center (OSTC).

Supplementary Materials

Supplemental Figure 1: assay of growth factor expression level of ADSC after storage in HBSS or UW solution for 16 hours. Results of RT-PCR to evaluate growth factor and cell surface marker mRNA expression of ADSCs (Supplemental Figure 1A). Full-length images of the blots used for Supplemental Figure 1A (Supplemental Figure 1B). *(Supplementary Materials)*

References

[1] A. J. Wagers and I. L. Weissman, "Plasticity of adult stem cells," *Cell*, vol. 116, no. 5, pp. 639–648, 2004.

[2] R. Tabatabaei Qomi and M. Sheykhhasan, "Adipose-derived stromal cell in regenerative medicine: a review," *World Journal of Stem Cells*, vol. 9, no. 8, pp. 107–117, 2017.

[3] W. P. Tang, T. Akahoshi, J. S. Piao et al., "Basic fibroblast growth factor-treated adipose tissue-derived mesenchymal stem cell infusion to ameliorate liver cirrhosis via paracrine hepatocyte growth factor," *Journal of Gastroenterology and Hepatology*, vol. 30, no. 6, pp. 1065–1074, 2015.

[4] K. Szoke and J. E. Brinchmann, "Concise review: therapeutic potential of adipose tissue-derived angiogenic cells," *Stem Cells Translational Medicine*, vol. 1, no. 9, pp. 658–667, 2012.

[5] C. Miyagi-Shiohira, K. Kurima, N. Kobayashi et al., "Cryopreservation of adipose-derived mesenchymal stem cells," *Cell Medicine*, vol. 8, no. 1-2, pp. 3–7, 2015.

[6] A. Seki, Y. Sakai, T. Komura et al., "Adipose tissue-derived stem cells as a regenerative therapy for a mouse steatohepatitis-induced cirrhosis model," *Hepatology*, vol. 58, no. 3, pp. 1133–1142, 2013.

[7] I. Ullah, R. B. Subbarao, and G. J. Rho, "Human mesenchymal stem cells - current trends and future prospective," *Bioscience Reports*, vol. 35, no. 2, article e00191, 2015.

[8] C. Miyagi-Shiohira, N. Kobayashi, I. Saitoh et al., "Evaluation of serum-free, xeno-free cryopreservation solutions for human adipose-derived mesenchymal stem cells," *Cell Medicine*, vol. 9, no. 1-2, pp. 15–20, 2017.

[9] M. Falah, A. Rayan, and S. Srouji, "Storage effect on viability and biofunctionality of human adipose tissue-derived stromal cells," *Cytotherapy*, vol. 17, no. 9, pp. 1220–1229, 2015.

[10] F. Moazami, H. Mirhadi, B. Geramizadeh, and S. Sahebi, "Comparison of soymilk, powdered milk, Hank's balanced salt solution and tap water on periodontal ligament cell survival," *Dental Traumatology*, vol. 28, no. 2, pp. 132–135, 2012.

[11] B. D. Souza, A. M. Alves, L. G. Santos, C. M. Simoes, W. T. Felippe, and M. C. Felippe, "Fibroblast viability after storage at 20 degrees C in milk, Hank's balanced salt solution and coconut water," *Brazilian Dental Journal*, vol. 27, no. 4, pp. 404–407, 2016.

[12] A. M. D'Alessandro, M. Kalayoglu, H. W. Sollinger, J. D. Pirsch, J. H. Southard, and F. O. Belzer, "Current status of organ preservation with University of Wisconsin solution," *Archives of Pathology & Laboratory Medicine*, vol. 115, no. 3, pp. 306–310, 1991.

[13] F. O. Belzer, M. Kalayoglu, A. M. D'Alessandro et al., "Organ preservation: experience with University of Wisconsin solution and plans for the future," *Clinical Transplantation*, vol. 4, no. 2, pp. 73–77, 1990.

[14] A. Katayama, H. Noguchi, T. Kuise et al., "Comparison of new preservation solutions, HN-1 and University of Wisconsin solution, in pancreas preservation for porcine islet isolation," *Cell Medicine*, vol. 6, no. 1-2, pp. 3–8, 2013.

[15] T. Eberl, T. Schmid, P. Hengster et al., "Protective effects of various preservation solutions on cultured endothelial cells," *The Annals of Thoracic Surgery*, vol. 58, no. 2, pp. 489–495, 1994.

[16] H. Yukawa, M. Watanabe, N. Kaji et al., "Monitoring transplanted adipose tissue-derived stem cells combined with heparin in the liver by fluorescence imaging using quantum dots," *Biomaterials*, vol. 33, no. 7, pp. 2177–2186, 2012.

[17] B. R. Weil, A. M. Abarbanell, J. L. Herrmann, Y. Wang, and D. R. Meldrum, "High glucose concentration in cell culture medium does not acutely affect human mesenchymal stem cell growth factor production or proliferation," *American Journal of Physiology. Regulatory, Integrative and Comparative Physiology*, vol. 296, no. 6, pp. R1735–R1743, 2009.

[18] N. Fillmore, A. Huqi, J. S. Jaswal et al., "Effect of fatty acids on human bone marrow mesenchymal stem cell energy metabolism and survival," *PLoS One*, vol. 10, no. 3, article e0120257, 2015.

[19] Y. M. Li, T. Schilling, P. Benisch et al., "Effects of high glucose on mesenchymal stem cell proliferation and differentiation," *Biochemical and Biophysical Research Communications*, vol. 363, no. 1, pp. 209–215, 2007.

15

Conditioned Medium from Human Amnion-Derived Mesenchymal Stem Cells Regulates Activation of Primary Hepatic Stellate Cells

Qingjie Fu, Shunsuke Ohnishi, and Naoya Sakamoto

Department of Gastroenterology and Hepatology, Hokkaido University Graduate School of Medicine, Sapporo, Japan

Correspondence should be addressed to Shunsuke Ohnishi; sonishi@pop.med.hokudai.ac.jp

Academic Editor: Toshio Miki

Mesenchymal stem cells (MSCs), or multipotent mesenchymal stromal cells, are present in almost all organs and tissues, including the amnion. Human amnion-derived mesenchymal stem cell (hAMSC) transplantation has been reported to ameliorate liver fibrosis in animal models. However, the mechanism for the prevention of liver fibrosis is poorly understood. In this study, we investigated the effects, and underlying mechanisms, of a conditioned medium obtained from hAMSC cultures (hAMSC-CM) on a primary culture of rat hepatic stellate cells (HSCs). We observed that in routine culture, hAMSC-CM in HSCs significantly inhibited the expression of alpha-smooth muscle actin (α-SMA), an activation marker of HSCs, and the production of collagen type 1 (COL1), a dominant component of the extracellular matrix (ECM) in the culture medium. In addition, hAMSC-CM upregulated the expression of ECM degradation-related genes, such as metalloproteinase- (*Mmp-*) 2, *Mmp-*9, *Mmp-*13, and tissue inhibitor of metalloproteinase- (*Timp-*) 1; however, it did not affect the expression of collagen type 1α1 (*Col1a1*). These regulatory effects on HSCs were concentration-dependent. A cell proliferation assay indicated that hAMSC-CM significantly suppressed HSC proliferation and downregulated the expression of cyclin B (*Ccnb*), a proliferation-related gene. Transforming growth factor-beta (TGF-β) treatment further activated HSCs and hAMSC-CM significantly inhibited the upregulation of *α-Sma* and *Col1a1* induced by TGF-β. These findings demonstrated that hAMSC-CM can modulate HSC function via secretory factors and provide a plausible explanation for the protective role of hAMSCs in liver fibrosis.

1. Introduction

Liver fibrosis, the precursor to cirrhosis, is a complex inflammatory and fibrogenic condition caused by chronic liver injury and an imbalance in extracellular matrix (ECM) synthesis and degradation mediated primarily by activated hepatic stellate cells (HSCs) [1]. Following liver injury, HSCs undergo an activation process and transform from quiescent, vitamin A-storing cells into highly proliferative, myofibroblast-like cells, upregulating collagen synthesis, especially collagen type 1α1 (COL1A1), and expressing alpha-smooth muscle actin (α-SMA), an activation marker of HSCs [2–4]. In addition, activated HSCs regulate ECM components by producing matrix metalloproteinases (MMPs), such as MMP-2, MMP-9, and MMP-13, and tissue inhibitors of metalloproteinases (TIMPs), such as TIMP-1 and TIMP-2 [1].

Mesenchymal stem cells (MSCs) are stromal cells that exhibit multilineage differentiation and self-renewal ability [5]. In addition, a variety of animal models as well as clinical trials have demonstrated the anti-inflammatory, antifibrotic, and antiapoptotic effects of MSCs in either MSC transplantation or MSC conditioned medium (CM) administration [6]. Although MSCs were first reported to be derived from bone marrow, they have been isolated from almost all tissues, including adipose tissue, the umbilical cord, dental pulp, and the amnion [7]. The advantages of human amnion-derived mesenchymal stem cells (hAMSCs) are that (i) they can be obtained in large numbers without invasive procedures and (ii) they have enormous proliferative capacity

[8]. Therefore, hAMSCs have attracted much attention in the cell therapy and regenerative medicine fields [9]. In a previous study, we found that hAMSC transplantation ameliorated liver fibrosis in rats, possibly through secretory factors from hAMSCs [10]. Thus, in this study, we investigated the effect of a conditioned medium obtained from hAMSC cultures (hAMSC-CM) on primary HSCs and also the underlying mechanisms of its antifibrotic effect *in vitro*.

2. Materials and Methods

2.1. Animals. The Animal Care and Use Committees of Hokkaido University approved the experimental protocol and animal care. Male Sprague–Dawley (SD) rats (400–450 g in weight) were procured from Japan SLC (Hamamatsu, Japan). They were housed in a temperature-controlled room (24°C) on a 12-hourly light–dark cycle and were provided with standard chow and water *ad libitum* until the time of the study.

2.2. Isolation and Expansion of hAMSCs. The Medical Ethical Committee of Hokkaido University, Graduate School of Medicine, Sapporo, Japan, approved the study. A pregnant woman provided written informed consent for use of her fetal membrane, which was obtained during her cesarean delivery. Isolation and expansion of hAMSCs were performed as described in a previous study [11]. The expanded hAMSCs were stored in liquid nitrogen until use.

2.3. Preparation of hAMSC-CM. We recovered cryopreserved hAMSCs and cultured them until the cells reached a subconfluent state (passage 6). After washing them with Hank's balanced salt solution without calcium, magnesium, or phenol red (HBSS (−); Nacalai Tesque, Kyoto, Japan), we further cultured the cells with serum-free minimum essential medium alpha (MEMα; Nacalai Tesque) for 48 h. Next, we collected hAMSC-CM and removed the debris by centrifugation at 1120 × *g* for 5 min. Serum-free MEMα incubated in a cell-free dish for 48 h was used as a standard medium (SM), and both SM and hAMSC-CM were stored at −80°C until use.

2.4. Isolation and Purification of HSCs. Previous studies have shown various methods of isolating HSCs [12–15]; we performed isolation after modifying several steps. The SD rats were anesthetized by intraperitoneal injection of 6.48 mg/100 g body weight of pentobarbital sodium (Kyoritsu Seiyaku, Tokyo, Japan). Each rat's liver was perfused via the portal vein using an 18 G needle (Terumo, Tokyo, Japan) that was fixed by sutures. Buffers were preheated to 42°C and pumped into the liver using a peristaltic pump.

2.4.1. Liver Perfusion and Enzymatic Digestion. Initially, the liver was perfused with 60 mL of HBSS (−) containing 1 mM ethylenediaminetetraacetic acid (EDTA; Thermo Fisher Scientific, Waltham, MA, USA) at 18 mL/min, and when the liver became distended, the inferior vena cava (IVC) was cut. We incised the diaphragm and clipped the intrathoracic IVC with a vascular clamp to ensure the buffers were drained completely via the abdominal IVC incision. Next, the liver was infused with 200 mL of HBSS (−) supplemented with 100 U/mL of collagenase II (Worthington Biochemical, Lakewood, NJ, USA) at 7.5 mL/min. The perfused liver was removed, minced using two tweezers in a sterile dish containing HBSS (−), and further digested in a flask containing 65 U/mL of collagenase II and 1% (*v*/*v*) deoxyribonuclease I (DNase I; Worthington Biochemical) with an initial concentration of 40 kU/mL. The flask was placed on a stir plate and shaken at 70 rpm/min for 20 min in an incubator at 37°C. The resulting cell suspension was filtered using first a 100 μm and then a 70 μm cell strainer and was centrifuged for 10 min at 600 × *g* and 4°C. The pellet was washed and resuspended using HBSS (−) containing 120 μL of DNase I and then centrifuged for 3 min at 50 × *g* and 4°C. Then, the supernatant was collected and centrifuged for 10 min at 400 × *g* and 4°C.

2.4.2. Density Gradient Centrifugation. The pellet was resuspended in HBSS (−) containing 120 μL of DNase I and, then, was mixed with Percoll (GE Healthcare Bio-Sciences, Uppsala, Sweden) to a final concentration of 30% (*v*/*v*) at 20°C. Next, 10 mL of a thoroughly mixed cell–Percoll suspension was pipetted into a 15 mL centrifugation tube, and 2 mL of HBSS (−) was gently overlaid on the suspension. Centrifugation was performed at 1470 × *g* and 20°C for 25 min with slow acceleration and deceleration. The interphase containing enriched HSCs between HBSS (−) and the 30% Percoll layer was harvested and washed using HBSS (−) for 8 min at 400 × *g* and 4°C.

2.4.3. Fluorescence-Activated Cell Sorting (FACS) for HSCs. The HSC pellet was resuspended in phenol red-free MEMα supplemented with 1.5% fetal bovine serum (FBS; Thermo Fisher Scientific, Carlsbad, LA, USA), and the suspension was filtered using a 40 μm cell strainer and adjusted to 6–8 × 10^6 cells/mL. A BD FACS Aria III Cell Sorter (BD Biosciences, San Jose, CA, USA) was used to perform HSC sorting. We used endogenous retinoid fluorescence of HSCs as a selection marker, performed excitation via a 375 nm laser, and measured the emission using a 450/20 nm band-pass filter at a Hoechst-blue channel. We used a 100 μm nozzle and a 2.0 neutral density filter, and the sample loading port was set to 4°C, 300 rpm. The sorting mode was set up in purity mode, and 2 μL/10^6 cells of 7-aminoactinomycin D solution (7-AAD; BD Biosciences) was added to the suspension immediately before sorting. The 15 mL collection tube was made of polypropylene and was coated with FBS overnight at 4°C. It contained 10 mL of Dulbecco minimal essential medium (DMEM; Nacalai Tesque) supplemented with 17% FBS. After sorting, the cells were centrifuged for 5 min at 400 × *g* and 4°C and cultured. Their purity was determined by flow cytometry with autofluorescence.

2.5. Culture Models. All the cells were cultured in a humidified atmosphere of 95% air and 5% CO_2 at 37°C. All the culture media were supplemented with 100 U/mL of penicillin and 100 μg/mL of streptomycin. A Luna automated cell counter (Logos Biosystems, Anyang, South Korea) was used to take a cell count.

Table 1: Sequences of primers.

Gene	Forward primers (5′–3′)	Reverse primers (5′–3′)
α-Sma	GACACCAGGGAGTGATGGTT	GTTAGCAAGGTCGGATGCTC
Col1a1	GATGGCTGCACGAGTCACAC	ATTGGGATGGAGGGAGTTTA
Mmp-2	CTTGCTGGTGGCCACATTC	CTCATTCCCTGCGAAGAACAC
Mmp-9	CGCTCATGTACCCCATGTATCA	TCAGGTTTAGAGCCACGACCAT
Mmp-13	TCGCATTGTGAGAGTCATGCCAACA	TGTGGTTCCAGCCACGCATAGTCA
Timp-1	GACCACCTTATACCAGCGTT	GTCACTCTCCAGTTTGCAAG
Timp-2	GGATGGACTGGGTCACAGAG	GCGCAAGAACCATCACTTCT
Ccnb-1	CCCTACCAAAACCTGTGGAC	CATCGGAGAAAGCCTGACAC
Ccnb-2	TGGAGAGTGAAATACTGGAAGTCA	TGAGAAGCACACGATGGAAG
Pdgfrb	GCACCGAAACAAACACACCTT	ATGTAACCACCGTCGCTCTC
Tgfbr1	ACCTTCTGATCCATCCGTT	CGCAAAGCTGTCAGCCTAG

2.5.1. Routine Culture of HSCs. Approximately 5×10^4 HSCs were seeded on 12-well plastic plates, on which the cells were automatically activated and proliferated [16]. They were cultured in 2 mL of stellate cell medium (SteCM; ScienCell, Carlsbad, CA, USA) supplemented with 2% FBS (ScienCell) and stellate cell growth supplement (SteCGS; ScienCell) for 48 h. Then, the HSCs were washed thrice using HBSS (−) and were cultured for 48 h with SM or hAMSC-CM. In addition, hAMSC-CM was mixed separately with the SM in two concentrations: 50% and 25% (*v*/*v*) of hAMSC-CM. These different concentrations of hAMSC-CM were also used for culturing washed HSCs for 48 h as described above.

2.5.2. Transforming Growth Factor-Beta (TGF-β) Treatment. Approximately 5×10^4 HSCs were cultured in 12-well plates in SteCM containing 2% FBS and SteCGS for 48 h and washed thrice using HBSS (−). Subsequently, the HSCs were treated with SM or hAMSC-CM supplemented with 5 ng/mL of transforming growth factor-beta 1 (TGF-β1; R&D Systems, Minneapolis, MN, USA) for 48 h. HSCs cultured in SM or hAMSC-CM served as negative controls.

2.6. Flow Cytometry Analysis of hAMSCs. Following the manufacturer' instructions, we harvested cultured hAMSCs with 0.5% trypsin/EDTA and stained them using a Human MSC Analysis Kit (BD Biosciences) containing phycoerythrin- (PE-) conjugated anticluster of differentiation 44 (anti-CD44), allophycocyanin- (APC-) conjugated anti-CD73, fluorescein-isothiocyanate- (FITC-) conjugated anti-CD90, and PerCP-Cy5.5-conjugated anti-CD105 antibodies, as well as a negative mixture comprising PE-conjugated anti-CD11b, anti-CD19, anti-CD34, anti-CD45, and anti-human leukocyte antigen–antigen D-related (HLA-DR) antibodies. All the cells were resuspended in HBSS (−), filtered using a 40 μm strainer, and then analyzed using a BD FACSCanto II Flow Cytometer (BD Biosciences).

2.7. Immunofluorescent Staining. HSCs cultured in SM and hAMSC-CM were washed thrice using HBSS (−), fixed in methanol for 10 min at 4°C, and then incubated in anti-rat α-SMA (1:500; Abcam, Cambridge, UK) in HBSS (−) containing 2% FBS for 1 h at 4°C. After washing, we incubated the cells in Alexa Flour 488-conjugated secondary antibody (1:1000; Cell Signaling Technology, Danvers, MA, USA) for 30 min at 4°C in the dark. Subsequently, we stained the nucleus with Hoechst 33342 (1:1000; Thermo Fisher Scientific) for 2 min at room temperature. Then, the cells were washed twice and analyzed using a FluoView FV10i confocal laser scanning microscope (Olympus, Tokyo, Japan); all the micrographs were taken under the same exposure time and laser intensity. ImageJ software (http://imagej.nih.gov/ij/) was used to measure fluorescence intensity.

2.8. Ribonucleic Acid (RNA) Isolation and Quantitative Reverse-Transcription Polymerase Chain Reaction (qRT-PCR). RNA of the cultured HSCs was extracted using a RNeasy Mini Kit (Qiagen, Hilden, Germany), and 20 ng of total RNA was reverse-transcribed into complementary deoxyribonucleic acid (cDNA) using a PrimeScript RT Reagent Kit with a genomic deoxyribonucleic acid (gDNA) Eraser (Takara Bio, Kusatsu, Japan) in a Veriti 96-well Thermal Cycler (Applied Biosystems, Waltham, MA, USA), incubated at 37°C for 15 min and 85°C for 15 s. Polymerase chain reaction (PCR) was carried out in a total reaction volume of 25 μL containing 5 μL of template cDNA, 12.5 μL of a Platinum SYBR Green PCR Mix (Invitrogen, Carlsbad, CA, USA), and 2 μL of a 10 μM corresponding primer mixture. PCR conditions, running on a StepOnePlus Real Time PCR System (Applied Biosystems), included predenaturation at 95°C for 20 s followed by 40 cycles at 95°C for 3 s and 60°C for 7 s. A melting curve was created to validate the specificity of the amplification products. A relative expression was determined using the standard curve method with platelet-derived growth factor receptor beta (*Pdgfrb*) used as an endogenous control [14]. Table 1 shows the primer sequences.

2.9. Proliferation Assay. Approximately 2×10^4 HSCs were cultured in a 96-well plate with SteCM containing 2% FBS and SteCGS for 48 h. Then, we changed the medium to SM or hAMSC-CM and cultured the cells further for 48 h. HSC proliferation was examined using a Cell Counting Kit-8 (CCK-8; Dojindo Laboratories, Kumamoto, Japan) at 0, 24, and 48 h after changing the medium; the medium without cells was used as a blank control. A GloMax-Multi+ Detection System (Promega, Fitchburg, WI, USA) was used to measure absorbance.

2.10. Collagen Type 1 (COL1) Assay. We evaluated the COL1 concentration in SM and hAMSC-CM using a rat COL1 enzyme-linked immunosorbent assay (ELISA) kit (MyBioSource, San Diego, CA, USA) according to the manufacturer's instructions. Cell-free SM and hAMSC-CM were incubated at the same time and taken as blank controls to determine the baseline.

2.11. Statistical Analysis. GraphPad Prism 7.0 (GraphPad Software, La Jolla, CA, USA) was used to perform the statistical analysis, and the data were expressed as mean ± standard deviation (SD). Intergroup differences were identified using one-way analysis of variance (ANOVA), followed by the Tukey test. Unpaired t-tests or Welch's test was used to identify pairwise differences. The differences were considered statistically significant at $P < 0.05$.

3. Results

3.1. Characterization of hAMSCs. We observed that cultured hAMSCs have a typical morphology of fibroblast-like cells (Figure 1(a)). Flow cytometry showed that hAMSCs exhibit high expression of CD44, CD73, CD90, and CD105 but no expression of CD11b, CD19, CD34, CD45, or HLA-DR (Figure 1(b)), which is consistent with a characteristic of MSCs [17, 18]. The high expression of MSC-specific marker *ITGA11* and low expression of fibroblast-specific marker *CD26* [19] in cultured hAMSCs indicated that fibroblast contamination is rarely observed in these hAMSCs (Supplementary Figure 1).

3.2. Isolation and Characterization of HSCs. First, we gated cells with high sideward scatter (SSC) and low forward scatter (FSC) [20], and 7-AAD was used to select living cells (Figure 2(a)). We used the forward scatter area/forward scatter height (FSC-A/FSC-H) to exclude doublets, and a high autofluorescence area was gated as HSCs (Figure 2(a)). FACS of HSCs resulted in a final purity of >98%, as defined by retinol-based autofluorescence (Figure 2(b)). The freshly isolated HSCs were irregularly round-shaped, and their cytoplasm was rich in lipid droplets. When excited at 352 nm, the vitamin A-rich lipid droplets emitted cyan intrinsic autofluorescence (Figure 2(c)). Postculturing for 2 days, HSCs became extended and presented an asteroid phenotype, accompanied by a reduction of lipid droplets (Figure 2(c)). HSCs were further activated by routine culture, and it was difficult to observe autofluorescence postculturing for 4 days (Figure 2(c)), suggesting that quiescent HSCs were activated by routine culture. Isolated HSCs proliferated well after seeding (Supplementary Figure 2A), and long-term culture showed that HSCs proliferated rapidly with good viability (Supplementary Figure 2B).

3.3. Effects of hAMSC-CM on Routinely Cultured HSCs. Next, we investigated whether hAMSC-CM inhibits the profibrogenic effects of HSCs, which is a key contributor for fibrosis. After culturing HSCs with hAMSC-CM for 48 h, immunofluorescence staining indicated that α-SMA expression in HSCs was much lower compared to HSCs cultured in SM (Figure 3(a)). Consistently, qRT-PCR showed that hAMSC-CM significantly decreased *α-Sma* expression (Figure 3(b)). Then, we examined the expression profile of fibrosis-related genes of HSCs. Compared to control HSCs, hAMSC-CM did not affect *Col1a1* expression (Figure 3(c)). On the other hand, although *Timp-2* expression did not vary, hAMSC-CM significantly upregulated the expression of *Mmp-2*, *Mmp-9*, *Mmp-13*, and *Timp-1* (Figure 3(c)). In addition, hAMSC-CM markedly increased the *Mmp-13*/*Timp-1* ratio, an index for evaluating the ECM accumulation degree [21] (Figure 3(d)), and decreased the concentration of COL1 in culture media, detected by ELISA (Figure 3(e)). Investigation of the effect of hAMSC-CM on HSC proliferation showed that hAMSC-CM reduced the gene expressions of cyclin B1 (*Ccnb-1*) and cyclin B2 (*Ccnb-2*); however, the reduction of *Ccnb-1* was not statistically significant (Figure 3(f)). The CCK-8 proliferation assay showed that hAMSC-CM significantly inhibited HSC proliferation at 48 h (Figure 3(g)). qRT-PCR and ELISA results indicated that the effect of hAMSC-CM on HSCs was concentration-dependent (Figures 3(b)–3(e)).

3.4. Effects of hAMSC-CM on TGF-β-Treated HSCs. TGF-β is the most efficient collagen synthesis factor on HSCs [22]; therefore, we investigated whether hAMSC-CM could reverse HSC activation and the progression of ECM accumulation after TGF-β1 stimulation. We observed that TGF-β1 upregulated TGF-β receptor 1 (*Tgfbr1*) expression, and the increased expression of *Tgfbr1* in hAMSC-CM was greater than that in SM (Figure 4(a)). TGF-β1 significantly increased *α-Sma* expression, while hAMSC-CM inhibited the increase in TGF-β1-induced *α-Sma* expression (Figure 4(b)). Although hAMSC-CM did not affect *Col1a1* expression in routine culture, it significantly suppressed TGF-β1-induced upregulation of *Col1a1* (Figure 4(c)). In addition, compared to SM, hAMSC-CM significantly increased *Mmp-2*, *Mmp-9*, *Mmp-13*, and *Timp-1* expression, although there was no change in *Timp-2* expression (Figure 4(c)). TGF-β1 significantly downregulated the *Mmp-13*/*Timp-1* relative ratio, which was increased, however, by hAMSC-CM, even in the presence of TGF-β1 (Figure 4(d)).

4. Discussion

Previous studies have shown that hAMSC transplantation ameliorates liver fibrosis *in vivo* [10, 23]. Given that HSCs play an important role in the development of liver fibrosis [24], we hypothesized that hAMSCs inhibit liver fibrosis by regulating the functions of HSCs with secretory factors. We found that (i) hAMSC-CM inhibits HSC activation, (ii) regulates ECM accumulation during HSC activation, and (iii) suppresses HSC proliferation.

Highly purified HSCs are required for mechanistic studies in liver fibrosis. Therefore, to improve their purity, we isolated HSCs with FACS-based sorting. A previous study has demonstrated that FACS can obtain unaffected, functional

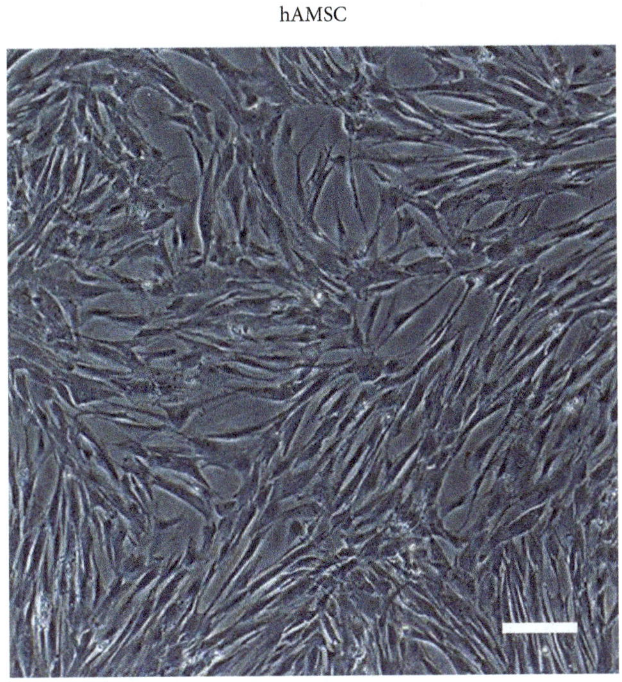

(a)

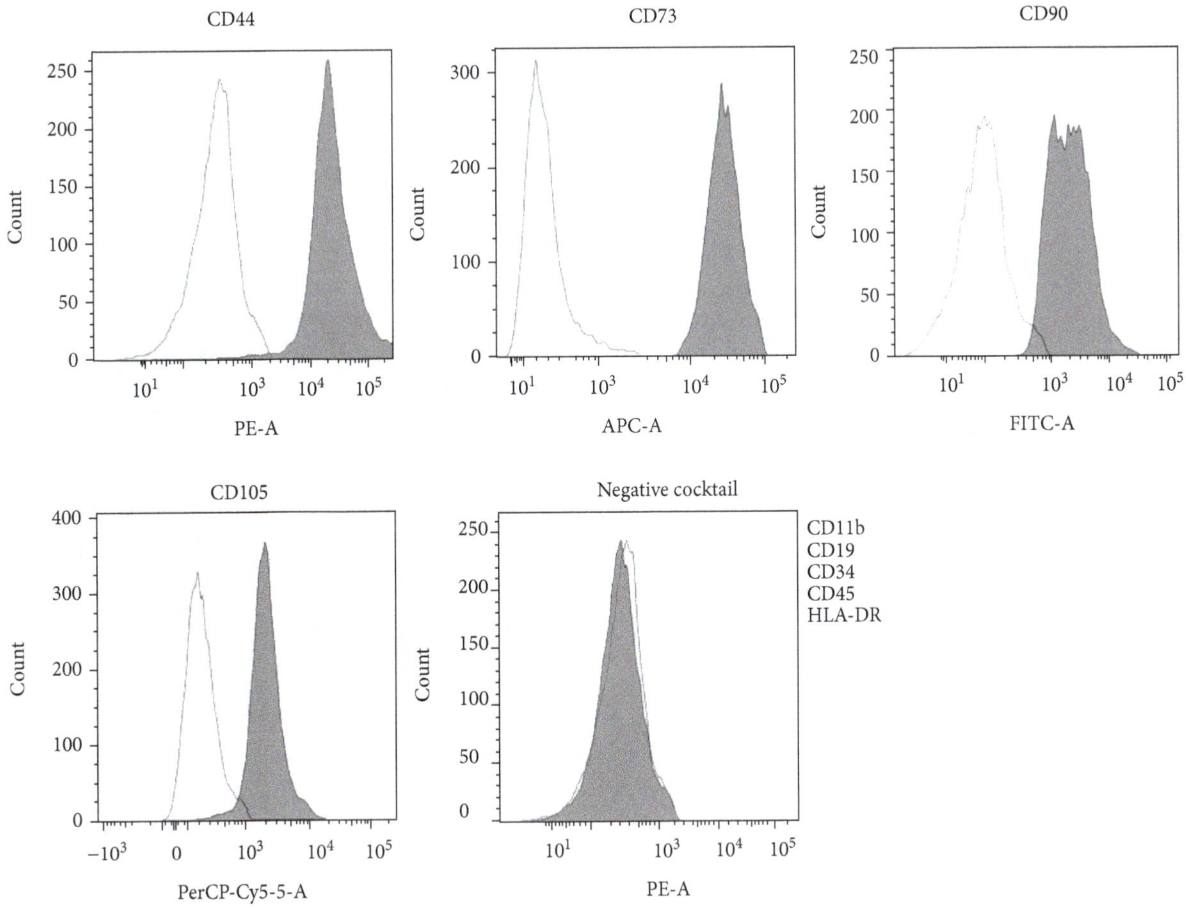

(b)

FIGURE 1: Characterization of cultured hAMSCs. (a) Morphology of cultured hAMSCs. Scale bar = 200 μm. (b) Flow cytometry analysis of cultured hAMSCs.

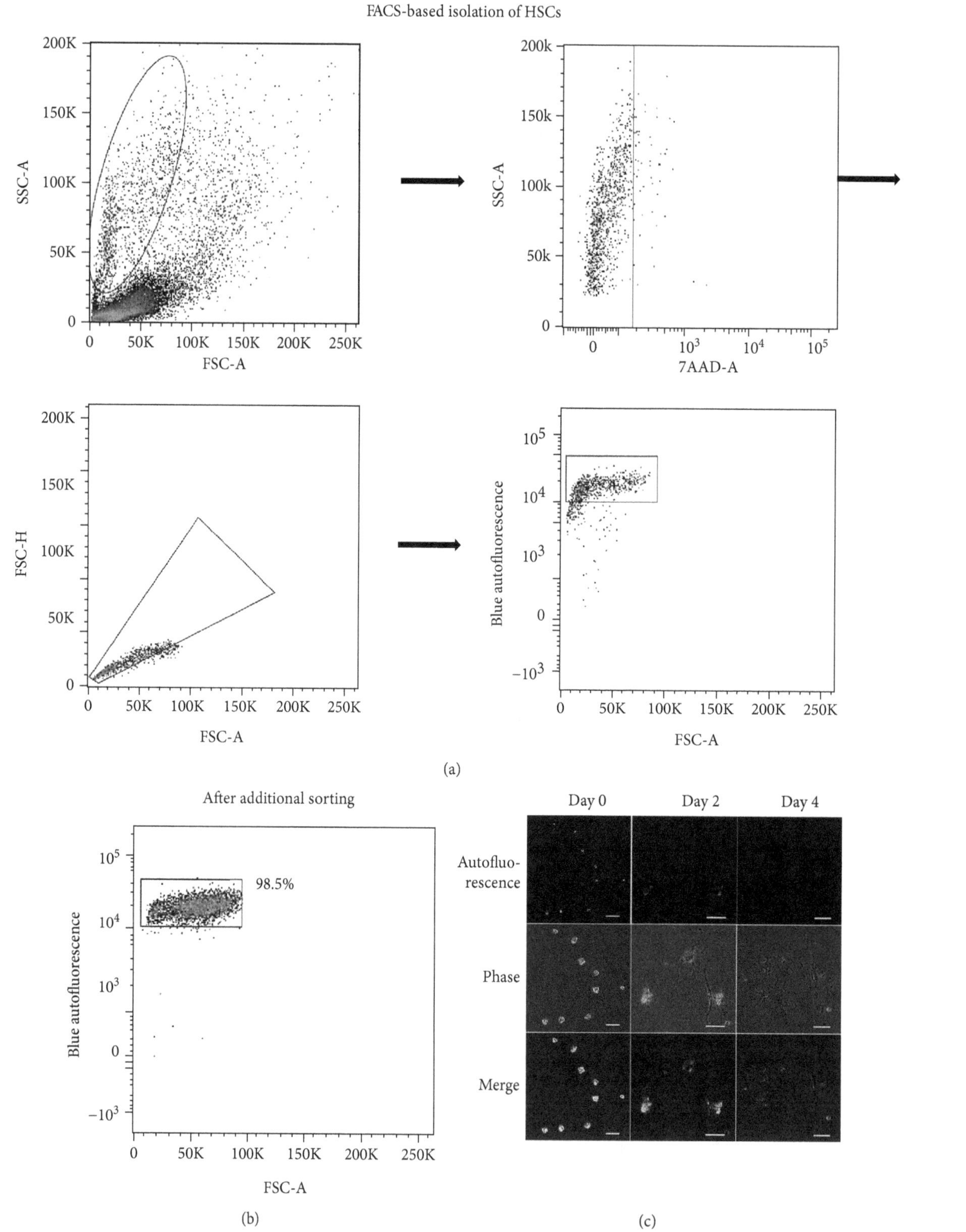

FIGURE 2: Gating strategy for HSC purification using FACS and HSC characterization. (a) Cells were gated on the basis of their FSC and SSC, viable cells were selected using 7-AAD, and doublets were excluded by FSC-A/FSC-H. Finally, HSCs were selected on the basis of the cyan light emission from retinol. (b) Purity of HSCs after FACS. (c) Primary HSCs are irregularly round-shaped, and retinol-rich lipid droplets emit cyan autofluorescence by a 352 nm laser. The HSCs cultured for 2 days became extended and presented an asteroid phenotype, whereas large numbers of lipid droplets were observed still. No autofluorescence could be detected after culturing HSCs for 4 days, and the cells extended further. FSC: forward scatter; SSC: sideward scatter; 7-AAD: 7-aminoactinomycin D; NUV: near ultraviolet. Scale bar = 50 μm.

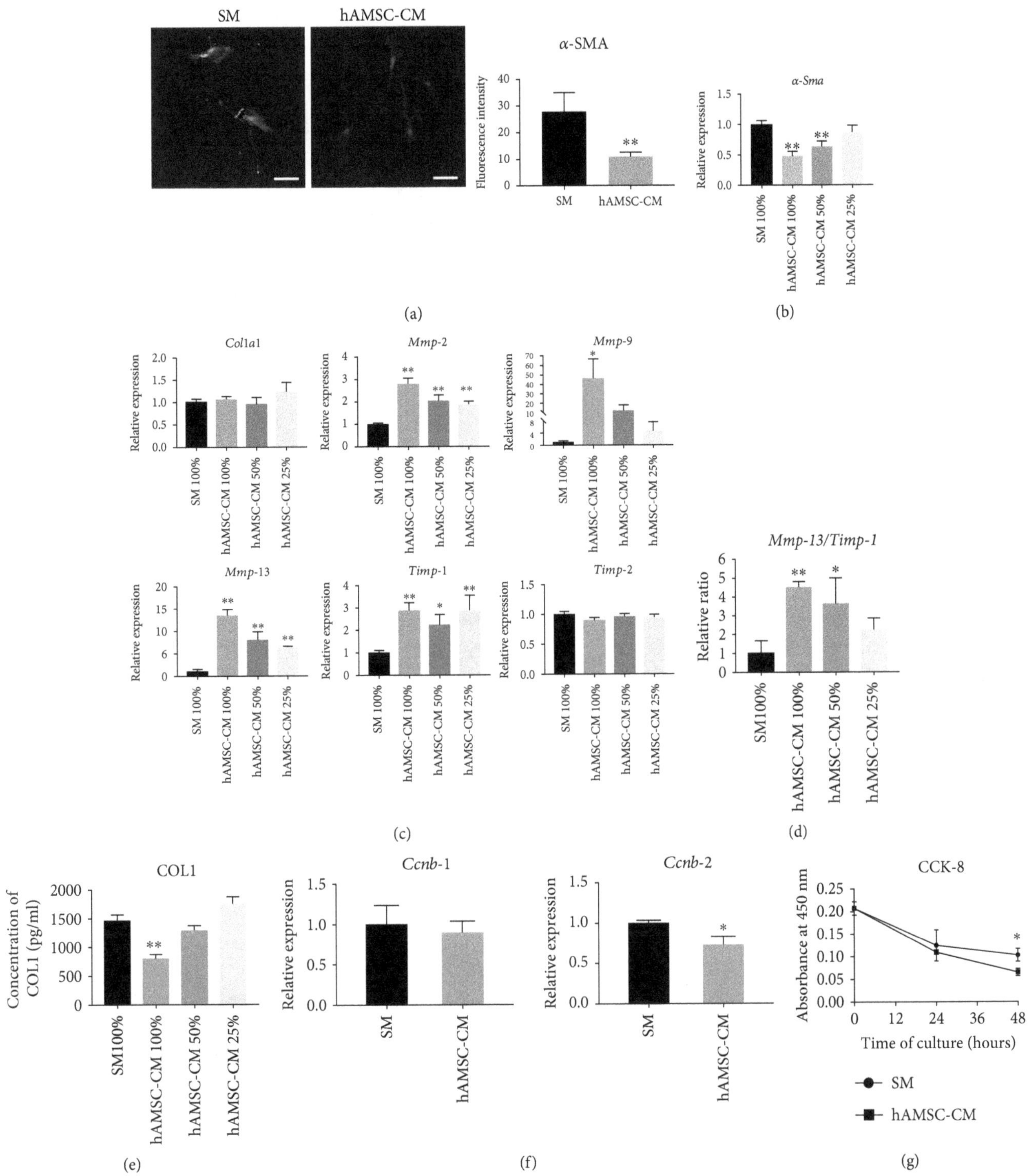

Figure 3: Effect of hAMSC-CM on primary HSC activation and proliferation and ECM accumulation in routine culture. (a) Immunofluorescence staining of α-SMA (green) in HSCs cultured in SM or hAMSC-CM for 48 h. Nuclei were stained by Hoechst 33342 (blue). Scale bar = 50 μm. Data are expressed as mean ± SD ($n = 28$ in the SM group and $n = 24$ in the hAMSC-CM group). $^{**}P < 0.01$ versus SM. (b) Expression of *α-Sma* in different concentrations of hAMSC-CM. Data are expressed as mean ± SD ($n = 3$). $^{**}P < 0.01$ versus SM 100%. (c) ECM-related gene expression analysis of HSCs cultured in SM or different concentrations of hAMSC-CM. The data are expressed as mean ± SD ($n = 3$). $^{*}P < 0.05$ and $^{**}P < 0.01$ versus SM 100%. (d) Relative *Mmp-13/Timp-1* expression ratio. Data are expressed as mean ± SD ($n = 3$). $^{*}P < 0.05$ and $^{**}P < 0.01$ versus SM 100%. (e) Expression of COL1 in culture media analyzed by ELISA. Data are expressed as mean ± SD ($n = 3$). $^{**}P < 0.01$ versus SM 100%. (f) Proliferation-related gene expression analysis for *Ccnb-1* and *Ccnb-2*. The data are expressed as mean ± SD ($n = 3$). $^{*}P < 0.05$ versus SM. (g) Detection of proliferation of HSCs cultured in SM or hAMSC-CM by CCK-8. The data are expressed as mean ± SD ($n = 3$ for each time point and culture condition). $^{*}P < 0.05$ versus SM.

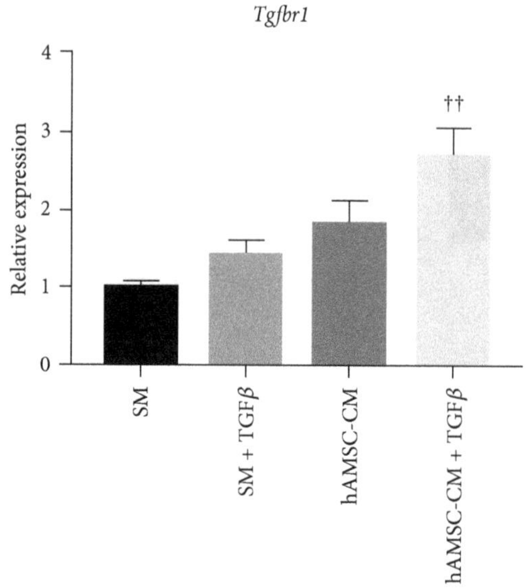

(a)

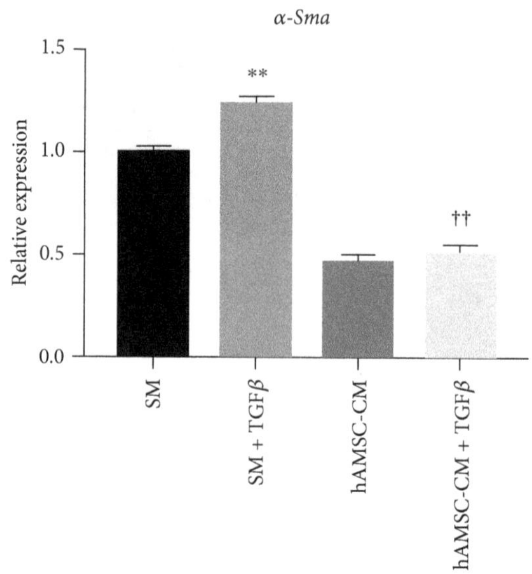

(b)

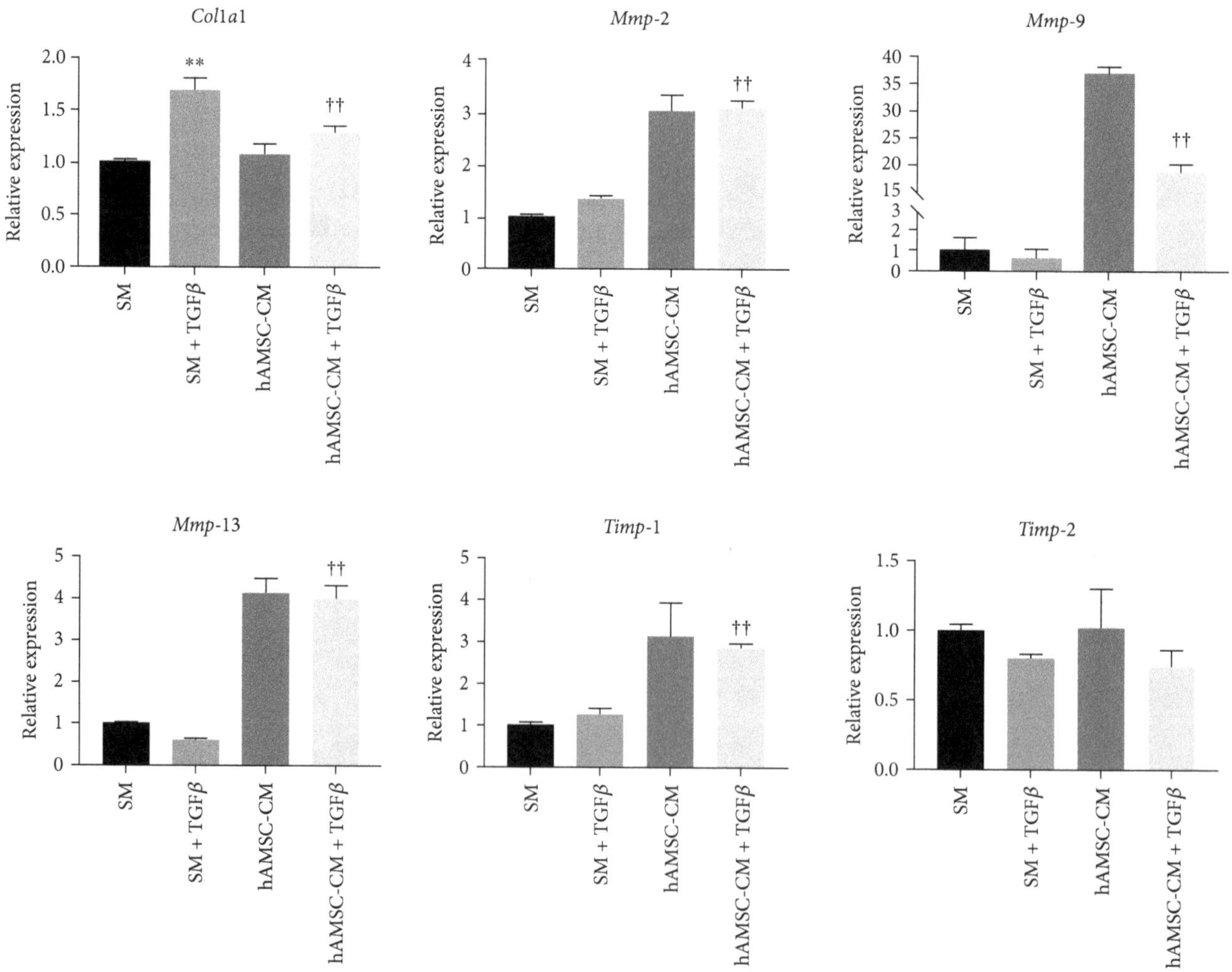

(c)

Figure 4: Continued.

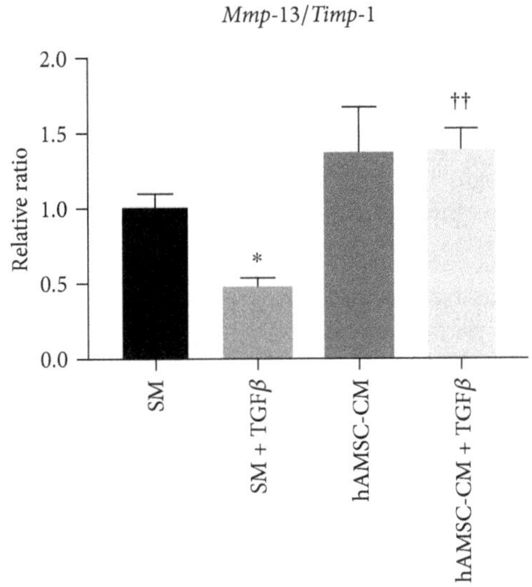

(d)

FIGURE 4: Effect of hAMSC-CM on TGF-β1-induced HSC activation. Gene expression analysis of HSCs with or without TGF-β1 in SM or hAMSC-CM, analyzed by qRT-PCR for (a) *Tgfbr1*, (b) *α-Sma*, and (c) ECM-related genes. (d) Relative *Mmp-13/Timp-1* expression ratio. Data are expressed as mean ± SD ($n = 3$). $^{*}P < 0.05$ and $^{**}P < 0.01$ versus SM; $^{\dagger\dagger}P < 0.01$ versus SM + TGF-β. qRT-PCR, quantitative reverse-transcription polymerase chain reaction.

HSCs with high purity [15], and we added 7-AAD to prevent interference by nonspecific autofluorescence of dead cells and to ensure that only viable HSCs were sorted. Previous studies reported several markers for HSCs such as desmin [25], glial fibrillary acidic protein (GFAP) [26], and CD38 [27]. However, the specificity of these markers is still questionable [27–29], and desmin staining in the present study showed that only 74.6% were positive (Supplementary Figure 3B). Therefore, we chose using autofluorescence to confirm the purity of isolated HSCs instead of using those markers. In addition, cell type-specific gene expression analysis and flow cytometry analysis indicated that isolated HSCs were rarely mixed with other kinds of cells in the liver (Supplement Figures 3A and 3B). In this study, we obtained highly purified HSCs; however, because of the different amounts of lipid droplets in every cell, FACS may isolate only HSCs full of lipid droplets.

After sorting HSCs, we cultured them in medium with FBS and growth supplement for 48 h to boost HSC adhesion and activation. FBS-free SM or hAMSC-CM was used in the subsequent culture because cytokines and factors present in FBS may mask the potential effects of hAMSC-CM.

HSCs are activated and proliferate rapidly in pathological conditions such as liver injury and transform into myofibroblast-like cells, which express *α*-SMA and secrete abundant collagen [30]. In this study, we demonstrated that hAMSC-CM can inhibit HSC activation, as indicated by the decreased α-SMA expression at both gene and protein levels.

Excessive ECM accumulation, namely, the disequilibrium of interstitial collagens, MMPs, and TIMPs, induces liver fibrosis. When HSCs are activated, large amounts of COL1, the key protein involved in liver fibrosis development, are secreted [31]. In this study, we showed that hAMSC-CM does not influence *Col1a1* expression but has a positive effect on *Mmps* and *Timps* in routine culture of HSCs. MMP-13 (the rodent equivalent of MMP-1) is a kind of collagenase and the main protease that can degrade COL1 in a fibrotic liver [30]. Although *Mmp-13* upregulation might imply that hAMSC-CM decreased the amount of COL1, an increase in *Timp-1* made the result indistinct. TIMP-1 is an MMP inhibitor and forms tight 1:1 inhibitory complexes with MMP-13 [32]. Thus, evaluating COL1 degradation with *Mmp-13/Timp-1* is considered more objective [21]. An increase in *Mmp-13/Timp-1* by hAMSC-CM in this study suggested that hAMSC-CM may downregulate the amount of COL1, as verified by a COL1 assay. On the other hand, studies have also reported that MMP-2 (gelatinase A) and MMP-9 (gelatinase B) bind to TIMP-2 and TIMP-1, respectively [33]. Although MMP-2 and MMP-9 barely cleave COL1, their upregulation may also benefit COL1 degradation by blocking of TIMPs. On the basis of the above-mentioned analysis, we believe that instead of inhibiting COL1 synthesis in routine culture of HSCs, hAMC-CM reduces ECM accumulation by promoting COL1 degradation.

TGF-β is the most efficient fibrogenic factor. Stimulated by TGF-β1, upregulation of COL1 and TIMP-1 and downregulation of MMPs lead to ECM deposition [34]. In this study, hAMSC-CM reversed this profibrogenic state and inhibited the increase in TGF-β1-induced *Col1a1* expression, accompanied by *Mmp-2*, *Mmp-9*, and *Mmp-13/Timp-1* ratio upregulation. Although studies have demonstrated that α-SMA expression does not involve the TGF-β signaling pathway [35], the view that TGF-β intensifies α-SMA expression *in vitro* is widely accepted [1, 36]. In this study, we observed that TGF-β1 augments *α-Sma* expression and hAMSC-CM inhibits TGF-β1-induced HSC activation. Interestingly, compared to TGF-β1, hAMSC-CM enhances *Tgfbr1* expression, which appears to be contrary to the antifibrogenic effects of hAMSC-CM. In addition, we found that hAMSC-CM contains TGF-β1 (data not shown), and *Tgfbr1* upregulation is most likely caused by additional exogenous TGF-β1. These results implied that hAMSC-CM exerts antifibrogenic functions by modifying downstream genes in the TGF-β signaling pathway or through the TGF-β-independent pathway. Further studies are required to clarify the underlying mechanism.

HSC activation is accompanied by massive cell proliferation, promoting ECM remodeling and portal resistance increase in liver fibrosis [30]. In this study, the CCK-8 proliferation assay indicated that hAMSC-CM reduces HSC proliferation. In addition, it downregulates the expression of *Ccnb-1* and *Ccnb-2* which are positive cell cycle regulators strongly associated with the G2/M phase. As previous research has clarified that TGF-β1 inhibits cell cycle progression by blocking the activation of cyclin-dependent kinases [37], it appeared that TGF-β1 existing in hAMSC-CM is involved in suppressing HSC proliferation.

Furthermore, in order to investigate whether the suppressive effect on HSCs is specific to hAMSC-CM, we cultured HSCs with CM obtained from skin fibroblasts (fibroblast-CM, Supplementary Figure 4). Although fibroblast-CM significantly enhanced *Col1a1* expression and suppressed *Timp-2* expression in HSCs, it increased the expression of *Mmps* and *Timp-1* and decreased the expression of *α-Sma* and *Ccnb* (Supplementary Figure 4). These results suggest that hAMSCs and fibroblasts have something in common in certain functions. However, because there are few studies demonstrating the similar functions of hAMSCs and fibroblasts, their common mechanism is unclear.

In the present study, we demonstrated the antiactivation effect of hAMSC-CM on HSCs *in vitro*; however, HSCs may display a significant difference *in vivo* [38].

5. Conclusion

In conclusion, hAMSC-CM inhibits activation and proliferation of primary HSCs and reduces the accumulation of ECM from HSCs. The results of this study provide mechanistic evidence that hAMSCs play an inhibitory role through paracrine signaling to HSCs. Although several clinical studies report the use of human MSCs in liver fibrosis, the application of MSCs is limited by their availability. Future studies are required to determine the active ingredients and their amounts in hAMSC-CM, which may provide a new approach to treating liver fibrogenesis.

Acknowledgments

This study was supported by a Grant-in-Aid for Scientific Research (B) from the Japan Society for the Promotion of Science (JSPS, 16H05282) and by Otsuka Toshimi Scholarship Foundation (NO. 17-S28). We are grateful to Dr. Hidetaka Hosono for the excellent technical assistance.

Supplementary Materials

Supplementary Figure 1: expressions of MSC-specific gene IGTA11 and fibroblast-specific gene CD26 were examined in hAMSCs and skin fibroblasts by quantitative reverse-transcription polymerase chain reaction. Gene expression was normalized to 18s rRNA. Data are shown as mean ± SD ($n = 3$). $^{**}P < 0.01$ versus hAMSC. Supplementary Figure 2: morphology of sorted HSCs in vitro. (A) Most of the seeded HSCs present an asteroid phenotype with remaining a great quantity of lipid droplets after 1 day of culture. Arrows indicate lipid droplets, and the inset at the upper right corner shows the lipid droplets close-up. Scale bar = 100 μm. (B) Sorted HSCs proliferated during culture and presented a fibroblast-like phenotype. Scale bar = 100 μm. Supplementary Figure 3: characterization of sorted HSCs. (A) Cell type-specific gene expression analysis of sorted HSCs and remaining cells. Beta-type platelet-derived growth factor receptor (Pdgfb) is a marker of HSCs, C-type lectin domain family 4f (Clec4f) is a marker for Kupffer cells, and albumin is a marker for hepatocytes. Data are expressed as mean ± SD ($n = 3$). $^{*}P < 0.05$ and $^{**}P < 0.01$ versus sorted HSCs. (B) Desmin (HSC marker), CD31 (endothelial cell marker), CD163 (Kupffer cell marker) expressions of sorted HSCs were analyzed by flow cytometry. Supplementary Figure 4: gene expressions of primary HSCs cultured in SM or skin fibroblast-CM. Data are expressed as mean ± SD ($n = 3$). $^{*}P < 0.05$ and $^{**}P < 0.01$ versus SM. Supplementary Table 1: sequences of primers. *(Supplementary Materials)*

References

[1] D. Schuppan, "Liver fibrosis: common mechanisms and antifibrotic therapies," *Clinics and Research in Hepatology and Gastroenterology*, vol. 39, Supplement 1, pp. S51–S59, 2015.

[2] C. Hellerbrand, "Hepatic stellate cells—the pericytes in the liver," *Pflügers Archiv*, vol. 465, no. 6, pp. 775–778, 2013.

[3] M. Sun and T. Kisseleva, "Reversibility of liver fibrosis," *Clinics and Research in Hepatology and Gastroenterology*, vol. 39, Suppl 1, pp. S60–S63, 2015.

[4] B. Parekkadan, D. van Poll, Z. Megeed et al., "Immunomodulation of activated hepatic stellate cells by mesenchymal stem cells," *Biochemical and Biophysical Research Communications*, vol. 363, no. 2, pp. 247–252, 2007.

[5] D. C. Ding, W. C. Shyu, and S. Z. Lin, "Mesenchymal stem cells," *Cell Transplantation*, vol. 20, no. 1, pp. 5–14, 2011.

[6] L. da Silva Meirelles, A. M. Fontes, D. T. Covas, and A. I. Caplan, "Mechanisms involved in the therapeutic properties of mesenchymal stem cells," *Cytokine & Growth Factor Reviews*, vol. 20, no. 5-6, pp. 419–427, 2009.

[7] R. Hass, C. Kasper, S. Böhm, and R. Jacobs, "Different populations and sources of human mesenchymal stem cells (MSC): a comparison of adult and neonatal tissue-derived MSC," *Cell Communication and Signaling*, vol. 9, no. 1, p. 12, 2011.

[8] S. Barlow, G. Brooke, K. Chatterjee et al., "Comparison of human placenta- and bone marrow-derived multipotent mesenchymal stem cells," *Stem Cells and Development*, vol. 17, no. 6, pp. 1095–1108, 2008.

[9] S. Ilancheran, A. Michalska, G. Peh, E. M. Wallace, M. Pera, and U. Manuelpillai, "Stem cells derived from human fetal

membranes display multilineage differentiation potential," *Biology of Reproduction*, vol. 77, no. 3, pp. 577–588, 2007.

[10] K. Kubo, S. Ohnishi, H. Hosono et al., "Human amnion-derived mesenchymal stem cell transplantation ameliorates liver fibrosis in rats," *Transplant Direct*, vol. 1, no. 4, article e16, 2015.

[11] S. Miyamoto, S. Ohnishi, R. Onishi et al., "Therapeutic effects of human amnion-derived mesenchymal stem cell transplantation and conditioned medium enema in rats with trinitrobenzene sulfonic acid-induced colitis," *American Journal of Translational Research*, vol. 9, no. 3, pp. 940–952, 2017.

[12] W. Liu, Y. Hou, H. Chen et al., "Sample preparation method for isolation of single-cell types from mouse liver for proteomic studies," *Proteomics*, vol. 11, no. 17, pp. 3556–3564, 2011.

[13] Q. Zhang, Y. Qu, Z. Li et al., "Isolation and culture of single cell types from rat liver," *Cells, Tissues, Organs*, vol. 201, no. 4, pp. 253–267, 2016.

[14] I. Mederacke, D. H. Dapito, S. Affò, H. Uchinami, and R. F. Schwabe, "High-yield and high-purity isolation of hepatic stellate cells from normal and fibrotic mouse livers," *Nature Protocols*, vol. 10, no. 2, pp. 305–315, 2015.

[15] M. Bartneck, K. T. Warzecha, C. G. Tag et al., "Isolation and time lapse microscopy of highly pure hepatic stellate cells," *Analytical Cellular Pathology*, vol. 2015, Article ID 417023, 13 pages, 2015.

[16] Y. Osawa, M. Hoshi, I. Yasuda, T. Saibara, H. Moriwaki, and O. Kozawa, "Tumor necrosis factor-α promotes cholestasis-induced liver fibrosis in the mouse through tissue inhibitor of metalloproteinase-1 production in hepatic stellate cells," *PLoS One*, vol. 8, no. 6, article e65251, 2013.

[17] M. Dominici, K. le Blanc, I. Mueller et al., "Minimal criteria for defining multipotent mesenchymal stromal cells. The International Society For Cellular Therapy position statement," *Cytotherapy*, vol. 8, no. 4, pp. 315–317, 2006.

[18] O. Parolini, F. Alviano, G. P. Bagnara et al., "Concise review: isolation and characterization of cells from human term placenta: outcome of the first international workshop on placenta derived stem cells," *Stem Cells*, vol. 26, no. 2, pp. 300–311, 2008.

[19] G. Kundrotas, "Surface markers distinguishing mesenchymal stem cells from fibroblasts," *Acta Medica Lituanica*, vol. 19, no. 2, pp. 75–79, 2012.

[20] A. Geerts, T. Niki, K. Hellemans et al., "Purification of rat hepatic stellate cells by side scatter-activated cell sorting," *Hepatology*, vol. 27, no. 2, pp. 590–598, 1998.

[21] U. Fearon, R. Mullan, T. Markham et al., "Oncostatin M induces angiogenesis and cartilage degradation in rheumatoid arthritis synovial tissue and human cartilage cocultures," *Arthritis and Rheumatism*, vol. 54, no. 10, pp. 3152–3162, 2006.

[22] D. Li and S. Friedman, "Liver fibrogenesis and the role of hepatic stellate cells: new insights and prospects for therapy," *Journal of Gastroenterology and Hepatology*, vol. 14, no. 7, pp. 618–633, 1999.

[23] D. Zhang, M. Jiang, and D. Miao, "Transplanted human amniotic membrane-derived mesenchymal stem cells ameliorate carbon tetrachloride-induced liver cirrhosis in mouse," *PLoS One*, vol. 6, no. 2, article e16789, 2011.

[24] C. Y. Zhang, W. G. Yuan, P. He, J. H. Lei, and C. X. Wang, "Liver fibrosis and hepatic stellate cells: etiology, pathological hallmarks and therapeutic targets," *World Journal of Gastroenterology*, vol. 22, no. 48, pp. 10512–10522, 2016.

[25] Y. Yokoi, T. Namihisa, H. Kuroda et al., "Immunocytochemical detection of desmin in fat-storing cells (Ito cells)," *Hepatology*, vol. 4, no. 4, pp. 709–714, 1984.

[26] A. L. Gard, F. P. White, and G. R. Dutton, "Extra-neural glial fibrillary acidic protein (GFAP) immunoreactivity in perisinusoidal stellate cells of rat liver," *Journal of Neuroimmunology*, vol. 8, no. 4–6, pp. 359–375, 1985.

[27] S. March, M. Graupera, M. Rosa Sarrias et al., "Identification and functional characterization of the hepatic stellate cell CD38 cell surface molecule," *The American Journal of Pathology*, vol. 170, no. 1, pp. 176–187, 2007.

[28] G. Ballardini, P. Groff, L. B. de Giorgi, D. Schuppan, and F. B. Bianchi, "Ito cell heterogeneity: desmin-negative Ito cells in normal rat liver," *Hepatology*, vol. 19, no. 2, pp. 440–446, 1994.

[29] T. Niki, P. J. de Bleser, G. Xu, K. van der Berg, E. Wisse, and A. Geerts, "Comparison of glial fibrillary acidic protein and desmin staining in normal and CCl_4-induced fibrotic rat livers," *Hepatology*, vol. 23, no. 6, pp. 1538–1545, 1996.

[30] S. L. Friedman, "Hepatic stellate cells: protean, multifunctional, and enigmatic cells of the liver," *Physiological Reviews*, vol. 88, no. 1, pp. 125–172, 2008.

[31] T. Tsuchida and S. L. Friedman, "Mechanisms of hepatic stellate cell activation," *Nature Reviews Gastroenterology & Hepatology*, vol. 14, no. 7, pp. 397–411, 2017.

[32] S. Iyer, S. Wei, K. Brew, and K. R. Acharya, "Crystal structure of the catalytic domain of matrix metalloproteinase-1 in complex with the inhibitory domain of tissue inhibitor of metalloproteinase-1," *Journal of Biological Chemistry*, vol. 282, no. 1, pp. 364–371, 2007.

[33] R. P. Mecham and W. C. Parks, *Matrix Metalloproteinases*, Academic Press - Elsevier Science, USA, 1998.

[34] F. Xu, C. Liu, D. Zhou, and L. Zhang, "TGF-β/SMAD pathway and its regulation in hepatic fibrosis," *The Journal of Histochemistry and Cytochemistry*, vol. 64, no. 3, pp. 157–167, 2016.

[35] S. Lindert, L. Wickert, I. Sawitza et al., "Transdifferentiation-dependent expression of α-SMA in hepatic stellate cells does not involve TGF-β pathways leading to coinduction of collagen type I and thrombospondin-2," *Matrix Biology*, vol. 24, no. 3, pp. 198–207, 2005.

[36] H. L. Reeves and S. L. Friedman, "Activation of hepatic stellate cells - a key issue in liver fibrosis," *Frontiers in Bioscience*, vol. 7, no. 1-3, pp. d808–d826, 2002.

[37] P. Mukherjee, S. L. Winter, and M. G. Alexandrow, "Cell cycle arrest by transforming growth factor β1 near G_1/S is mediated by acute abrogation of prereplication complex activation involving an Rb-MCM interaction," *Molecular and Cellular Biology*, vol. 30, no. 3, pp. 845–856, 2010.

[38] S. De Minicis, E. Seki, H. Uchinami et al., "Gene expression profiles during hepatic stellate cell activation in culture and in vivo," *Gastroenterology*, vol. 132, no. 5, pp. 1937–1946, 2007.

16

3D Culture of Bone Marrow-Derived Mesenchymal Stem Cells (BMSCs) Could Improve Bone Regeneration in 3D-Printed Porous Ti6Al4V Scaffolds

Lingjia Yu,[1] Yuanhao Wu,[2] Jieying Liu,[2] Bo Li,[1,3] Bupeng Ma,[2] Yaqian Li,[2] Zhenfei Huang,[1] Yu He,[1] Hai Wang,[1] Zhihong Wu,[2,4] and Guixing Qiu[1]

[1]*Department of Orthopaedic Surgery, Peking Union Medical College Hospital, Peking Union Medical College and Chinese Academy of Medical Sciences, Beijing 100730, China*
[2]*Central Laboratory, Peking Union Medical College Hospital, Peking Union Medical College and Chinese Academy of Medical Sciences, Beijing 100730, China*
[3]*Department of Orthopaedic Surgery, Fourth Clinical Medical College of Peking University, Beijing Jishuitan Hospital, Beijing 100035, China*
[4]*Beijing Key Laboratory for Genetic Research of Bone and Joint Disease, Beijing, China*

Correspondence should be addressed to Hai Wang; wanghai907@hotmail.com and Zhihong Wu; wuzh3000@126.com

Academic Editor: Alain Chapel

Mandibular bone defect reconstruction is an urgent challenge due to the requirements for daily eating and facial aesthetics. Three-dimensional- (3D-) printed titanium (Ti) scaffolds could provide patient-specific implants for bone defects. Appropriate load-bearing properties are also required during bone reconstruction, which makes them potential candidates for mandibular bone defect reconstruction implants. However, in clinical practice, the insufficient osteogenesis of the scaffolds needs to be further improved. In this study, we first encapsulated bone marrow-derived mesenchymal stem cells (BMSCs) into Matrigel. Subsequently, the BMSC-containing Matrigels were infiltrated into porous Ti6Al4V scaffolds. The Matrigels in the scaffolds provided a 3D culture environment for the BMSCs, which was important for osteoblast differentiation and new bone formation. Our results showed that rats with a full thickness of critical mandibular defects treated with Matrigel-infiltrated Ti6Al4V scaffolds exhibited better new bone formation than rats with local BMSC injection or Matrigel-treated defects. Our data suggest that Matrigel is able to create a more favorable 3D microenvironment for BMSCs, and Matrigel containing infiltrated BMSCs may be a promising method for enhancing the bone formation properties of 3D-printed Ti6Al4V scaffolds. We suggest that this approach provides an opportunity to further improve the efficiency of stem cell therapy for the treatment of mandibular bone defects.

1. Introduction

Mandibular bone defects caused by tumor resection, infection, trauma, or surgery are so common that they consume a large amount of medical resources [1]. Although mandibular reconstructive surgery has been performed for more than a century, the regeneration of critically sized bone defects remains challenging in maxillofacial surgery [2, 3]. Autogenous bone grafting derived from the iliac crest and fibula is the most common procedure for reconstructing mandibular bone defects. However, several limitations restrict its clinical use, including the limited sources of donor tissue, additional surgery, lack of an accurate fit with the defect site, and high rate of donor site infection [4]. Allogeneic bone grafting has also been widely used, but the associated disease transmission and immunogenicity cannot be neglected [5].

Regenerative approaches that avoid autogenous and allogeneic grafts by employing tissue-engineering bone substitutes may provide superior alternative strategies for effective bone reconstruction. Tissue engineering is the use of cells and materials in combination to improve or replace biological tissue, which involves the use of a tissue scaffold. It is well known that the ideal mandibular ramus bone reconstruction implants should have a 3D porous structure with desirable porosity for new bone ingrowth, nutrient diffusion, cell proliferation, capillary infiltration, and appropriate mechanical properties [6].

A large number of tissue-engineering biomaterials, such as collagen, hydroxyapatite (HA), and tricalcium phosphates (TCP), have been developed, but their insufficient mechanical properties and fast degradation rate are unable to meet the clinical demand [7]. With the enormous advantages of 3D printing technology in precision medicine, the 3D-printed porous Ti scaffold showed a superior biocompatibility, high strength-to-weight ratio, lower elastic modulus, and good anticorrosion resistance [8]. However, the inherently insufficient osteogenesis of the Ti makes it difficult for the bone cells to grow into the Ti scaffold. Therefore, scaffolds combined with autologous stem cell tissue have attracted much attention [9, 10]. The major concern with graft cell therapy is the survival rate of cells, which might be improved by the proper 3D extracellular environment [11, 12]. The interaction between stem cells and their surrounding environment is critical for cell behavior. 3D culture may represent a more physiological environment than 2D culture for stem cells, while 2D culture has a dramatically reduced differentiation capacity [13].

In this study, we prepared a 3D-printed porous Ti6Al4V scaffold with customized shape and structure and loaded the Matrigel encapsulating BMSCs into the Ti6Al4V scaffold. This device was designed to provide suitable mechanical properties and a 3D stem cell culture environment. The advantages of our 3D-printed scaffold are the accurate outline dimensions and complex internal morphology of the mandibular ramus, which might meet with the patients' individual requirements [14]. Matrigel has been chosen in our study as the extracellular matrix (ECM) for BMSCs. The ECM is a network tissue that provides mechanical support for stem cells and is essential for stem cells *in vivo*, and it can affect stem cell fate by mediating cell attachment and migration. Several hydrogels, including collagen and laminin, have been produced as an ECM for the 3D culture of stem cells, but Matrigel is regarded as one of the most promising materials that simulates ECM functions [11, 15]. Matrigel can rapidly form a 3D structured hydrogel at 37°C and support cell morphogenesis and differentiation as well as proliferation. It has also been used as a suitable scaffold for supporting stem cells in the treatment of cardiac infarction and arterial injury animal models [16, 17]. Several studies have also reported that on-top Matrigel culture could promote BMSCs osteodifferentiation *in vitro* [18, 19]. However, to date, there have been few reports on the proliferation, osteogenic differentiation, and osteogenesis effects of 3D-cultured BMSCs in Matrigel combined with the Ti6Al4V scaffold *in vivo*.

The goal of this study was to investigate the effects of BMSCs 3D cultured in Matrigel *in vitro* via a cell transplantation viability assay and osteodifferentiation study. Moreover, the efficacy of the combinational strategy of BMSCs, Matrigel, and 3D-printed Ti6Al4V scaffold was evaluated in a full-thickness critical mandibular defect animal model. The experimental process is schematically depicted in Figure 1.

2. Methods

2.1. 3D-Printed Ti6Al4V Scaffolds. The Ti6Al4V scaffolds were produced as previously reported [5] with minor modifications. Briefly, the scaffolds were produced with Ti6Al4V powder (ASTM B348, grade 23) using selective laser melting (SLM; Concept Laser, Lichtenfels, Germany). The scaffolds were disk shaped with a 5 mm diameter, 1 mm height, 200 μm strut width, and 600 μm pore size. The porosity was 87.4% for animal experiments. All samples underwent a post-production heat treatment and were verified by micro-CT (SHIMADZU, inspeXio SMX-90CT Plus, Japan).

2.2. 2D Cell Culture. Briefly, human BMSCs (passage 1) were purchased from 307-Ivy Translation Medicine Center (Beijing, China) and grown in hMSC basal media (HUXMA-90011, Cyagen, USA) supplemented with 10% fetal bovine serum (Cyagen, USA) and 1% penicillin-streptomycin (Cyagen, USA) and glutamine (Cyagen, USA) at 37°C with 5% CO_2 and saturated humidity. We used 0.25% trypsin without EDTA (Solarbio Science & Technology Co. Ltd., Beijing, China) to digest cells when the cells had grown to a confluence of 70–80% in the flask (431464U, Corning, USA). The media were changed every two days, and cells at passage 3–5 were used for the following experiments. The BMSC phenotypes are identified (S Figure 2).

2.3. Cell Encapsulation in Matrigel. The BMSCs were encapsulated into the Matrigel according to a published method [20]. Briefly, Matrigel was diluted to 8 mg/ml with ice-cold phosphate-buffered saline (PBS), pH 7.4. The pre-chilled culture plates (96-well and 6-well plates) were coated with a thin layer of phenol red-free Matrigel and incubated for 20 mins at 37°C to form a layer of gel on the surface of the plates. The BMSCs were trypsinized to a single cell suspension and pelleted by centrifugation at 800 rpm for 5 mins (Sorvall, ST 16R, Thermo Fisher Scientific, USA). The BMSCs were suspended in the Matrigel at 1×10^6 cells/ml. The mixture of cells and Matrigel was added to the precoated plates and further incubated at 37°C for 30 mins to allow the Matrigel to form a gel. Finally, an appropriate volume of serum-free culture media was added to the plates, and the medium was changed every two days.

2.4. Cell Morphology. The BMSCs incubated in the 2D plates and 3D Matrigel for 48 h were observed under an optical microscope (TE2000-U, Eclipse, Nikon) and then fixed in 4% paraformaldehyde (Aspen, China). After rinsing 3 times with PBS, the cells were stained with TRITC phalloidin (40734ES75, Yeasen, China) for 30 mins at room temperature in the dark. Then, the nuclei were counterstained with diamidine-phenylindole-dihydrochloride (DAPI) (D1306, Thermo Fisher Scientific, USA) for 5 mins, and fluorescent

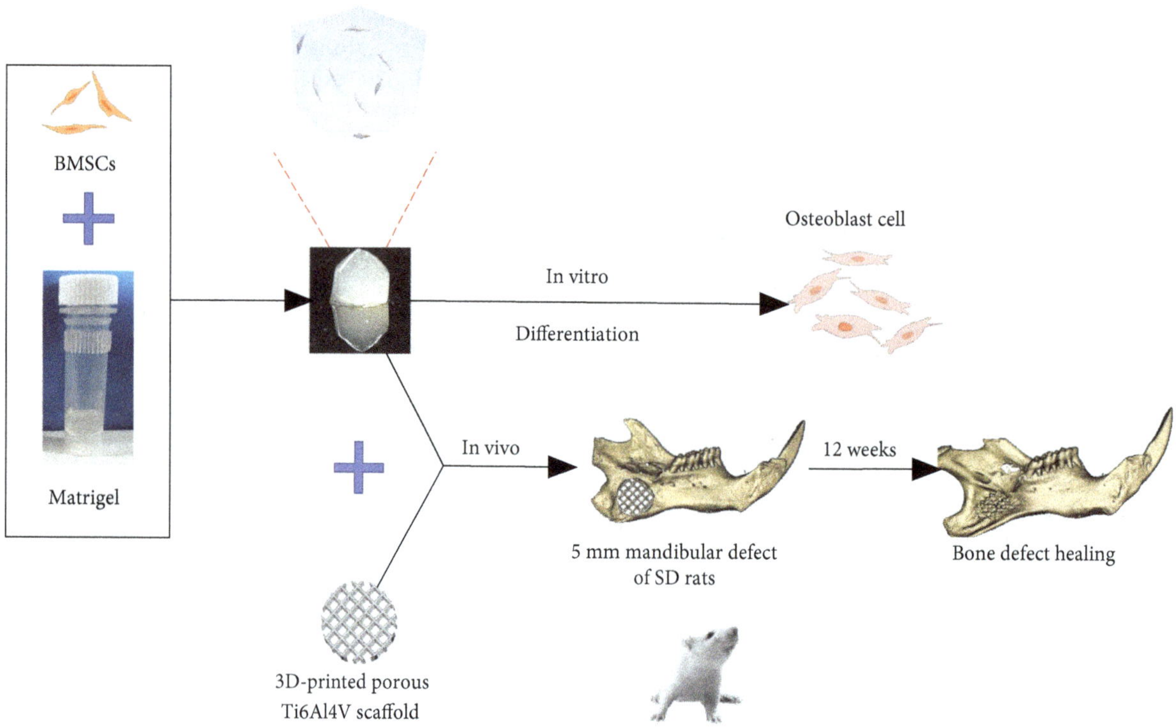

FIGURE 1: A schematic of the experimental design both *in vivo* and *in vitro*. A schematic of the bone differentiation process of BMSCs encapsulated in the Matrigel *in vitro* and the Ti6Al4V scaffold-Matrigel-BMSC complex device enhancing bone repair *in vivo*.

images were captured with a confocal fluorescence microscope system (Leica SP2, Leica, Germany).

2.5. Cell Viability and Proliferation. A LIVE/DEAD assay was performed to evaluate cell viability in the Matrigel and 2D plates. The LIVE/DEAD Viability/Cytotoxicity Assay kit (L3224, Invitrogen™, USA) provides a two-color fluorescence cell viability assay with calcein AM and ethidium homodimer (EthD-1). After culturing in the 2D plates or 3D Matrigel for 5 days, the BMSCs were incubated with 10 μM calcein AM and 10 μM EthD-1 solution at 37°C for 40 mins in the dark. The samples were then imaged under fluorescence microscopy (80i, Eclipse, Nikon). Live cells were stained green, while the dead cells were stained red. The stained cell areas were calculated with 6 different regions of interest (ROI) fields for each sample ($n = 3$) from immunofluorescence imaging using ImageJ 1.50i software (National Institutes of Health, USA).

The proliferation rates of cells cultured in Matrigel were detected by CCK-8 kits (Dojindo, Tokyo, Japan) after BMSCs were encapsulated in the Matrigel for 1, 3, 5, or 7 days. BMSCs cultured on 2D plates with normal media served as the control.

2.6. Osteodifferentiation Studies. BMSCs were encapsulated in the Matrigel and cultured with osteogenic media for 7 or 14 days (cell density 1×10^6 cells/ml). Similar to 2D plate culture, BMSCs were seeded into the 6-well plates (same cell density as described above) with either normal media or osteogenic media (HUXMA-90021, Cyagen, USA), which contains 1×10^{-6} M dexamethasone, 50 μg/ml ascorbic acid, and 1×10^{-12} M β-glycerophosphate. The osteogenic differentiation of BMSCs in Matrigel was assessed by ALP activity assay and Alizarin Red S staining. Briefly, 3 volumes of ice-cold PBS-EDTA was added to the Matrigel and vibrated on ice gently for 30 min until the Matrigel dissolved completely. Then, the cells were pelleted at 100×g for 5 min followed by lysing with 0.2% Triton X-100. The alkaline phosphatase (ALP) activity assay was performed following the manufacturer's instructions (Beyotime, China) in the presence of the substrate p-nitrophenyl phosphate (pNPP). The final ALP activity was normalized as pNPP production (nM) per total intracellular protein content (mg) per min (nmol/min/mg protein) (determined by MicroBCA protein assay kits, Thermo Fisher Scientific).

After incubation for 14 days, all cells were stained with a 0.1% Alizarin Red S (Sigma-Aldrich, USA) for calcium deposits, and an optical microscope (TE2000-U, Eclipse, Nikon) was used to take photographs. To quantify the orange-red coloration of ARS, 10% acetic acid (Sigma Aldrich, USA) was added to the plates. After centrifuging and neutralizing with 10% ammonium hydroxide (Sigma-Aldrich, USA), 100 μl of each sample was added to 96-well plates, and the OD405 was read using a microplate reader (Varioskan Flash, Thermo Fisher Scientific).

2.7. Western Blotting Analyses. BMSCs were encapsulated and cultured with osteogenic media in Matrigel or cultured in the 6-well plates with either normal media or osteogenic media as described above. Total proteins were isolated from these cells after incubation for 14 days. An equal amount of protein (50 μg protein/lane) was separated by sodium

Table 1: Primer pair sequences for the studied genes.

Gene	Sequences: Forward (5′-3′)	Sequences: Reverse (3′-5′)	Annealing temperature (°C)
GAPDH	GTCAAGGCTGAGAACGGGAA	AAATGAGCCCCAGCCTTCTC	58
COL-1	CCTCGCTTTCCTTCCTCTCC	GTCAAGGCTGAGAACGGGAA	58
Runx2	CATGTCCCTCGGTATGTCCG	ACTCTGGCTTTGGGAAGAGC	58
OPN	ATCTCCTAGCCCCACAGACCC	CACACTATCACCTCGGCCATC	58
ALP	TCCTGTTGACACCCCAAACC	GGAAACGCAGGATTTCCCAC	58
OCN	CTCACACTCCTCGCCCTATTG	CGCCTGGGTCTCTTCACTAC	58

dodecyl sulfate polyacrylamide gel electrophoresis (SDS-PAGE) and transferred to polyvinylidene difluoride (PVDF) membranes. The membranes were incubated in 5% skimmed milk for 1 hour at room temperature and overnight at 4°C with primary rabbit antibodies. All antibodies were purchased from Abcam Inc. (UK). GAPDH was used as the control. Bands were visualized using an ECL chemiluminescent kit (WP20005, Invitrogen™, USA) and quantitated by Quantity One (Bio-Rad, Hercules, USA).

2.8. Real-Time Quantitative PCR. RT-PCR was used to assess the osteogenic mRNA expression of BMSCs. At day 7 and day 14, RNA was extracted from encapsulated BMSCs cultured with osteogenic media in Matrigel or 6-well plates (cultured with either normal media or osteogenic media). Briefly, total RNA was extracted with TRIZOL reagent (Invitrogen™, USA) and reverse transcribed into cDNA using a cDNA synthesis kit (Thermo Fisher Scientific, USA) according to the manufacturer's protocol. PCR conditions comprised an initial step of denaturation for 1 min at 95°C, followed by a total of 40 cycles of 15 s at 95°C, 20 s at 58°C, and 20 s at 72°C. The expression levels of osteoblastic markers, including Col-1, Runx2, OPN, ALP, and OCN, were calculated based on the $2^{-\Delta\Delta Ct}$ method by normalizing values to the housekeeping gene GAPDH. The primer sequences of selected genes are listed in Table 1.

2.9. Surgical Procedures. Forty-eight male SD rats weighing 250–300 g were purchased from the Laboratory Animal Center of Peking Union Medical College Hospital (PUMCH) and were used for animal experiments. All experimental procedures were approved by the Institutional Animal Care and Use Committee (IACUC) of PUMCH. All the rats were anesthetized with ketamine hydrochloride (6 mg/100 g) and a 5 mm full-thickness standardized defect was made with a stainless-steel punch on the mandibular ramus of SD rats (S Figure 1A and B). All rats were randomly divided into four groups ($n = 12$ each group): (1) bare scaffold (BS); (2) scaffold with injected BMSCs + PBS (SC); (3) scaffold + Matrigel (SM); and (4) scaffold + BMSC-loaded Matrigel (SMB). For the BS group, the bare scaffold was carefully pressed to fit into the defect. For the SC group, 1×10^6 BMSCs were resuspended in 250 μl PBS and then injected into the scaffold after implantation. For the SMB group and the SM group, Matrigel with or without 1×10^6 encapsulated BMSCs was added to fill the scaffold before implantation (S Figure 1C and D). Finally, the wounds were closed with sutures. Soft gel food was provided, and penicillin was intramuscularly injected for three days postsurgery.

2.10. Micro-CT Evaluation. At 6 and 12 weeks postoperatively, the mandibles were harvested. The mandibles were first fixed in 4% paraformaldehyde and then dehydrated in a graded ethanol solution from 70%–100% and embedded in methyl methacrylate. Micro-CT scans were performed using inspeXio SMX-90CT Plus micro-CT (SHIMADZU, Japan) with a resolution of 10 μm (voltage: 90 kV, current: 110 μA, 1.0 mm Al filter). The volume of newly formed hard tissue within the defect area was assessed through MIMICS 15.0 (Materialise, Belgium), and bone regeneration was expressed as bone volume (BV), total volume (TV), and percent bone volume (BV/TV).

2.11. Histological Analysis. An interlocked diamond saw (Leica Microtome, Wetzlar, Germany) was used to obtain 200 μm thick sections. After polishing to a thickness of 50 μm, these sections were stained in 1.2% trinitrophenol solution as well as 1% acid fuchsin solution (Van Gieson staining). The stained sections were observed under an optical microscope (TE2000-U, Eclipse, Nikon). The red represents new bone formation, the blue indicates fibrous tissue, and the black is the metal.

2.12. Statistical Analysis. All the values were expressed as the mean ± standard deviation (SD). Statistical significance was measured using Student's *t*-test and one-way analysis of variance (ANOVA). Statistical significance was defined as P value < 0.05.

3. Results

3.1. Cell Culture and Morphology. The cells in the 2D plate showed a spindle-like morphology and were well spread in the wells. Compared with 2D plate culture, the BMSCs in the Matrigel exhibited more connections with surrounding cells, and separated cell clusters can be seen (Figures 2(a) and 2(b)). The cell adhesion and connection behavior were investigated by fluorescent staining of F-actin (by rhodamine-phalloidin, shown as red) and nuclei (by DAPI, shown as blue), respectively. The BMSCs within the Matrigel formed a more complex network and interactions between them than did the 2D plate culture (Figures 2(c) and 2(d)). For

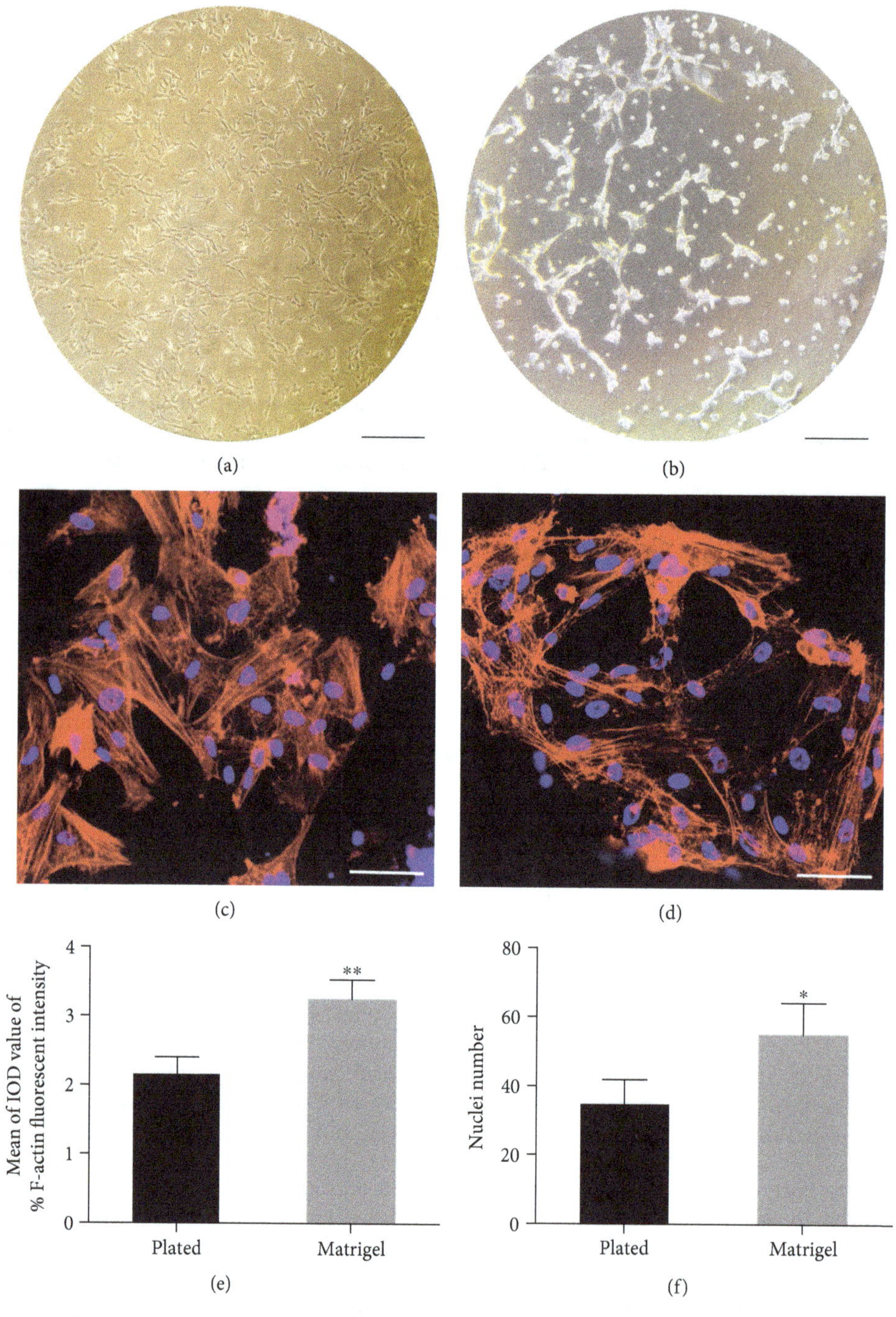

Figure 2: Representation of passage 4 BMSCs on 2D culture plates (a) and in Matrigel 3D culture (b) (scale bar: 300 μm). Representative images of fluorescent staining for F-actin and nuclei (c and d). Blue: DAPI stain, red: rhodamine-phalloidin (scale bar 50 μm). The fluorescent quality of F-actin (e) and the nuclei number (f) was analyzed and compared using ImageJ 1.50i, and the mean of the IOD value was considered as the level of fluorescence intensity. $^{*}p < 0.05$, $^{**}p < 0.01$.

quantitative analysis of cell adhesion and interaction behavior, the cell nuclei number and fluorescent intensity were measured using ImageJ software. The results showed that both the fluorescent intensity of F-actin and the cell nuclei number in the 3D Matrigel group were significantly higher than in the 2D plated culture (Figures 2(e) and 2(f)) (fluorescent intensity of F-actin $P < 0.01$ and nuclei number $P < 0.05$). This result indicated that the 3D Matrigel culture environment could promote BMSC adherence and interaction with surrounding cells.

3.2. Cell Proliferation and Biocompatibility. Figures 3(a) and 3(b) show the LIVE/DEAD staining images after culturing for 5 days in Matrigel or 2D plates. Almost no dead cells can be seen in either group. The fluorescence intensity of the cells calculated by ImageJ software showed that

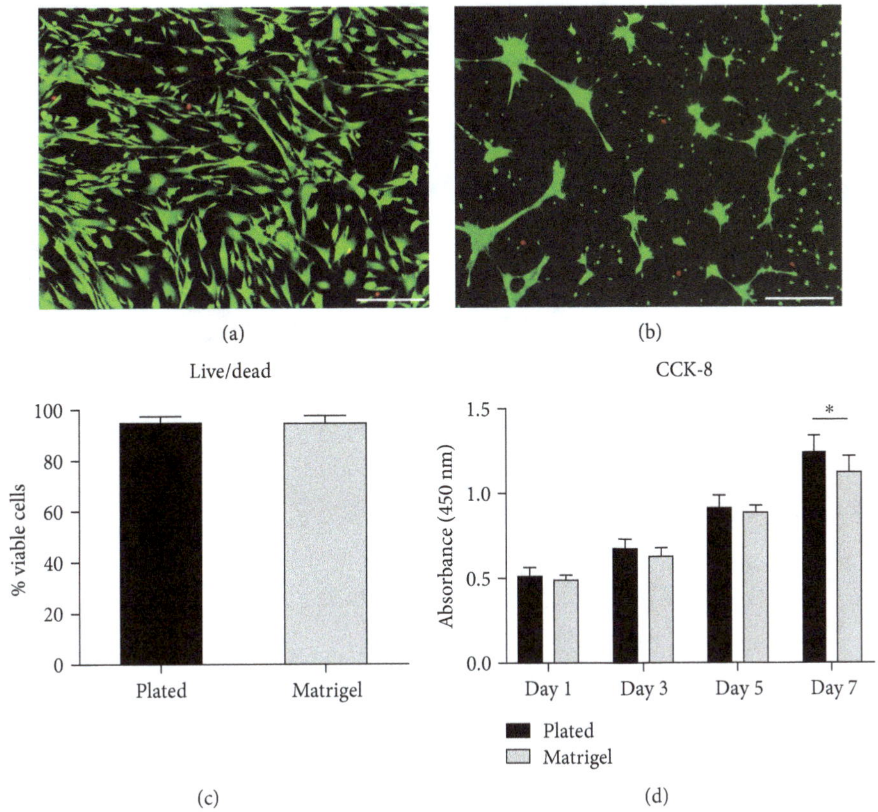

FIGURE 3: Representative images of the live/dead assay of BMSCs cultured on 2D plates (a) and encapsulated within the Matrigel (b) at 5 days (scale bar: 150 μm). The quantitative results of the live/dead assay of BMSCs (c). A CCK8 assay was used to assess BMSC proliferation over 7 days (d). $^{*}p < 0.05$.

no differences were found between the two groups (Figure 3(c)). BMSC proliferation was investigated by CCK-8 assay at day 1, 3, 5, and 7 after incubation. The cell viability steadily increased both in 2D plate culture and 3D Matrigel encapsulated culture during the incubation period (Figure 3(d)). These results indicate that the Matrigel can support BMSC proliferation and showed a negligible reduction in cell viability.

3.3. ALP Activity and ARS Staining. Alkaline phosphatase plays an important role in the matrix mineralization process. We evaluated the bone differentiation capability of BMSCs by ALP activity after 7 and 14 days of incubation. With increasing incubation time, the ALP activity of the experimental groups gradually increased. It should be noted that there was no significant difference between 2D culture induced by osteogenic media and 3D Matrigel culture at day 7. However, at day 14, the ALP activity in the Matrigel group was significantly higher than that in the other two groups ($P < 0.001$) (Figure 4).

Alizarin Red S was used to identify the calcium deposition of the BMSCs after incubation in 2D plates and 3D Matrigel. Figures 5(a)–5(c) show the deposition of the mineralized matrix on day 14. After extraction with acetic acid, a quantitative analysis of the formed calcium nodes was undertaken by colorimetric detection (Figure 5(d)). The results showed that the osteogenic medium significantly improved

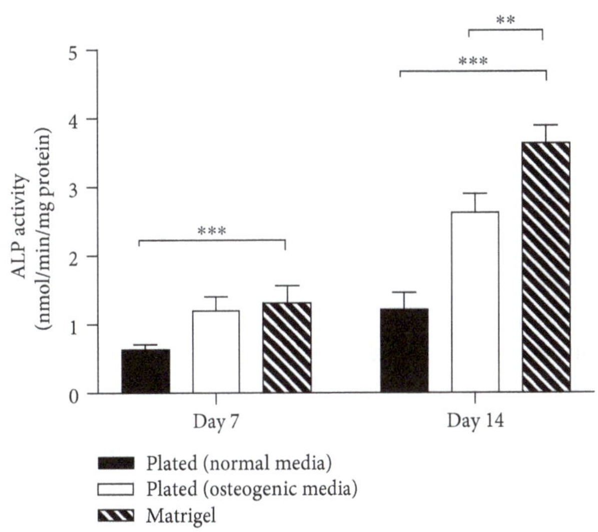

FIGURE 4: ALP activity of BMSCs cultured on 2D plates with standard medium or with osteogenic medium and BMSCs encapsulated in 3D Matrigel after culture for 7 and 14 days. $^{**}p < 0.01$, $^{***}p < 0.001$.

the cellular mineralization ability, and when compared to the 2D plates with an osteogenic medium, cells in the 3D Matrigel exhibited nearly 1.5 times higher calcium node deposition. These results indicated that 3D Matrigel culture could promote osteogenic differentiation of BMSCs.

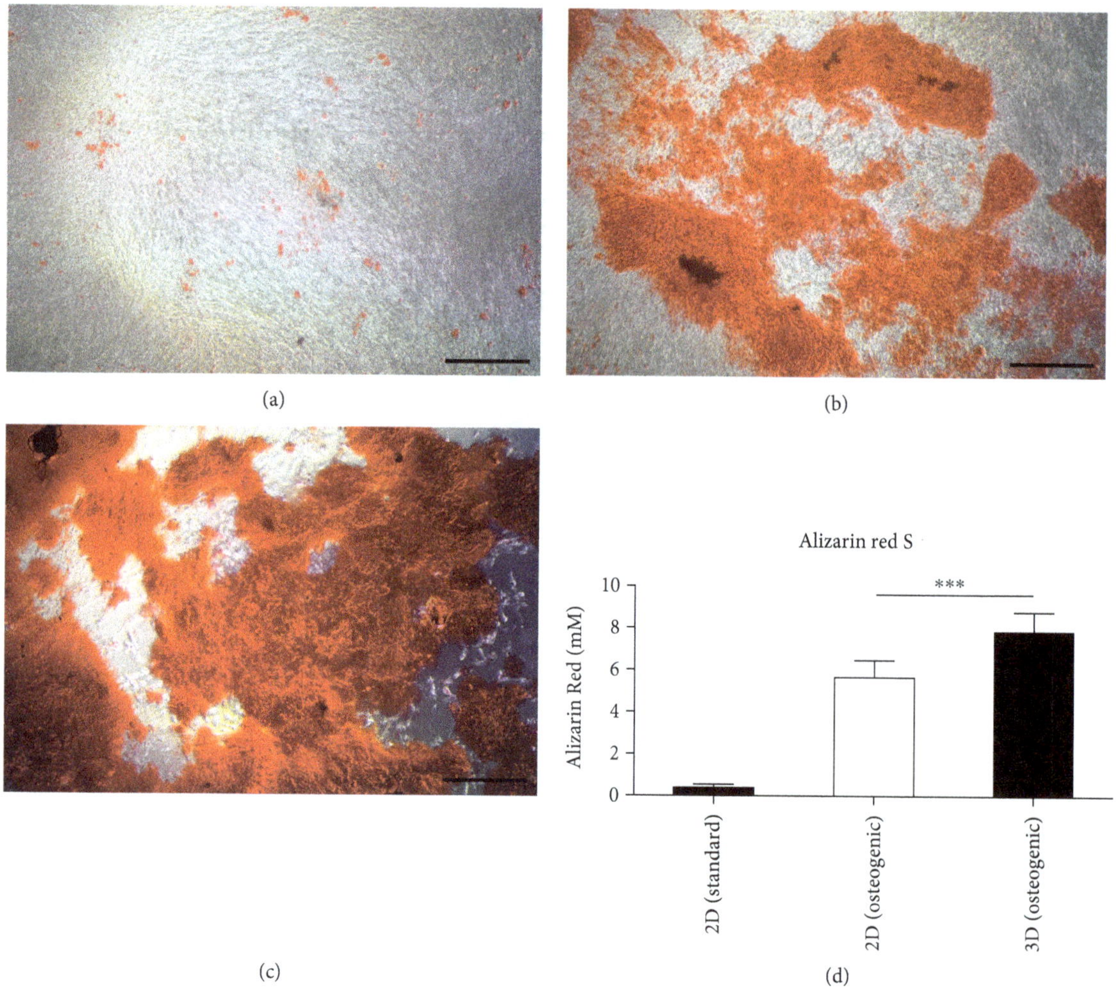

FIGURE 5: The amount of the mineralized matrix deposited was determined by Alizarin Red S staining and quantification on day 14. BMSC 2D culture with standard medium (a), BMSC 2D culture with osteogenic medium (b), BMSCs cultured in 3D Matrigel (c), and quantitative levels of calcium accumulation (d). $^{***}p < 0.001$.

3.4. Induction of BMSC Differentiation by Matrigel. Western blot assays were used to evaluate osteogenesis markers, including Col-1, Runx2, OPN, ALP, and OCN, while GAPDH was used as a housekeeping gene. After 14 days of culture in Matrigel with the osteogenic medium, the expression level of all osteogenic-related proteins, such as Col-1, Runx2, and OCN ($P < 0.001$) and OPN and ALP ($P < 0.05$), in BMSCs was much higher when compared to the cells cultured in 2D plates with the osteogenic medium. All these proteins were significantly higher in 3D Matrigel-cultured BMSCs compared to those cultured in 2D standard medium ($P < 0.001$) (Figures 6(a) and 6(b)).

The RT-PCR test was performed on day 7 and day 14 to evaluate the mRNA expression levels of Col-1, Runx2, OPN, ALP, and OCN. On day 7, 3D-cultured BMSCs showed higher mRNA expression of Col-1 ($P < 0.05$), ALP ($P < 0.01$), and OCN ($P < 0.001$) than 2D-cultured BMSCs with the osteogenic medium. Similarly, RT-PCR analysis confirmed the same results as those observed by Western blotting on day 14, which showed significantly upregulated expression of Col-1 ($P < 0.001$), Runx2 ($P < 0.001$), OPN ($P < 0.001$), ALP ($P < 0.01$), and OCN ($P < 0.05$) in the 3D Matrigel group (Figures 6(c)–6(g)). These results confirmed the osteogenic differentiation ability of Matrigel at both the protein and mRNA levels.

3.5. Micro-CT Analysis. No complications were observed in the 48 SD rats, and all skin wounds were healed within 5 days. At 6 and 12 weeks after implantation, micro-CT was used to detect the newly formed bone within the scaffold. As shown in Figure 7, the BS group without Matrigel and stem cells showed rare bone formation. The Matrigel alone and the BMSC injection resulted in only minor neo-bone formation. However, the SMC group exhibited accelerated bone regeneration and showed clear enhancement of the repair as determined by a quantitative analysis of BV/TV (Figure 7(i)).

3.6. Histological Evaluation. Histological analyses were used to characterize mineralized formation in all defects. At the end of 6 and 12 weeks, the rats were euthanized, and the implant site tissue was harvested for Van Gieson staining.

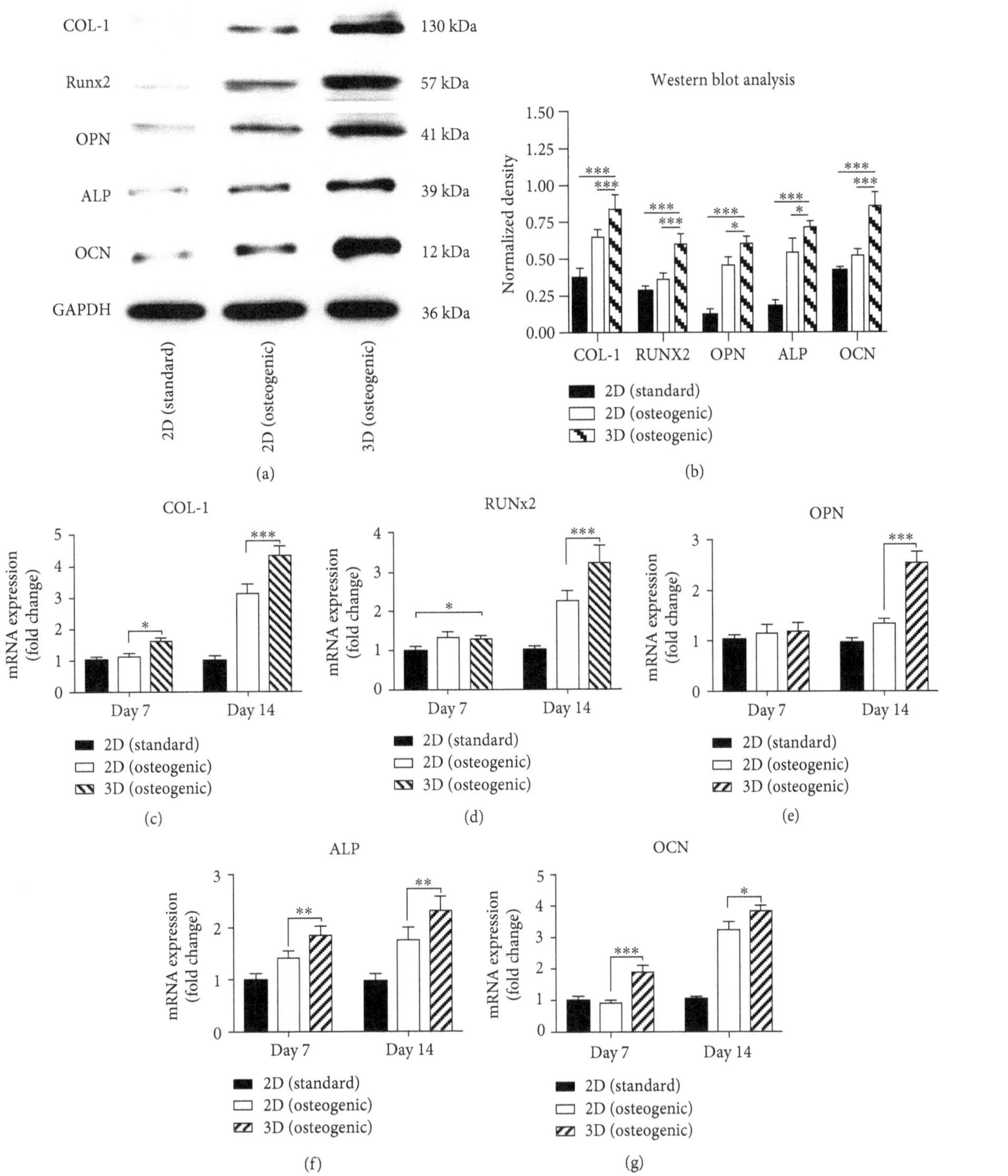

Figure 6: Western blot analysis was used to determine the expression of COL-I, Runx2, OPN, ALP, and OCN in BMSCs (a). Quantification of the density of Western blots in each group (b). The real-time polymerase chain reaction (RT-PCR) measurements of the COL-1 (c), Runx2 (d), OPN (e), ALP (f), and OCN (g) genes. These values are ratios relative to GAPDH and the mean relative quantity (RQ) ± square deviation (SD). $^{*}p < 0.05$, $^{**}p < 0.01$, $^{***}p < 0.001$.

The histological analysis results corresponded with those observed by micro-CT. The amount of the new bone was significantly higher in the SMC group compared with that in the other three groups both at 6 and 12 weeks, and the pores of the Ti6Al4V scaffold were filled with the newly formed bone. The newly formed bone was found rarely in the BS group. In the SM group, the new bone was only found at the surface of the scaffold and not inside. In the SC group, only a few newly formed bones were detected within the scaffold (Figure 8).

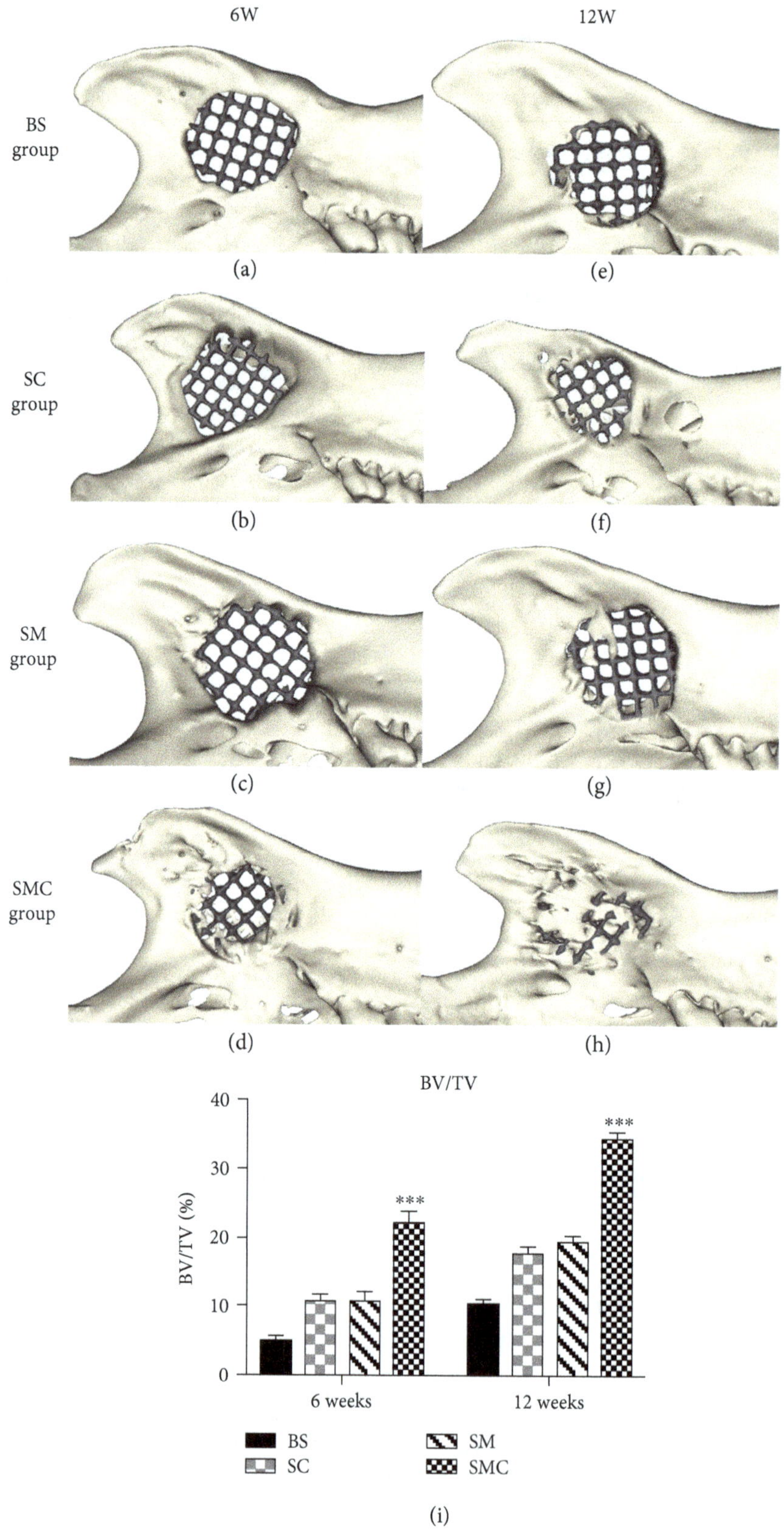

FIGURE 7: The volume of regenerated bone reconstruction based on ex vivo micro-CT scans at 6 and 12 weeks (a–h). The percent bone volume BV/TV was calculated by MIMICS 15.0 (Materialise, Belgium) (i). $^{***}p < 0.001$.

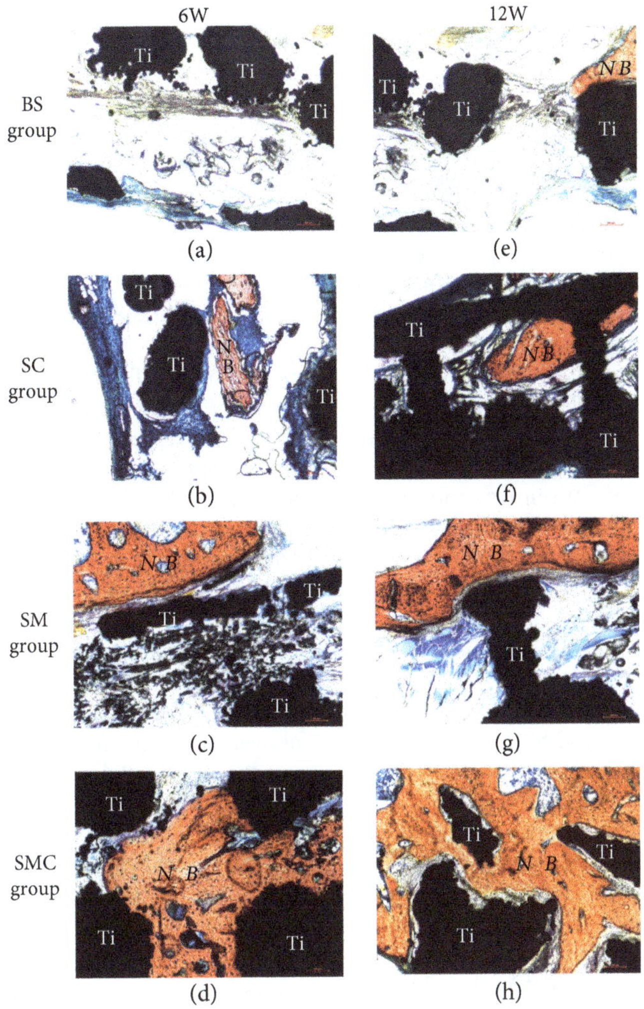

FIGURE 8: Histological analysis of osteointegration ability of four groups using Van Gieson staining at 6 weeks (a, b, c, and d) and 12 weeks (e, f, g, and h). BS group (a, e); SC group (b, f); SM group (c, g); SMC group (d, h). (red represents new bone formation (NB), blue indicates fibrous tissue, and black is the metal (Ti)) (scale bar: 100 μm).

4. Discussion

Over the past decade, great progress has been made in the surgical techniques and clinical outcomes of mandibular defect repair. However, mandibular bone regeneration remains a major unsolved problem. The lack of osteogenic cells in the surgical bed continues to be a pitfall in every mandibular reconstruction [21]. In this study, Matrigel was chosen to provide an excellent BMSC 3D culture environment for bone regeneration, and the combination of 3D-printed Ti6Al4V scaffold can serve as a complementary component to provide robust bone structure and customized shape.

4.1. Matrigel Increases BMSC Osteogenic Activity In Vitro. Critical mandibular defects need a considerable number of BMSCs. However, BMSCs are scarce in tissue [22]. Thus, BMSC grafts are considered to be a promising method for treating mandibular bone defects. Keeping BMSCs viable and promoting bone differentiation is a major concern. In the present study, BMSCs were encapsulated in Matrigel for 3D culture, and BMSCs grown on 2D plates either in normal or osteogenic media were used as controls. Interestingly, the BMSCs grown in Matrigel showed a higher level of ALP activity, calcium deposition, and osteogenic-related protein and gene expression than those cultured on 2D plates with or without osteogenic media. A previous study showed that stem cells grown on Matrigel-coated surfaces had higher osteogenic activity [19]. This is because of the ECM properties of Matrigel, which can promote the osteogenic differentiation of BMSCs directly. The ECM has already been reported to provide structural support for cells and physical and biochemical cues to regulate cell phenotype [23, 24]. BMSCs cultured in Matrigel can interact with multiple ECM components within the Matrigel, such as laminin and TGF-β. The laminin can regulate osteogenic differentiation via the integrin signaling pathway [25], and TGF-β is an important osteogenic growth factor.

Moreover, 3D culture in Matrigel strongly mimics the physiological condition *in vivo*. Many studies have reported that 3D culture provides an optimal environment for cellular adhesion and communication [23, 26]. The 3D constructs represent a completely different environment, due to different signaling pathway activity compared to 2D culture. Grayson et al. [27] reported that BMSCs express more integrin in 3D culture compared to that in 2D culture. Thus, 3D culture might activate the integrin-BMP/Smad pathway in BMSCs [28]. However, traditional 2D-cultured stem cells are grown on plastic surfaces, which helps them to retain proliferation potential but dramatically reduces differentiation capacity [23]. Previous reports have proposed that culturing BMSCs in a 3D hydrogel system could reduce their stemness properties and differentiate them into other lineages, such as osteogenic or myogenic commitment [9, 29]. This agrees with the results of the CCK-8 assay, where the BMSCs cultured in the Matrigel proliferated less than those on the 2D plates (Figure 3(d)). Therefore, some researchers have reported that the differentiation capability of stem cells is enhanced in a 3D culture system both *in vivo* and *in vitro* [30, 31]. In the present study, we also found that the 3D Matrigel culture could promote cell adhesion and that the Matrigel served as an artificial 3D microenvironment to regulate BMSC bone differentiation *in vitro*. However, the underlying mechanisms require further exploration.

4.2. Scaffold-Matrigel-BMSC Complex Enhances Bone Repair In Vivo. The reconstruction of the mandible is different from midface or calvaria repair because it demands load-bearing ability. Ti has been attractive for clinical use because of its excellent load-bearing properties, biocompatibility, and high corrosion resistance [32]. Today, with the help of digital medicine and computer-aided technology, a 3D-printed porous Ti scaffold could mimic bone tissue morphology and mechanical behavior functionally and aesthetically, thus helping to reconstruct mandibular bone defects [33, 34]. The 3D-printed implants can reconstruct complex defective sections anatomically using a mirror image of the unaffected side [34, 35]. In this study, 3D-printed Ti6Al4V scaffolds with more than 80% porosity can accommodate new bone and provide an adequate biological fixation. However, three major factors were found to restrict bone regeneration, including the lack of stem cells, the bioinert properties of Ti, and the intrusion of the surrounding muscle into the scaffold. To solve these problems, BMSC-loaded Matrigels were prepared and incorporated into the 3D-printed porous Ti6Al4V scaffold. Therefore, we hypothesized that by combining cell therapy and 3D-printed scaffolds, the device might provide a robust bone substitute with biological activity for bone regeneration.

To evaluate the hypothesis, a mandibular ramus defect model of 5 mm was established to fully investigate the bone repair of BMSC-loaded Matrigel + porous Ti6Al4V scaffold *in vivo*. The micro-CT and histological analysis results both confirmed the bone repair capability of our device. In the animal model, a defect diameter greater than 5 mm is a critical size that cannot spontaneously heal [36–38]. The graft BMSCs could help bone formation within the scaffold. After 12 weeks of device implantation, both micro-CT and histological analysis showed that the bare scaffold group has rare bone formation (Figures 7(e) and 8(e)). However, in the scaffold + injected BMSCs group, few new bones formed within the scaffold (Figures 7(f) and 8(f)). This indicated that the BMSC-injection grafting method could partially help new bone formation, but the low survival rate of grafted BMSCs, which results from acute inflammation and mechanical damage, is the major obstacle [11]. Therefore, we encapsulated BMSC in Matrigel because Matrigel can retain BMSC viability, enhance the osteogenic potential of BMSCs, and prevent surrounding muscle intrusion into the scaffold. Cao et al. [39] used longitudinal bioluminescence imaging to assess cell signals in the Matrigel and found that Matrigel supported stem cell engraftment superior to cells alone or other matrices (collagen I and Puramatrix) up to 5 months. Thus, we believe that BMSCs may promote bone repair up to 5 months. Rosová et al. [40] and Chen et al. [41] reported that hypoxic conditions could improve BMSC survival and tissue regenerative potential *in vivo*, and the Matrigel hydrogel microenvironment is moderately hypoxic. Similarly, in our scaffold + Matrigel group, Matrigel without BMSCs inside only formed new bone on the surface of the scaffold, not inside (Figures 7(g) and 8(g)). However, in the scaffold + BMSC-loaded Matrigel group, BMSC viability showed a dramatic increase, and a large amount of new bone tissue formed around and within the scaffold (Figures 7(h) and 8(h)). This method not only solved the abovementioned disadvantages of the Ti scaffold but also produced a scaffold-Matrigel-BMSC complex with appropriate bioactivity and mechanical properties that enhanced bone repair *in vivo*. However, the long-term function of BMSCs in the *in vivo* model need further investigation before clinical usage.

In conclusion, this combination device was shown to be a complementary treatment modality for both Ti scaffold- and hydrogel-based cell therapy by avoiding the bioinertia of Ti scaffold and the weak mechanical properties of Matrigel. We believe that this device might be a promising method with high stem cell therapy efficiency for the treatment of mandibular bone defects. For further applications, a clinical trial is needed in the near future.

Acknowledgments

This work was supported by the Peking Union Medical College Graduate Student Innovation fund (no. 2017-1002-2-13), the Fundamental Research Funds for Central Public Welfare Research Institutes, Chinese Academy of Medical Sciences (no. 2016ZX310177-7), and the National High-Tech R&D Program of China (863 Program, 2015AA020316, 2015AA033601).

Supplementary Materials

Figure 1: the surgical procedure for the rat mandibular defect model. Exposure of the mandibular ramus (A). 5 mm full-thickness standardized defect was made (B). Porous titanium scaffold was pressed into the defect (C). Gross appearance of the mandibular defect (D). Supplementary Figure 2: BMSC phenotypes were identified. CD34− cells accounted for 0.05% of total cells. CD44+ cells accounted for 98.65% of total cells. CD45− cells accounted for 0.23% of total cells. CD73+ cells accounted for 99.73% of total cells. CD90+ cells accounted for 95.69% of total cells. CD105+ cells accounted for 97.32% of total cells. HLA-ABC+ cells accounted for 99.87% of total cells. HLA-DR− cells accounted for 0.04% of total cells. *(Supplementary Materials)*

References

[1] L. Larsson, A. M. Decker, L. Nibali, S. P. Pilipchuk, T. Berglundh, and W. V. Giannobile, "Regenerative medicine for periodontal and peri-implant diseases," *Journal of Dental Research*, vol. 95, no. 3, pp. 255–266, 2016.

[2] A. J. Abbasi, A. Azari, S. Z. Mohebbi, and A. Javani, "Mandibular rami implant: a new approach in mandibular reconstruction," *Journal of Oral and Maxillofacial Surgery*, vol. 75, no. 12, pp. 2550–2558, 2017.

[3] B. T. Goh, S. Lee, H. Tideman, and P. J. W. Stoelinga, "Mandibular reconstruction in adults: a review," *International Journal of Oral and Maxillofacial Surgery*, vol. 37, no. 7, pp. 597–605, 2008.

[4] X. Wang, X. Wu, H. Xing et al., "Porous Nanohydroxyapatite/collagen scaffolds loading insulin PLGA particles for restoration of critical size bone defect," *ACS Applied Materials & Interfaces*, vol. 9, no. 13, pp. 11380–11391, 2017.

[5] B. Yin, P. Ma, J. Chen et al., "Hybrid macro-porous titanium ornamented by degradable 3D gel/nHA micro-scaffolds for bone tissue regeneration," *International Journal of Molecular Sciences*, vol. 17, no. 4, p. 575, 2016.

[6] H. Shao, M. Sun, F. Zhang et al., "Custom repair of mandibular bone defects with 3D printed bioceramic scaffolds," *Journal of Dental Research*, vol. 97, no. 1, pp. 68–76, 2018.

[7] J. Van der Stok, E. M. M. Van Lieshout, Y. El-Massoudi, G. H. Van Kralingen, and P. Patka, "Bone substitutes in the Netherlands - a systematic literature review," *Acta Biomaterialia*, vol. 7, no. 2, pp. 739–750, 2011.

[8] S. Raisian, H. R. Fallahi, K. S. Khiabani, M. Heidarizadeh, and S. Azdoo, "Customized titanium mesh based on the 3D printed model vs. manual intraoperative bending of titanium mesh for reconstructing of orbital bone fracture: a randomized clinical trial," *Reviews on Recent Clinical Trials*, vol. 12, no. 3, pp. 154–158, 2017.

[9] K. Shou, Y. Huang, B. Qi et al., "Induction of mesenchymal stem cell differentiation in the absence of soluble inducer for cutaneous wound regeneration by a chitin nanofiber-based hydrogel," *Journal of Tissue Engineering and Regenerative Medicine*, vol. 12, no. 2, pp. e867–e880, 2018.

[10] Y. Duan, W. Ma, D. Li, T. Wang, and B. Liu, "Enhanced osseointegration of titanium implants in a rat model of osteoporosis using multilayer bone mesenchymal stem cell sheets," *Experimental and Therapeutic Medicine*, vol. 14, no. 6, pp. 5717–5726, 2017.

[11] M. Uemura, M. M. Refaat, M. Shinoyama, H. Hayashi, N. Hashimoto, and J. Takahashi, "Matrigel supports survival and neuronal differentiation of grafted embryonic stem cell-derived neural precursor cells," *Journal of Neuroscience Research*, vol. 88, no. 3, pp. 542–551, 2010.

[12] T. Führmann, R. Y. Tam, B. Ballarin et al., "Injectable hydrogel promotes early survival of induced pluripotent stem cell-derived oligodendrocytes and attenuates longterm teratoma formation in a spinal cord injury model," *Biomaterials*, vol. 83, pp. 23–36, 2016.

[13] A. Braccini, D. Wendt, C. Jaquiery et al., "Three-dimensional perfusion culture of human bone marrow cells and generation of osteoinductive grafts," *Stem Cells*, vol. 23, no. 8, pp. 1066–1072, 2005.

[14] S. E. Kim, K. M. Shim, K. Jang, J. H. Shim, and S. S. Kang, "Three-dimensional printing-based reconstruction of a maxillary bone defect in a dog following tumor removal," *In Vivo*, vol. 32, no. 1, pp. 63–70, 2018.

[15] L. Qian and W. M. Saltzman, "Improving the expansion and neuronal differentiation of mesenchymal stem cells through culture surface modification," *Biomaterials*, vol. 25, no. 7-8, pp. 1331–1337, 2004.

[16] Q. Xiao, L. Zeng, Z. Zhang et al., "Sca-1^{+} progenitors derived from embryonic stem cells differentiate into endothelial cells capable of vascular repair after arterial injury," *Arteriosclerosis, Thrombosis, and Vascular Biology*, vol. 26, no. 10, pp. 2244–2251, 2006.

[17] P. Zhang, H. Zhang, H. Wang, Y. Wei, and S. Hu, "Artificial matrix helps neonatal cardiomyocytes restore injured myocardium in rats," *Artificial Organs*, vol. 30, no. 2, pp. 86–93, 2006.

[18] B.-J. Kang, H.-H. Ryu, S.-S. Park et al., "Effect of matrigel on the osteogenic potential of canine adipose tissue-derived mesenchymal stem cells," *Journal of Veterinary Medical Science*, vol. 74, no. 7, pp. 827–836, 2012.

[19] M. B. Eslaminejad, F. Bagheri, and E. Zomorodian, "Matrigel enhances *in vitro* bone differentiation of human marrow-derived mesenchymal stem cells," *Iranian Journal of Basic Medical Sciences*, vol. 13, no. 1, pp. 187–194, 2010.

[20] G. Y. Lee, P. A. Kenny, E. H. Lee, and M. J. Bissell, "Three-dimensional culture models of normal and malignant breast epithelial cells," *Nature Methods*, vol. 4, no. 4, pp. 359–365, 2007.

[21] K. Fu, Y. Liu, N. Gao, J. Cai, W. He, and W. Qiu, "Reconstruction of maxillary and orbital floor defect with free fibula flap and whole individualized titanium mesh assisted by computer techniques," *Journal Oral and Maxillofacial Surgery*, vol. 75, no. 8, pp. 1791.e1–1791.e9, 2017.

[22] M. F. Pittenger, A. M. Mackay, S. C. Beck et al., "Multilineage potential of adult human mesenchymal stem cells," *Science*, vol. 284, no. 5411, pp. 143–147, 1999.

[23] Q. Zhang, S. Lin, J. Liao, and X. Cai, "Physical cues drive chondrogenic differentiation," *Current Stem Cell Research & Therapy*, vol. 13, no. 7, pp. 576–582, 2018.

[24] A. Cheng, S. A. Cain, P. Tian et al., "Recombinant extracellular matrix protein fragments support human embryonic stem cell chondrogenesis," *Tissue Engineering Part A*, vol. 24, no. 11-12, pp. 968–978, 2018.

[25] S. Viale-Bouroncle, M. Gosau, and C. Morsczeck, "Laminin regulates the osteogenic differentiation of dental follicle cells via integrin-α2/-β1 and the activation of the FAK/ERK signaling pathway," *Cell and Tissue Research*, vol. 357, no. 1, pp. 345–354, 2014.

[26] D. Gupta, D. M. Grant, K. M. Zakir Hossain, I. Ahmed, and V. Sottile, "Role of geometrical cues in bone marrow-derived mesenchymal stem cell survival, growth and osteogenic differentiation," *Journal of Biomaterials Applications*, vol. 32,

no. 7, pp. 906–919, 2018.

[27] W. L. Grayson, T. Ma, and B. Bunnell, "Human mesenchymal stem cells tissue development in 3D PET matrices," *Biotechnology Progress*, vol. 20, no. 3, pp. 905-912, 2004.

[28] H. Liu, H. Peng, Y. Wu et al., "The promotion of bone regeneration by nanofibrous hydroxyapatite/chitosan scaffolds by effects on integrin-BMP/Smad signaling pathway in BMSCs," *Biomaterials*, vol. 34, no. 18, pp. 4404–4417, 2013.

[29] P. C. Tseng, T. H. Young, T. M. Wang, H. W. Peng, S. M. Hou, and M. L. Yen, "Spontaneous osteogenesis of MSCs cultured on 3D microcarriers through alteration of cytoskeletal tension," *Biomaterials*, vol. 33, no. 2, pp. 556–564, 2012.

[30] X.-. F. Tian, B. C. Heng, Z. Ge et al., "Comparison of osteogenesis of human embryonic stem cells within 2D and 3D culture systems," *Scandinavian Journal of Clinical and Laboratory Investigation*, vol. 68, no. 1, pp. 58–67, 2009.

[31] S. N. Rath, P. Nooeaid, A. Arkudas et al., "Adipose- and bone marrow-derived mesenchymal stem cells display different osteogenic differentiation patterns in 3D bioactive glass-based scaffolds," *Journal of Tissue Engineering and Regenerative Medicine*, vol. 10, no. 10, pp. E497–E509, 2016.

[32] F. Suska, G. Kjeller, P. Tarnow et al., "Electron beam melting manufacturing technology for individually manufactured jaw prosthesis: a case report," *Journal of Oral and Maxillofacial Surgery*, vol. 74, no. 8, pp. 1706.e1–1706.e15, 2016.

[33] T. Schouman, M. Schmitt, C. Adam, G. Dubois, and P. Rouch, "Influence of the overall stiffness of a load-bearing porous titanium implant on bone ingrowth in critical-size mandibular bone defects in sheep," *Journal of the Mechanical Behavior of Biomedical Materials*, vol. 59, pp. 484–496, 2016.

[34] D. Luo, Q. Rong, and Q. Chen, "Finite-element design and optimization of a three-dimensional tetrahedral porous titanium scaffold for the reconstruction of mandibular defects," *Medical Engineering & Physics*, vol. 47, pp. 176–183, 2017.

[35] Y. Leiser, D. Shilo, A. Wolff, and A. Rachmiel, "Functional reconstruction in mandibular avulsion injuries," *The Journal of Craniofacial Surgery*, vol. 27, no. 8, pp. 2113–2116, 2016.

[36] W. Zhang, Z. Zhang, S. Chen, L. Macri, J. Kohn, and P. C. Yelick, "Mandibular jaw bone regeneration using human dental cell-seeded tyrosine-derived polycarbonate scaffolds," *Tissue Engineering Part A*, vol. 22, no. 13-14, pp. 985–993, 2016.

[37] L. B. Kaban, J. Glowacki, and J. E. Murray, "Repair of experimental mandibular bony defects in rats," *Surgical Forum*, vol. 30, pp. 519–521, 1979.

[38] X. Wang, H. Xing, G. Zhang et al., "Restoration of a critical mandibular bone defect using human alveolar bone-derived stem cells and porous nano-HA/collagen/PLA scaffold," *Stem Cells International*, vol. 2016, Article ID 8741641, 13 pages, 2016.

[39] F. Cao, A. H. Sadrzadeh Rafie, O. J. Abilez et al., "In vivo imaging and evaluation of different biomatrices for improvement of stem cell survival," *Journal of Tissue Engineering and Regenerative Medicine*, vol. 1, no. 6, pp. 465–468, 2007.

[40] I. Rosová, M. Dao, B. Capoccia, D. Link, and J. A. Nolta, "Hypoxic preconditioning results in increased motility and improved therapeutic potential of human mesenchymal stem cells," *Stem Cells*, vol. 26, no. 8, pp. 2173–2182, 2008.

[41] J. Chen, Y. Yang, L. Shen et al., "Hypoxic preconditioning augments the therapeutic efficacy of bone marrow stromal cells in a rat ischemic stroke model," *Cellular and Molecular Neurobiology*, vol. 37, no. 6, pp. 1115–1129, 2017.

17

Differentiation Potential of Human Wharton's Jelly-Derived Mesenchymal Stem Cells and Paracrine Signaling Interaction Contribute to Improve the In Vitro Maturation of Mouse Cumulus Oocyte Complexes

Martin Maldonado, Tianhua Huang, Jianying Chen, and Ying Zhong

Reproductive Medicine & Genetics, Chengdu Jinjiang Hospital for Maternal & Child Health Care, Chengdu 610066, China

Correspondence should be addressed to Ying Zhong; yzhong2014@126.com

Academic Editor: Hua Tan

In vitro maturation (IVM) in cumulus oocyte complexes (COCs) can be improved by the presence of human Wharton's jelly-derived MSCs (hWJ-MSCs), under specific culture conditions. COCs were cultured in twelve different culture systems, composed of four stock media, stock media conditioned with hWJ-MSCs, and stock media in which the oocytes were indirectly cocultured with the hWJ-MSCs. The rates of maturation to meiosis II were compared among the groups. G2-PLUS and coculture with DMEM-F12 were the most efficient systems for the maturation of COCs. The fertilization rate and rate of development to the blastocyst stage were compared between these two groups. Moreover, hWJ-MSC-conditioned media showed no benefits for the COC-IVM. The analysis of OCT4 expression of hWJ-MSCs in G1-PLUS, TYH, and G2-PLUS showed a downregulation of OCT4 by 25.9, 24.7, and 6.6%, respectively, compared to that in hWJ-MSCs cultured in DMEM-F12. Finally, we have demonstrated that two prerequisites appeared to be necessary for the hWJ-MSCs to improve the IVM of COCs: hWJ-MSCs' differentiation potential and the presence of coordinated paracrine interaction between the stem cells and COCs. Under the appropriate conditions, the paracrine factors produced in the coculture system with DMEM-F12 may help to develop synthetic media for successful in vitro culture of COCs.

1. Background

In vitro maturation (IVM) in cumulus oocyte complexes (COCs) can be improved by the presence of human Wharton's jelly-derived MSCs (hWJ-MSCs), under specific culture conditions.

Mesenchymal stem cells (MSCs) are attractive candidates for cell-based therapeutic strategies, primarily due to their intrinsic ability to self-renew and undergo multipotential differentiation and because they are amenable to genetic manipulation [1–3].

In a coculture, MSCs not only provide a target cell source with multipotent differentiation capacity but can also act as assisting cells to promote tissue homeostasis, metabolism, growth, and repair [4]. Their incorporation into coculture systems seems to be important for creating complex tissues or organs by cell-to-cell contact or/and through the delivery of soluble factors to the target cells.

Among the different types of MSCs, human Wharton's jelly-derived MSCs (hWJ-MSCs) appear to offer the best clinical advantages due to their unique beneficial characteristics [5]. hWJ-MSCs reprogram resident cells to favor tissue regeneration, attenuate wound inflammation, and inhibit fibrosis [6, 7]. They interact with host cells and influence the stem cell niche through differentiation and/or paracrine signaling mechanisms [6, 8, 9]. They are poor antigen-presenting cells; do not express MHC class II or the costimulatory molecules CD40, CD40L, CD80, and CD86 [10, 11]; and are not prone to undergo malignant transformation [12, 13].

Many attempts have been made to grow immature oocytes *in vitro* [14–16]. The culture conditions used for *in vitro* maturation (IVM), which include various media types and hormone supplements, as well as the presence of cumulus cells, can significantly influence maturation rates and subsequent embryo development [14, 17–19].

Furthermore, during ovarian follicular development, several growth factors and cytokines act as intraovarian regulators *in vivo*, and in the follicle, the action of gonadotrophins is modulated by locally produced paracrine and autocrine growth factors [20, 21].

Scientific evidence indicates that the secretion of trophic, soluble, or immunomodulatory factors, known as paracrine signals, may represent the most important underlying mechanism of MSC effects [9, 22, 23].

Given the appropriate stimuli and local environment, MSCs not only can develop into various cell types in vitro and regenerate tissues in vivo, but they can also secrete a variety of cytokines and growth factors, such as MCP-1, VEGF-A, EGF, FGF-2, IL-6, LIF, and TGF-β [2, 24].

Since cytokines and growth factors are known to stimulate meiotic progress and the processes associated with IVM, the aim of the present study was to determine whether IVM in cumulus oocyte complexes (COCs) could be improved by the presence of hWJ-MSCs through nonspecific release of cytokines and soluble factors using conditioned medium or by paracrine signaling from hWJ-MSCs using indirect coculture conditions. However, the success of IVM of COCs in coculture also depends on the choice of a suitable medium to allow oocyte maturation and the survival and potency of the hWJ-MSCs. In this work, we have opted to use DMEM-F12, a defined combination of nutrients, growth factors, and hormones that supports stemness and the differentiation potential of MSCs; two commercially available culture media for culture of human embryos from after fertilization until the 8-cell stage (G1-PLUS); a medium for culture of human embryos from the 8-cell stage on day three until the blastocyst stage (G2-PLUS); and TYH, first reported as a medium for in vitro fertilization (IVF) of mouse eggs with epididymal spermatozoa, by Yoda et al. [25] and Toyoda et al. [26] in 1971.

2. Methods

2.1. Animals. Male and female Kunming mice were maintained in a specific-pathogen-free animal facility in individual ventilated cages and housed at 23°C under a 12-hour dark/light cycle. Water and food were given *ad libitum*. All animal work was performed using protocols approved by the Institutional Review Board of the Chengdu Jinjiang Maternity and Child Health Hospital.

The health conditions of mice were monitored daily. Prior to the experimental endpoint, mice experienced minimal pain or stress during routine handling and hormone administration.

No ill or dead mice were observed prior to the experimental endpoint. Mice were euthanized by cervical dislocation.

2.2. Oocyte Handling. Mouse COCs were retrieved from 6- to 8-week-old Kunming mice (Chengdu Da Suo Biology and Technology Company) by ovary puncture with a 28 G sterile needle under a stereomicroscope. COCs were isolated 48 hours after an intraperitoneal injection of 10 IU of pregnant mare serum gonadotropin (PMSG, Sigma Chemical Co., St. Louis, MO). G-MOPS™ PLUS was used for handling and manipulation of the oocytes outside the incubator. Groups of oocytes were separated and cultured in 12 different culture systems and divided into 3 experimental stages. The first experimental stage included the following stock media preparations: (a) DMEM-F12 (Gibco; Thermo Fisher Scientific Inc., Waltham, MA, USA), (b) G1-PLUS (Vitrolife), (c) G2-PLUS (Vitrolife), and (d) TYH medium (Table S1). The second experimental stage included the following types of hWJ-MSC-conditioned media: (e) conditioned-DMEM-F12, (f) conditioned-G1-PLUS, (g) conditioned-G2-PLUS, and (h) conditioned-TYH. The third experimental stage included the following types of coculture with hWJ-MSCs: (i) coculture in DMEM-F12, (j) coculture in G1-PLUS, (k) coculture in G2-PLUS, and (l) coculture in TYH. The maturation status was evaluated after 24 hours of in vitro culture at 37°C in 6% CO_2. Oocytes with polar bodies were considered mature MII oocytes.

For all the experimental assays in this study, DMEM-F12 was supplemented with 10% fetal bovine serum (FBS, Thermo Fisher Scientific).

2.3. Isolation and Culture of hWJ-MSCs. Protocols for sampling the human umbilical cord were approved by the Institutional Review Board of Chengdu Jinjiang Hospital for Maternal & Child Health Care, according to the principles expressed in the Declaration of Helsinki. All participants provided their written consent to participate in this study. Human umbilical cords were obtained from consenting patients delivering full-term infants by cesarean section. The procedures for culture of hWJ-MSCs were consistent with those of Huang et al., with minor modifications [27]. Briefly, the arteries and veins of each tissue were mechanically removed, and the subamniotic region of the Wharton jelly was transferred to a sterile container and diced into small fragments. The explants were transferred into 100 mm plates with fresh growth media containing DMEM-F12 (Gibco)/FBS. The cells were left undisturbed for 7 days in a 37° humidified incubator with 5% CO_2 to allow migration of cells from the explants. Thereafter, the tissue was removed, and the hWJ-MSCs were evenly redistributed by digesting them with TrypLE (Gibco). Fresh media (4-5 ml) were added every 2/3 days. Then, the cells (±90% confluence) were digested and replated at a 1 : 5 ratio.

We have previously assessed the phenotypic properties of hWJ-MSCs based on the immune response-related surface markers CD80, CD86, CD40, CD40L, HLA-1, and HLA-DR [12].

2.4. Preparation of Conditioned Media. hWJ-MSCs (80% confluence) were cultured for 24 hours with each one of the following media types: (a) DMEM-F12, (b) G1-PLUS, (c) G2-PLUS, or (d) TYH. Thereafter, the media were collected and immediately used for COC IVM.

2.5. Indirect Coculture of COCs with hWJ-MSCs. hWJ-MSCs were plated in 24.5 mm, 3 μm Transwel culture plates (Corning™, Inc.). COCs were allocated on the permeable polycarbonate membrane and coincubated with the hWJ-MSCs for 24 hours in the following media conditions: (a) hWJ-MSC-COCs-DMEM-F12, (b) hWJ-MSC-COCs-G1-PLUS, (c) hWJ-MSC-COCs-G2-PLUS, or (d) hWJ-MSC-COCs-TYH.

2.6. Quantitative Real-Time Polymerase Chain Reaction (qPCR) Assay. The OCT4 expression of hWJ-MSCs in the 4 coculture systems were analyzed by qPCR. The cells were homogenized, and the RNA was extracted with the TaKaRa MiniBEST Universal RNA Extraction Kit (TaKaRa Bio Inc.). The total RNA concentration and O.D. were assayed by UV spectrophotometry. Genomic DNA elimination was performed with TaKaRa RR047Q. qPCR was performed with 200 ng of target cDNA; OCT4 (forward, GTGTTCAGC CAAAAGACCATCT; reverse, GGCCTGCATGAGGGTT TCT) and β-actin (Table S2), which was used as a reference gene (forward, CCTCATGAAGATCCTCACCGA; reverse, TTGCCAATGGTGATGACCTGG), were evaluated using relative quantification with SYBR Premix Ex Taq™ (Takara RR420Q) using an ABI 7500 (Applied Biosystems, Foster City, CA). The data analyzed was collected from 3 different experiments and the samples were run in triplicate.

2.7. IVM and IVF. IVM, with standard and conditioned media, was performed in 50 μl microdrops of medium containing 10 COCs per microdrop, under mineral oil submersion for 24 hours at 37°C with 6% CO_2. For coculture, groups of ±50 COCs were cultured with hWJ-MSCs in the various combinations of media, as explained in Section 2.5. The oocytes were monitored for IVM by confocal microscopy at 0 and 24 hours.

IVF then was performed as follows. Briefly, epididymis tissues from Kunming mice were isolated and subjected to small cuts with scissors. The growth medium (1 ml of G2-PLUS or DMEM-F12) was added, and the mixture was incubated for 7 min at 37°C. Then, the supernatant was centrifuged at 650 ×g for 5 min and discarded. The remaining pellet was resuspended by pipetting with 1 ml of medium and incubated at 37°C for 1 hour (capacitation). A second centrifugation was performed, and 700 μl of the 800 μl of supernatant was discarded. The remaining volume contained the activated spermatozoa. Groups of oocytes ($n = 20$) were inseminated in 80 μl microdrops of the activated spermatozoa in G2-PLUS medium (under equilibrated mineral oil at 37°C in air with 6% CO_2). For IVF in coculture conditions, groups of oocytes ($n = 20$) were inseminated in 80 μl microdrops previously cultured with hWJ-MSCs in DMEM-F12 medium. At the time of insemination, the DMEM-F12 medium was replaced with the activated spermatozoa in DMEM-F12 medium. A portion of the oocytes from each treatment was incubated without spermatozoa to evaluate the incidence of spontaneous activation (data not shown). Six hours after insemination, the oocytes were gently cleaned by pipetting, and presumptive zygotes obtained from COCs were separately cultured *in vitro* for 5 days in G2-PLUS medium or cocultured with hWJ-MSCs in DMEM-F12 medium (37°C, in air with 6% CO_2). The proportion of the embryos at each stage was recorded at 24 hours, 48 hours, and after 5 days of *in vitro* culture.

2.8. Statistical Analysis. Statistical analysis was performed using Microsoft Office Excel 2010. The oocyte maturation, fertilization, and embryonic development rates were calculated using the Pearson chi-squared test. The qPCR data was analyzed with the two-tailed paired Student's t-test. A P value < 0.05 was considered to indicate statistical significance.

3. Results

3.1. IVM and IVF of COCs. A total of 2422 immature oocytes met the eligibility criteria for this study. The developmental competency of COCs is listed in Table 1.

Among the 12 culture systems analyzed in this work, G2-PLUS and coculture-DMEM-F12 were the most effective media conditions for IVM. Both showed no significant differences in their ability to improve oocyte maturation and were statistically different from the rest of the systems.

When the groups were compared according to media type (Figure 1), we noticed that conditioning DMEM-F12 (Figure 1(a)) and G2-PLUS (Figure 1(c)) with hWJ-MSCs yielded negative outcomes compared to those from stock media, suggesting that the release of unspecific soluble factors from hWJ-MSCs may have an adverse effect on the oocyte maturation. In conditioned-G1-PLUS (Figure 1(b)), IVM was not significantly different from the stock media. Moreover, no improvement was noted in conditioned-TYH culture (Figure 1(d)).

On the other hand, the coculture system in G1- and G2-PLUS media appeared to have detrimental effects on IVM (Figures 1(b) and 1(c)) compared to the effects of culture in stock media. Coculture in TYH showed no significant differences with stock media conditions (Figure 1(d)). However, the IVM of COCs in coculture with hWJ-MSC-DMEM-F12 was significantly improved compared to IVM in stock DMEM-F12 (Figure 1(a)).

We also analyzed the fertilization and developmental rates of oocytes cultured in G2-PLUS and cocultured with DMEM-F12 media. Although we noticed a modest improvement in the rate of development to the blastocyst stage in the coculture with DMEM-F12, the result was not significant at $P < 0.05$ (Table 1). Oocytes, either cultured in G2-PLUS or cocultured in DMEM-F12 media, cleaved and likely did not experience developmental arrest at the pronuclear stage.

3.2. Analysis of OCT4 Expression. The POU transcription factor OCT4 (Table S2), encoded by POU5F1, is critical for sustaining the self-renewal capacity of adult somatic stem cells [28, 29] and is considered a master regulator of pluripotency

Table 1: Developmental competency of COCs among the different culture systems.

Culture media	Total number of COCs	Polar bodies (number)	Polar bodies (%)	Number of cleaved oocytes (%)	Number of blastocyst stage (%)
DMEM-F12	199	81	40.7		
G1-PLUS	204	85	41.6		
G2-PLUS	199	115	57.8*	61 (53.04)	7 (11.48)
TYH	198	71	35.9		
Conditioned-DMEM-F12	200	56	28		
Conditioned-G1-PLUS	206	79	38.4		
Conditioned-G2-PLUS	204	69	33.8		
Conditioned-TYH	202	81	40.1		
Coculture-DMEM-F12	205	115	56.1*	58 (50.43)	8 (13.79)
Coculture-G1-PLUS	203	51	25.1		
Coculture-G2-PLUS	206	66	32		
Coculture-TYH	196	74	37.7		

Oocytes with polar bodies were considered mature MII oocytes. The fertilization rate and rate of development to the blastocyst stage were compared between G2-PLUS and coculture-DMEM-F12. *Both showed no significant differences in their ability to improve oocyte maturation and were statistically different from the rest of the systems. The data were analyzed by the chi-squared test. A value of $P < 0.05$ was considered statistically significant.

that controls lineage commitment [30]. We analyzed OCT4 expression of hWJ-MSCs, by qPCR in the 4 different stock media with the aim of verifying whether the specific media affected hWJ-MSC potency. Our data confirmed that the expression of OCT4 in hWJ-MSCs cultured on G1-PLUS, TYH, and G2-PLUS was downregulated by 25.9, 24.7, and 6.6%, respectively, compared to that in hWJ-MSCs cultured in DMEM-F12 (Figure 2). We also confirmed that the expression of OCT4 from hWJ-MSCs was not affected by the presence of COCs when cultured in DMEM-F12.

4. Discussion

Culture conditions, including the formulation of the base medium, supplementations, and the in vitro physical environment (such as the oxygen tension and presence of cumulus cells), all influence multiple events that are crucial to oocyte maturation and subsequent embryonic development [31, 32].

The culture media types have been shown to modulate not only the metabolism of oocytes [33] but also the maturation to MII, the kinetics of cell cycle progression, and spindle/chromatin organization [34, 35].

Scientific evidence suggests that gonadotropins, epidermal growth factor, and essential and nonessential amino acids improve the maturation of porcine oocytes [36, 37]. Human menopausal gonadotropin, pregnant mare serum gonadotropin, follicle-stimulating hormone (FSH), and luteinizing hormone, pyruvic acid, estradiol (E2), recombinant FSH, insulin, transferrin, and selenium have been included in the IVM media for human oocyte maturation [38–40]. Undefined protein sources, such as fetal bovine serum, human maternal serum, synthetic human serum, and human follicular and peritoneal fluid have also been used to supplement maturation media [41–43].

Although taurine and calcium lactates have been suggested as necessary components for IVM of mouse COCs [30], the two most efficient culture media (G2-PLUS and DMEM-F12) tested in this work lacked these compounds.

It is evident that there is no consensus on the adequate supplementation media for oocyte maturation as the postulated compounds and combinations stated above have yielded suboptimal results, thus reinforcing the idea that the in vitro culture conditions lack some crucial components.

One of the shortcomings in the type of culture system used to date has been the absence of somatic cell support.

The role of stem cells in coculture reaches beyond that of simply providing a favorable cell source with multipotent differentiation capacity. Whether serving in target or assisting roles, stem cells are pivotal in tissue growth, metabolism, maturation, and repair [44, 45].

Many kinds of exogenous growth factors are secreted by MSCs, some of which are important components of the follicle developmental microenvironment for appropriate "oocyte capacitation" or oocyte cytoplasmic development prior to maturation [20].

The present work supported the idea that remote cell signaling from hWJ-MSCs positively affects meiotic progression of COCs maintained in the same microenvironment with DMEM-F12, resulting in a defined combination of nutrients, growth factors, and hormones that supports oocyte maturation and the differentiation potential of MSCs.

Our data also suggest that the paracrine factors produced by hWJ-MSCs in DMEM-F12 helped cocultured COCs to reach levels of nuclear and cytoplasmic maturation similar to those seen in culture with G2-PLUS, a blastocyst culture medium with superior efficiency for IVM of immature oocytes [30]. However, the specific compounds produced by the hWJ-MSCs, such as cytokines and soluble and growth factors that might be involved in the regulation of oocyte maturation, need to be identified.

In addition, the beneficial effect of coculture did not require any direct contact between the hWJ-MSCs and COCs during IVM and IVF, as previously reported for

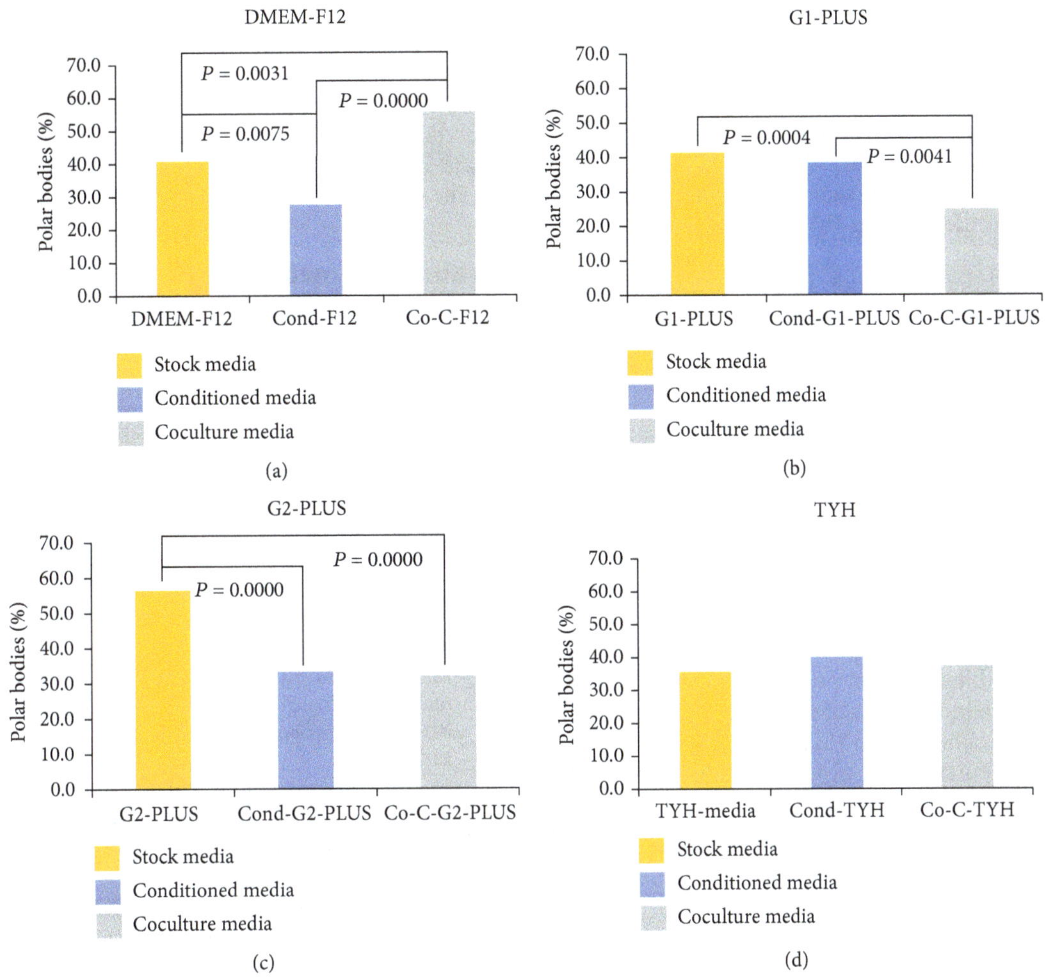

FIGURE 1: Comparison of IVM for COCs cultured in the same media: DMEM-F12 (a), G1-PLUS (b), G2-PLUS (c), and TYH (d). The data were analyzed by the chi-squared test. A value of $P < 0.05$ was considered statistically significant.

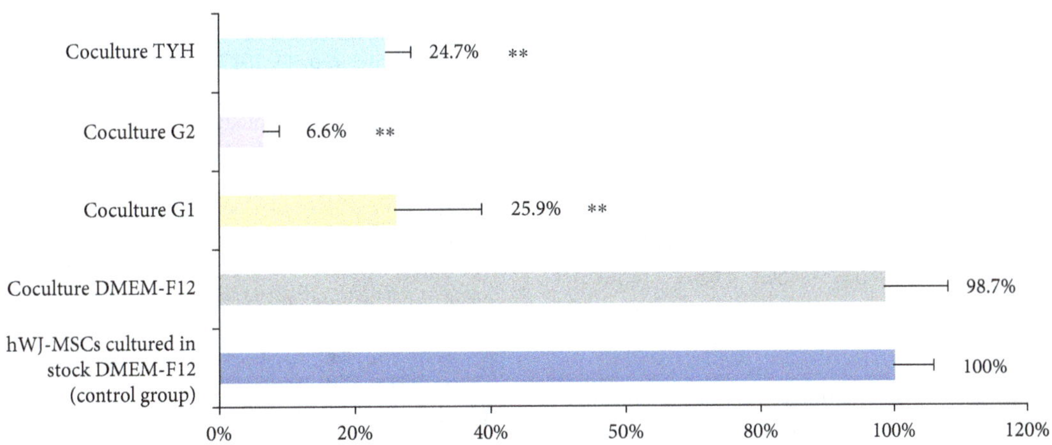

FIGURE 2: qPCR analysis of OCT4 in hWJ-MSCs cultured under the 4 coculture conditions. In G1-PLUS, TYH, and G2-PLUS, OCT4 expression was downregulated to 25.9, 24.7, and 6.6%, respectively, compared to the OCT4 level in hWJ-MSCs cultured in DMEM-F12. The expression of OCT4 from hWJ-MSCs was not affected by the presence of COCs when cultured in DMEM-F12 (control group). The data was analyzed with the two-tailed paired Student's *t*-test. A P value < 0.05 was considered to indicate statistical significance. $^{**}(P < 0.01)$ is the statistical significance compared with coculture-DMEM-F12.

bovine and mouse oocytes [46, 47], supporting the idea that cell-cell interaction occurs via soluble factors triggered by remote cell signaling.

The scientific evidence suggests that some of the positive effects of soluble factors secreted by hWJ-MSCs might be due to antioxidant properties, especially since it is now recognized that exogenous antioxidants improve maturation *in vitro* in the cat [48] and specifically support the MI to MII transition in pig oocytes [49].

The above statements appear to be consistent with our results showing that the hWJ-MSC-conditioned medium had no positive effect on the IVM of COCs and suggest that coordinated paracrine signaling communication is required between the assisting (hWJ-MSCs) and the target cells (COCs).

We evaluated the fertilization rate and extended culture up to the blastocyst stage to detect the maturation and developmental competence of the oocytes, which should be better indicators than molecular markers or detailed morphological studies.

We also verified that oocytes, either cultured in G2-PLUS or cocultured in DMEM-F12 media, cleaved and likely did not experience developmental arrest at the pronuclear stage. Nonetheless, further studies should be conducted to ascertain the implantation and pregnancy potential of these embryos, and detailed analysis of their chromosomal status or genomic imprinting pattern should be performed.

OCT4 is a critical transcription factor for regulating the self-renewal and differentiation properties of ESCs [50] and its downregulation induces loss of pluripotency and dedifferentiation to the trophectoderm [51].

hWJ-MSCs constitutively express the early embryonic transcription factors Nanog, OCT4, Sox-2, Rex-1, and LIN28, indicating their multipotency and high self-renewal capacity [52, 53].

Moreover, the expression of the pluripotency genes, OCT4, Nanog, and Sox-2, was also reported for WJ-MSCs [52, 54, 55], although it was much lower than that in ESC [53]. Modest expression of pluripotency genes might explain why WJ-MSCs are not tumorigenic.

In our work, we have opted to analyze the pluripotency gene OCT4 as a tool for the identification of cell differentiation since up- or downregulation of OCT4 indicates loss of differentiation potential and stemness regardless of the expression of the other markers of pluripotency expressed in these cells.

We have already suggested that specific MSC media compositions are necessary for the hWJ-MSCs to positively interact with COCs and improve IVM, which is also correlated with the expression of OCT4 and consequently with the differentiation potential of the hWJ-MSCs. However, further investigation with different commercially available media formulations that support MSC culture will be required to support this idea.

Importantly, cell-cell interactions are seldom unidirectional, with both cell populations being affected in a coculture system. However, the rate at which COCs were cocultured with hWJ-MSCs in this study demonstrated that oocytes had no effect on the OCT4 expression of hWJ-MSCs; thus, the potency of the stem cells remained unaffected.

5. Conclusion

Our findings support the concept of cross-talk between hWJ-MSCs and COCs in indirect coculture. We have demonstrated that two prerequisites appear to be necessary for hWJ-MSCs to improve COC IVM: stem cell differentiation potential and paracrine signaling interaction with the COCs. The paracrine factors produced by hWJ-MSCs in the coculture system with the DMEM-F12 medium may guide the development of synthetic media for successful in vitro culture of COCs.

Acknowledgments

This work was supported by the Chengdu Jinjiang Hospital for Maternal & Child Health Care, Chengdu, China.

References

[1] R. J. Deans and A. B. Moseley, "Mesenchymal stem cells: biology and potential clinical uses," *Experimental Hematology*, vol. 28, no. 8, pp. 875–884, 2000.

[2] A. I. Caplan and J. E. Dennis, "Mesenchymal stem cells as trophic mediators," *Journal of Cellular Biochemistry*, vol. 98, no. 5, pp. 1076–1084, 2006.

[3] M. Kassem, M. Kristiansen, and B. M. Abdallah, "Mesenchymal stem cells: cell biology and potential use in therapy," *Basic & Clinical Pharmacology & Toxicology*, vol. 95, no. 5, pp. 209–214, 2004.

[4] N. K. Paschos, W. E. Brown, R. Eswaramoorthy, J. C. Hu, and K. A. Athanasiou, "Advances in tissue engineering through stem cell-based co-culture," *Journal of Tissue Engineering and Regenerative Medicine*, vol. 9, no. 5, pp. 488–503, 2015.

[5] A. Bongso and C. Y. Fong, "The therapeutic potential, challenges and future clinical directions of stem cells from the Wharton's jelly of the human umbilical cord," *Stem Cell Reviews*, vol. 9, no. 2, pp. 226–240, 2013.

[6] M. Maldonado, T. Huang, L. Yang, L. Xu, and L. Ma, "Human umbilical cord Wharton jelly cells promote extra-pancreatic insulin formation and repair of renal damage in STZ-induced diabetic mice," *Cell Communication and Signaling*, vol. 15, no. 1, p. 43, 2017.

[7] W. M. Jackson, L. J. Nesti, and R. S. Tuan, "Mesenchymal stem cell therapy for attenuation of scar formation during wound healing," *Stem Cell Research & Therapy*, vol. 3, no. 3, p. 20, 2012.

[8] H. Li and X. Fu, "Mechanisms of action of mesenchymal stem cells in cutaneous wound repair and regeneration," *Cell and Tissue Research*, vol. 348, no. 3, pp. 371–377, 2012.

[9] A. M. Hocking and N. S. Gibran, "Mesenchymal stem cells: paracrine signaling and differentiation during cutaneous wound repair," *Experimental Cell Research*, vol. 316, no. 14, pp. 2213–2219, 2010.

[10] M. L. Weiss, C. Anderson, S. Medicetty et al., "Immune properties of human umbilical cord Wharton's jelly-derived cells," *Stem Cells*, vol. 26, no. 11, pp. 2865–2874, 2008.

[11] S. Liu, M. Yuan, K. Hou et al., "Immune characterization of mesenchymal stem cells in human umbilical cord Wharton's jelly and derived cartilage cells," *Cellular Immunology*, vol. 278, no. 1-2, pp. 35–44, 2012.

[12] Q. Tang, Q. Chen, X. Lai et al., "Malignant transformation potentials of human umbilical cord mesenchymal stem cells both spontaneously and via 3-methycholanthrene induction," *PLoS One*, vol. 8, no. 12, article e81844, 2013.

[13] A. Bongso, C. Y. Fong, and K. Gauthaman, "Taking stem cells to the clinic: major challenges," *Journal of Cellular Biochemistry*, vol. 105, no. 6, pp. 1352–1360, 2008.

[14] H. Miki, N. Ogonuki, K. Inoue, T. Baba, and A. Ogura, "Improvement of cumulus-free oocyte maturation in vitro and its application to microinsemination with primary spermatocytes in mice," *Journal of Reproduction and Development*, vol. 52, no. 2, pp. 239–248, 2006.

[15] N. Mousset-Simeón, P. Jouannet, L. Le Cointre, C. Coussieu, and C. Poirot, "Comparison of three in vitro culture systems for maturation of early preantral mouse ovarian follicles," *Zygote*, vol. 13, no. 2, pp. 167–175, 2005.

[16] S. Lenie, R. Cortvrindt, T. Adriaenssens, and J. Smitz, "A reproducible two-step culture system for isolated primary mouse ovarian follicles as single functional units," *Biology of Reproduction*, vol. 71, no. 5, pp. 1730–1738, 2004.

[17] H. Nakano and H. Kubo, "Study of the in vitro maturation of mouse oocytes induced by microinjection of maturation promoting factor (MPF)," *Journal of Assisted Reproduction and Genetics*, vol. 17, no. 1, pp. 67–73, 2000.

[18] B. C. A. Heng and N. S. Chye, "Investigations of oocyte in vitro maturation within a mouse model," *Zygote*, vol. 12, no. 1, pp. 1–18, 2004.

[19] R. De La Fuente, M. J. O'Brien, and J. J. Eppig, "Epidermal growth factor enhances preimplantation developmental competence of maturing mouse oocytes," *Human Reproduction*, vol. 14, no. 12, pp. 3060–3068, 1999.

[20] R. B. Gilchrist and J. G. Thompson, "Oocyte maturation: emerging concepts and technologies to improve developmental potential in vitro," *Theriogenology*, vol. 67, no. 1, pp. 6–15, 2007.

[21] M. Sakaguchi, T. Dominko, N. Yamauchi, M. L. Leibfried-Rutledge, T. Nagai, and N. L. First, "Possible mechanism for acceleration of meiotic progression of bovine follicular oocytes by growth factors in vitro," *Reproduction*, vol. 123, no. 1, pp. 135–142, 2002.

[22] G. Ren, X. Chen, F. Dong et al., "Concise review: mesenchymal stem cells and translational medicine: emerging issues," *Stem Cells Translational Medicine*, vol. 1, no. 1, pp. 51–58, 2012.

[23] K. Khosrotehrani, "Mesenchymal stem cell therapy in skin: why and what for?," *Experimental Dermatology*, vol. 22, no. 5, pp. 307–310, 2013.

[24] M. Heil, T. Ziegelhoeffer, B. Mees, and W. Schaper, "A different outlook on the role of bone marrow stem cells in vascular growth: bone marrow delivers software not hardware," *Circulation Research*, vol. 94, no. 5, pp. 573-574, 2004.

[25] Y. Yoda, M. Yokoyama, and T. Hosi, "Studies on the fertilization of mouse eggs in vitro. I. In vitro fertilization of eggs by fresh epididymal sperm," *The Japanese Journal of Animal Reproduction*, vol. 16, no. 4, pp. 147–151, 1971.

[26] Y. Toyoda, M. Yokoyama, and T. Hosi, "Studies on the fertilization of mouse eggs in vitro. II. Effects of in vitro preincubation of spermatozoa on time of sperm penetration of mouse eggs in vitro," *The Japanese Journal of Animal Reproduction*, vol. 16, no. 4, pp. 152–157, 1971.

[27] P. Huang, L. M. Lin, X. Y. Wu et al., "Differentiation of human umbilical cord Wharton's jelly-derived mesenchymal stem cells into germ-like cells in vitro," *Journal of Cellular Biochemistry*, vol. 109, pp. 747–754, 2010.

[28] M. H. Tai, C. C. Chang, M. Kiupel, J. D. Webster, L. K. Olson, and J. E. Trosko, "Oct4 expression in adult human stem cells: evidence in support of the stem cell theory of carcinogenesis," *Carcinogenesis*, vol. 26, no. 2, pp. 495–502, 2005.

[29] J. H. Kim, M. K. Jee, S. Y. Lee et al., "Regulation of adipose tissue stromal cells behaviors by endogenic Oct4 expression control," *PLoS One*, vol. 4, no. 9, article e7166, 2009.

[30] M. Kim, S. J. Hong, J. H. Lee, C. K. Min, K. J. Hwang, and R. W. Park, "Comparison of in vitro maturation media of immature oocytes: the effectiveness of blastocyst culture media," *Fertility and Sterility*, vol. 95, no. 2, pp. 554–557, 2011.

[31] J. J. M. van de Sandt, A. C. Schroeder, and J. J. Eppig, "Culture media for mouse oocyte maturation affect subsequent embryonic development," *Molecular Reproduction and Development*, vol. 25, no. 2, pp. 164–171, 1990.

[32] M. L. Sutton, R. B. Gilchrist, and J. G. Thompson, "Effects of in-vivo and in-vitro environments on the metabolism of the cumulus-oocyte complex and its influence on oocyte developmental capacity," *Human Reproduction Update*, vol. 9, no. 1, pp. 35–48, 2003.

[33] R. Roberts, S. Franks, and K. Hardy, "Culture environment modulates maturation and metabolism of human oocytes," *Human Reproduction*, vol. 17, no. 11, pp. 2950–2956, 2002.

[34] N. A. Cekleniak, C. M. H. Combelles, D. A. Ganz, J. Fung, D. F. Albertini, and C. Racowsky, "A novel system for in vitro maturation of human oocytes," *Fertility and Sterility*, vol. 75, no. 6, pp. 1185–1193, 2001.

[35] A. Trounson, C. Anderiesz, and G. Jones, "Maturation of human oocytes in vitro and their developmental competence," *Reproduction*, vol. 121, no. 1, pp. 51–75, 2001.

[36] M. M. Bevers and F. Izadyar, "Role of growth hormone and growth hormone receptor in oocyte maturation," *Molecular and Cellular Endocrinology*, vol. 197, no. 1-2, pp. 173–178, 2002.

[37] J. Y. Hong, H. Y. Yong, B. C. Lee, W. S. Hwang, J. M. Lim, and E. S. Lee, "Effects of amino acids on maturation, fertilization and embryo development of pig follicular oocytes in two IVM media," *Theriogenology*, vol. 62, no. 8, pp. 1473–1482, 2004.

[38] X. Zhang, A. Zerafa, J. Wong, D. T. Armstrong, and F. Khamsi, "Human menopausal gonadotropin during in vitro maturation of human oocytes retrieved from small follicles enhances in vitro fertilization and cleavage rates," *Fertility and Sterility*, vol. 59, no. 4, pp. 850–853, 1993.

[39] K. Cha, H. Chung, D. Lee et al., "Obstetric outcome of patients with polycystic ovary syndrome treated by in vitro maturation and in vitro fertilization-embryo transfer," *Fertility and Sterility*, vol. 83, no. 5, pp. 1461–1465, 2005.

[40] E. Isachenko, G. Rahimi, V. Isachenko, and F. Nawroth, "In-vitro maturation of germinal-vesicle oocytes and cryopreservation in metaphase I/II: a possible additional option to preserve fertility during ovarian tissue cryopreservation," *Reproductive BioMedicine Online*, vol. 8, no. 5, pp. 553–557, 2004.

[41] R.-C. Chian, W. M. Buckett, A. K. A. Jalil et al., "Natural-cycle in vitro fertilization combined with in vitro maturation of immature oocytes is a potential approach in infertility treatment," *Fertility and Sterility*, vol. 82, no. 6, pp. 1675–1678, 2004.

[42] A. L. Mikkelsen, "Strategies in human in-vitro maturation and their clinical outcome," *Reproductive BioMedicine Online*, vol. 10, no. 5, pp. 593–599, 2005.

[43] K. Y. Cha, J. J. Koo, J. J. Ko, D. H. Choi, S. Y. Han, and T. K. Yoon, "Pregnancy after in vitro fertilization of human follicular oocytes collected from nonstimulated cycles, their culture in vitro and their transfer in a donor oocyte program," *Fertility and Sterility*, vol. 55, no. 1, pp. 109–113, 1991.

[44] N. I. Kalinina, V. Y. Sysoeva, K. A. Rubina, Y. V. Parfenova, and V. A. Tkachuk, "Mesenchymal stem cells in tissue growth and repair," *Acta Naturae*, vol. 3, no. 4, pp. 30–37, 2011.

[45] N. Sato, L. Meijer, L. Skaltsounis, P. Greengard, and A. H. Brivanlou, "Maintenance of pluripotency in human and mouse embryonic stem cells through activation of Wnt signaling by a pharmacological GSK-3-specific inhibitor," *Nature Medicine*, vol. 10, no. 1, pp. 55–63, 2004.

[46] A. M. Luciano, V. Lodde, M. S. Beretta, S. Colleoni, A. Lauria, and S. Modina, "Developmental capability of denuded bovine oocyte in a co-culture system with intact cumulus-oocyte complexes: role of cumulus cells, cyclic adenosine $3',5'$-monophosphate, and glutathione," *Molecular Reproduction and Development*, vol. 71, no. 3, pp. 389–397, 2005.

[47] L. Ge, D. Han, G. C. Lan et al., "Factors affecting the in vitro action of cumulus cells on the maturing mouse oocytes," *Molecular Reproduction and Development*, vol. 75, no. 1, pp. 136–142, 2008.

[48] P. Comizzoli, D. E. Wildt, and B. S. Pukazhenthi, "Overcoming poor in vitro nuclear maturation and developmental competence of domestic cat oocytes during the non-breeding season," *Reproduction*, vol. 126, no. 6, pp. 809–816, 2003.

[49] Y. Tao, B. Zhou, G. Xia, F. Wang, Z. Wu, and M. Fu, "Exposure to L-ascorbic acid or α-tocopherol facilitates the development of porcine denuded oocytes from metaphase I to metaphase II and prevents cumulus cells from fragmentation," *Reproduction in Domestic Animals*, vol. 39, no. 1, pp. 52–57, 2004.

[50] J. Nichols, B. Zevnik, K. Anastassiadis et al., "Formation of pluripotent stem cells in the mammalian embryo depends on the POU transcription factor Oct4," *Cell*, vol. 95, no. 3, pp. 379–391, 1998.

[51] H. Niwa, J. Miyazaki, and A. G. Smith, "Quantitative expression of Oct-3/4 defines differentiation, dedifferentiation or self-renewal of ES cells," *Nature Genetics*, vol. 24, no. 4, pp. 372–376, 2000.

[52] C. K. Tong, S. Vellasamy, B. Chong Tan et al., "Generation of mesenchymal stem cell from human umbilical cord tissue using a combination enzymatic and mechanical disassociation method," *Cell Biology International*, vol. 35, no. 3, pp. 221–226, 2011.

[53] C.-Y. Fong, L.-L. Chak, A. Biswas et al., "Human Wharton's jelly stem cells have unique transcriptome profiles compared to human embryonic stem cells and other mesenchymal stem cells," *Stem Cell Reviews and Reports*, vol. 7, no. 1, pp. 1–16, 2011.

[54] J. H. Yoon, E. Y. Roh, S. Shin et al., "Comparison of explant-derived and enzymatic digestion-derived MSCs and the growth factors from Wharton's jelly," *BioMed Research International*, vol. 2013, Article ID 428726, 8 pages, 2013.

[55] U. Nekanti, L. Mohanty, P. Venugopal, S. Balasubramanian, S. Totey, and M. Ta, "Optimization and scale-up of Wharton's jelly-derived mesenchymal stem cells for clinical applications," *Stem Cell Research*, vol. 5, no. 3, pp. 244–254, 2010.

18

Notch Signaling Activation Enhances Human Adipose-Derived Stem Cell Retinal Differentiation

Yuqiang Huang,[1] Tsz Kin Ng,[1,2,3] Chong-Bo Chen,[1] Bing Huang,[1] Jiajian Liang,[1] Chi Pui Pang,[1,3] and Mingzhi Zhang[1]

[1]*Joint Shantou International Eye Center of Shantou University and the Chinese University of Hong Kong, Shantou, Guangdong, China*
[2]*Shantou University Medical College, Shantou, Guandong, China*
[3]*Department of Ophthalmology and Visual Sciences, The Chinese University of Hong Kong, Hong Kong*

Correspondence should be addressed to Mingzhi Zhang; zmz@jsiec.org

Academic Editor: Susanna Miettinen

Retinal disease treatment by stem cell-based replacement relies on stem cell differentiation into retinal cells. We previously demonstrated that human periodontal ligament-derived stem cells can be directed into retinal lineage upon induction. Here, we report the transdifferentiation potential of human adipose-derived stem cells (ASCs) into retinal lineage and its enhancement by Notch signaling modulation. Human ASCs, isolated from abdominal fat, expressed mesenchymal but not hematopoietic stem cell markers, and they can differentiate into adipocytes, chondrocytes, and osteoblasts *in vitro*. Upon noggin/Dkk-1/IGF-1 induction, the treated ASCs showed elevated expression of retinal progenitor, retinal ganglion, and photoreceptor cell markers as well as the glutamate-evoked calcium response, which was not observed in the noninduced cells. Compared to the regular induction treatment, Notch signaling activation by JAG1 enhanced the expression of retinal progenitor and precursor markers without affecting the glutamate-evoked calcium response. In contrast, Notch signaling inhibition by DAPT showed more retinal ganglion cells, but delayed the response to glutamate stimulation. In summary, our results revealed that human ASCs possess a retinal transdifferentiation potential upon noggin/Dkk-1/IGF-1 induction, which can further be enhanced by Notch signaling activation.

1. Introduction

Retinal diseases, including age-related macular degeneration, glaucoma, diabetic retinopathy, and retinitis pigmentosa, are the leading causes of irreversible blindness and visual impairment, affecting more than 300 million people worldwide. The human retina has limited intrinsic regenerative capability, and current treatment regimens are not sufficient for functional repair of the diseased retinal cells. Stem cell-based replacement, which relies on the differentiation of stem cells into retinal cells, could be a potential strategy for retinal disease treatment [1, 2].

Retinal progenitor cells (RPCs), embryonic stem cells (ESCs), and induced pluripotent stem cells (iPSCs) have been intensively studied for retinal cell synthesis [3, 4]. Yet, the studies on human adult stem cells, which can be conveniently obtained for autologous transplantation, for retinal differentiation are limited. We have established protocols to direct human periodontal ligament-derived stem cells (PDLSCs) into retinal lineage by inhibiting the bone morphogenetic protein (BMP) and Wnt signaling pathways with supplementation of insulin-like growth factor 1 (IGF-1) [5, 6]. We postulate that our retinal differentiation strategy can be generally applied to different types of adult stem cells.

Adipose tissue, derived from the mesoderm, can safely be obtained by liposuction and contains an abundance of adipose-derived stem cells (ASCs). Human ASCs possess a multilineage differentiation potential with a low risk of inducing autoimmunity and teratoma formation [7]. They can express retinal and retinal pigment epithelial (RPE) cell markers when cultured in RPE-conditioned medium [8, 9]. Moreover, ASCs can also be induced to retinal cells *in vitro* with ectopic expression of paired box protein-6 (*PAX6*) gene in a fibronectin-supplemented medium [10]. These suggested that human ASCs should possess a transdifferentiation potential towards retinal lineage.

Apart from the BMP, Wnt, and IGF-1 signaling pathways, the Notch signaling pathway is also involved in different developmental processes, including retinogenesis and neurogenesis, controlling cell fate decisions [11, 12]. Previous studies showed that Notch signaling activation promotes RPC proliferation and prevents RPC differentiation into retinal cells [12]. Moreover, Notch-1 signaling is involved in the regulation of photoreceptor development at early and late stages of retinal development [13]. Inactivation or removal of Notch-1 from RPCs increases photoreceptor precursor production in mice [14]. Similarly, inhibition of Notch promotes the generation of photoreceptor precursors from human iPS-derived RPCs [15]. In addition, reducing Notch expression increases retinal ganglion cell (RGC) genesis [16]. Nevertheless, Notch-1^+ progenitor cells express both Atoh7 and Otx2, suggesting a role of Notch1 signaling in the differentiation of RGCs and photoreceptors [17]. However, the role of Notch signaling in the retinal differentiation of human adult stem cells remains elusive. Herein, we hypothesize that Notch signaling modulation can enhance the transdifferentiation of human adult stem cells towards retinal lineage. This study determined the transdifferentiation potential of human ASCs into retinal lineage by noggin/Dkk-1/IGF-1 induction. We also delineated the role of Notch signaling in human ASCs' retinal differentiation.

2. Materials and Methods

2.1. Isolation and Maintenance of Human Adipose-Derived Stem Cells. Human ASCs were obtained from liposuction of abdominal fat in 3 healthy subjects after informed written consent. This study was approved by the Ethnic Committee of Human Study in the Joint Shantou International Eye Center of Shantou University and the Chinese University of Hong Kong. Briefly, after specimen collection from donors, the excess muscle tissues, nonfat tissues, and blood trace were first removed from the adipose tissue, which was then minced and centrifuged. The floating tissue was separated and digested with type I collagenase at 37°C for 2 hours. After enzyme blockage, the digested tissue was filtered through a 100 μm nylon mesh and centrifuged. Human ASCs were maintained in ADSC-BM medium (Lonza) supplemented with 10% fetal bovine serum (FBS; Gibco), 1% glutamine, and 0.1% antibiotics GA-1000. The medium was replenished every 3 days, and the cells were passaged when reaching 60–70% confluence. Human ASCs at passages 3–5 were used in this study.

2.2. Stem Cell Marker Expression in Human Adipose-Derived Stem Cells. The isolated human ASCs were characterized by the expressions of mesenchymal stem cell (MSC: CD44, CD73, CD90, and CD105) and hematopoietic stem cell (HSC: CD14, CD34, and CD45) markers using flow cytometry according to the manufacturer's protocol (BD Biosciences). Briefly, human ASCs were dissociated from culture dishes by 0.05% trypsin/EDTA, washed twice with cold stain buffer (BD Biosciences), and resuspended in cold stain buffer at a concentration of 2×10^7 cells/mL. The cell suspension was incubated with respective antibodies (Supplementary Table 1) or isotype controls for 30 min on ice covered with aluminum foil to avoid light. After antibody probing, the cells were washed twice with stain buffer and analyzed by the Accuri C6 Flow Cytometer (BD Biosciences) with at least 10,000 events. The percentage of positive cells was calculated with respect to the isotype control cells.

2.3. Mesenchymal Lineage Differentiation of Human Adipose-Derived Stem Cells. Adipogenesis differentiation of human ASCs was induced by the adipocyte differentiation basal medium supplemented with 10% adipocyte supplement (StemPro, Gibco) for 14 days. The treated cells were fixed with 4% (*w*/*v*) paraformaldehyde (pH 7.4; Sigma-Aldrich) and stained with Oil Red O reagent for 10 min at ambient temperature.

Osteogenesis differentiation of human ASCs was induced by the osteocyte/chondrocyte differentiation basal medium containing with 10% osteocyte supplement (StemPro, Gibco) for 14 days. For alkaline phosphatase activity detection, the cells were fixed in ice-cold acetone and incubated with NBT/BCIP solution for 20 min. For calcium deposition analysis, the cells were fixed in 4% paraformaldehyde and stained with Alizarin Red S (Sigma-Aldrich) for 2-3 min.

Chondrogenesis differentiation of human ASCs was induced by the osteocyte/chondrocyte differentiation basal medium with 10% chondrocyte supplement (StemPro, Gibco) on a Matrigel coating for 14 days. The resulting chondrogenic pellets were fixed in 4% (*w*/*v*) paraformaldehyde (pH 7.4), dehydrated, and imbedded in OCT. The imbedded cell pellets were cryosectioned and stained with Alcian blue (Sigma-Aldrich) staining for 30 min.

The negative control was the ASCs without the addition of the adipocyte, osteocyte, or chondrocyte supplements.

2.4. Retinal Induction of Human Adipose-Derived Stem Cells. Retinal induction treatment was divided into the negative control group and 3 induction groups. For the negative control group, the cells were treated with 10% FBS-supplemented 1 : 1 Dulbecco's Modified Eagle Medium: nutrient mixture F-12 (DMEM/F12; Gibco) medium in the ultralow attachment culture dish (Corning) for 3 days and then in the Matrigel-coated (Gibco) culture dish for 21 days. For the retinal induction groups, a three-stage noggin/Dkk-1/IGF-1 induction approach was adopted. Firstly, human ASCs (5×10^5 cells) were aggregated in the ultralow attachment culture dish with the induction medium 1 (IM1; DMEM/F12 medium supplemented with 10% knock-out serum replacement (Gibco), 1x B27 supplement (Gibco), 1 ng/mL noggin (PeproTech), 1 ng/mL dickkopf-related protein 1 (Dkk-1; PeproTech), and 5 ng/mL IGF-1 (PeproTech)) for 3 days. The aggregated cells were then transferred to the Matrigel-coated culture dish and treated with the induction medium 2 (IM2; DMEM/F12 medium supplemented with 1x B27 supplement, 1x N2 supplement (Gibco), 10 ng/mL noggin, 10 ng/mL Dkk-1, 10 ng/mL IGF-1, and 5 ng/mL basic fibroblast growth factor (bFGF; PeproTech)) for 7 days. Afterwards, the culture medium was replaced by the induction medium 3 (IM3; DMEM/F12 medium supplemented with 1x B27 supplement, 1x insulin-transferrin-selenium (ITS; Gibco), 10 ng/mL noggin, 10 ng/mL Dkk-1, 10 ng/mL IGF-1, and 5 ng/mL bFGF) and further treated for 2 weeks. To delineate the role of Notch signaling regulation in human ASCs' retinal differentiation, JAG1 (20 μM; Notch signaling activator) and γ-secretase inhibitor (DAPT, 10 μM; Notch signal inhibitor) were supplemented into IM3 and treated for 2 weeks. Medium was replenished every 3 days. The treated cells were collected at Days 0, 10, 17, and 24 for further analyses.

2.5. RNA and Protein Isolation. After medium aspiration, the treated cells were directly lysed with the addition of 350 μL Buffer RP1 supplemented with 3.5 μL of β-mercaptoethanol (Sangon Biotech). RNA and protein were extracted simultaneously according to the manufacturer's protocol (NucleoSpin RNA/Protein, Macherey-Nagel). RNA was eluted by the RNase-free water, whereas the protein pellet was dissolved in protein solving buffer containing TCEP. The extracted RNA and protein samples were stored at −80°C before respective gene expression and immunoblotting analyses.

2.6. Gene Expression Analysis. Total RNA concentration was measured by a NanoDrop ND-1000 spectrophotometer (Thermo Fisher Scientific). Total RNA (1 μg) was reverse transcribed into complementary DNA (cDNA) using the PrimeScript RT reagent Kit (TaKaRa) in a thermal cycler (S1000 Thermal Cycler, Bio-Rad). The expression of RPC (*PAX6* and *NES*), RGC (*ATOH7* and *TUBB3*), photoreceptor (*CRX*, *NRL*, *RHO*, and *RCVRN*), and Notch signaling (*NOTCH1* and *HES1*) markers was evaluated by the QuantiNova SYBR Green PCR Kit (Qiagen) with specific primers (Supplementary Table 2) in a LightCycler480 (Roche). A housekeeping gene (*ACTB*) was used for normalization.

2.7. Immunofluorescence Analysis. The treated human ASCs on the Matrigel-coated coverslips were fixed with the freshly prepared 4% (*w*/*v*) paraformaldehyde in PBS (pH 7.4) for 15 min at ambient temperature. The fixed cells were rinsed three times in PBS, and the remaining free aldehyde was quenched by 50 mM ice-cold NH_4Cl solution. After washing, the cells were permeated and blocked by PBS supplemented with 0.15% (*w*/*v*) saponin, 1% (*w*/*v*) bovine serum albumin (BSA), 1% (*v*/*v*) normal goat serum (NGS), 0.01% Triton X-100, and 0.01% Tween-20 for 10 min. After blocking, the cells were incubated with primary antibodies (Supplementary Table 1; diluted in PBS containing 0.425% saponin, 1% BSA, 1% NGS, 0.0015% Triton X-100, and 0.0015% Tween-20) for 18 hours at 4°C. The cells were then incubated with the respective fluorophore-conjugated secondary antibody and 0.1% (*v*/*v*) DAPI (diluted in PBS containing 1% BSA and 1% NGS) for 1 hour at ambient temperature. The cells were mounted, and the fluorescence signals were visualized under a confocal microscope (TCS SP5, Leica). Nine fields were imaged and means of the 3 independent human ASC samples from different treatment groups were compared.

2.8. Immunoblotting Analysis. Total protein was quantified by the BCA protein assay. An equal amount of total protein (20 μg) was heat denatured, resolved by 12.5% SDS-polyacrylamide gel electrophoresis, and transferred to the PVDF membrane. After blocking with 5% nonfat milk, the blot was probed with primary antibodies for RPC (PAX6) and photoreceptor (RHO) markers (Supplementary Table 1) for 18 hours at 4°C, followed by the respective horseradish peroxidase- (HRP-) conjugated secondary antibodies. The signals were detected by enhanced chemiluminescence (Santa Cruz Biotechnology, Inc.) and imaged by the ChemiDoC XRS$^+$ system (Bio-Rad). GAPDH was used as a housekeeping protein for normalization.

2.9. Glutamate-Evoked Calcium Response. Spontaneous intracellular calcium transient was evaluated using fluo-4-acetoxymethyl ester (Fluo-4 AM; Invitrogen). Briefly, the treated or control human ASCs at Day 24 were incubated in Hanks' balanced salt solution (HBSS, Ca^{2+}/Mg^{2+}-free; Gibco) containing 5 μM Fluo-4 AM and 0.1% pluronic F-127 (Invitrogen) for 30 min at room temperature. After washing with HBSS, 1 mM glutamate (Sigma-Aldrich) was added, and fluorescence images were immediately captured using a confocal microscope (Leica TCS SP5), with the excitation wavelength at 495 nm and emission wavelength at 515 nm, every 1 second in a total of 5 min under a 20x objective lens. Fluorescence intensity at specific time intervals was measured on a total of 50 cells in triplicate experiments (at least 10 cells in each sample). The cellular change of fluorescence (F; $\%\Delta F/F_{\text{baseline}}$) of each region was calculated as $(F_{\text{treated}} - F_{\text{baseline}})/F_{\text{baseline}} \times 100\%$. The Ca^{2+} fluorescence ratio was converted into Ca^{2+} concentration using the equation $[Ca^{2+}]_i = KR/\{K/([Ca^{2+}]_{\text{rest}} + 1) - R\}$, where K is the dissociation constant of Fluo-4 AM (400 nM), R is the fluorescence ratio ($\Delta F/F_{\text{baseline}}$), and $[Ca^{2+}]_{\text{rest}}$ is the resting Ca^{2+} concentration (100 nM in neuronal cells).

2.10. Statistical Analysis. The data were presented as mean ± standard deviation (SD) from the 3 independent cell lines. All statistical analyses were performed using a commercially available software (SPSS, version 20.0; SPSS Inc., Chicago, IL). Independent *t*-test and one-way analysis of variance (ANOVA) with post hoc Tukey's test were used to compare the means among the treatment groups. Significance was defined as $p < 0.05$.

3. Results

3.1. Characterization of Human Adipose Tissue-Derived Stem Cells. Human ASCs were first characterized by the expression of MSC (CD44, CD73, CD90, and CD105) and HSC (CD14, CD34, and CD45) markers. Flow cytometry analysis showed that CD44 expression was found in 99.10 ± 1.01%, CD73 in 97.07 ± 2.56%, CD90 in 99.90 ± 0.24%, and CD105 in 99.45 ± 0.39% of human ASCs (Figure 1(a)). In contrast,

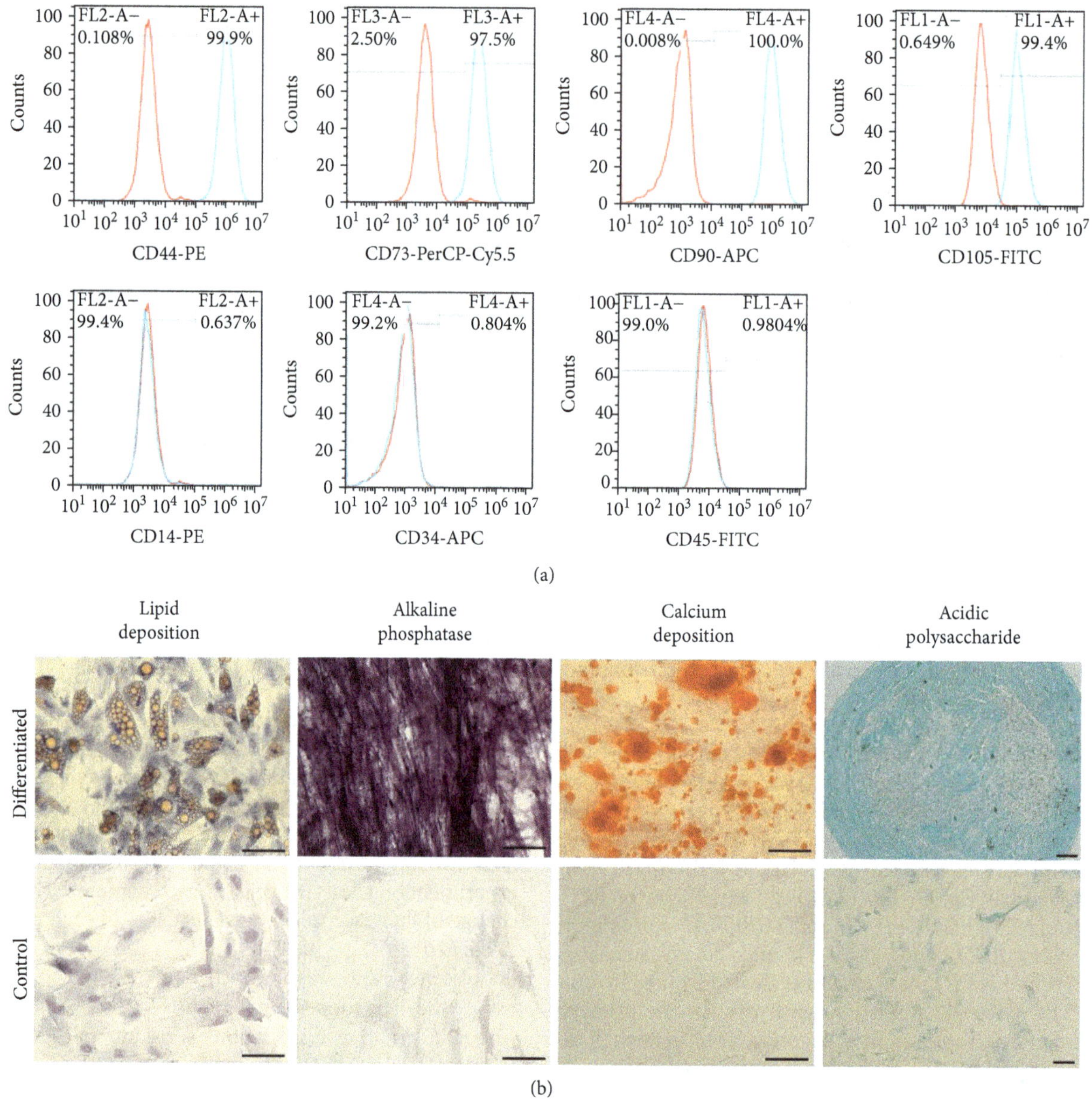

FIGURE 1: Characterization of human adipose-derived stem cells. (a) Human ASCs were characterized by flow cytometry based on the expression of mesenchymal stem cell (CD44, CD73, CD90, and CD105) and hematopoietic stem cell (CD14, CD34, and CD45) markers. The red histograms refer to the isotype controls, and the blue histograms refer to the human ASC samples for the test. (b) ASCs were differentiated into adipocytes, osteoblasts, and chondrocytes upon induction. Adipogenesis differentiation was evaluated by Oil Red O staining (red) and hematoxylin counterstain (blue), and the yellowish lipid depositions were observed in the differentiated cells. For the osteogenesis differentiation, the NBT/BCIP and Alizarin Red S staining demonstrated that the differentiated cells possess strong alkaline phosphatase activity (blue) and reddish calcium deposition, respectively. Chondrogenesis differentiation was evaluated by Alcian blue staining, and the production of acidic polysaccharide (light blue) can be observed in the differentiated cells. Scale bar: 100 μm.

$0.17 \pm 0.23\%$ of human ASCs were positive for CD14, $1.42 \pm 1.40\%$ for CD34, and $2.53 \pm 1.41\%$ for CD45. To determine the differentiation ability of the isolated ASCs, adipogenesis, osteogenesis, and chondrogenesis of human ASCs were evaluated. More than 90% of human ASCs could differentiate into adipocytes with yellowish lipid deposition (Figure 1(b)). Moreover, human ASCs could also differentiate into osteoblasts, indicated by intensive alkaline phosphatase activity and the reddish calcium deposition, as well as chondrocytes, indicated by the light blue staining of acidic polysaccharide. Our results indicated that human ASCs isolated from abdominal fat were predominantly functional MSCs.

3.2. Retinal Differentiation of Human Adipose Tissue-Derived Stem Cells. Human ASCs were treated with retinal induction medium for 24 days (Figure 2(a)). A sphere-like structure was observed on Day 3 under the low adherent culture. On the Matrigel-coated surface, the aggregated ASCs migrated out from the rosette and exhibited

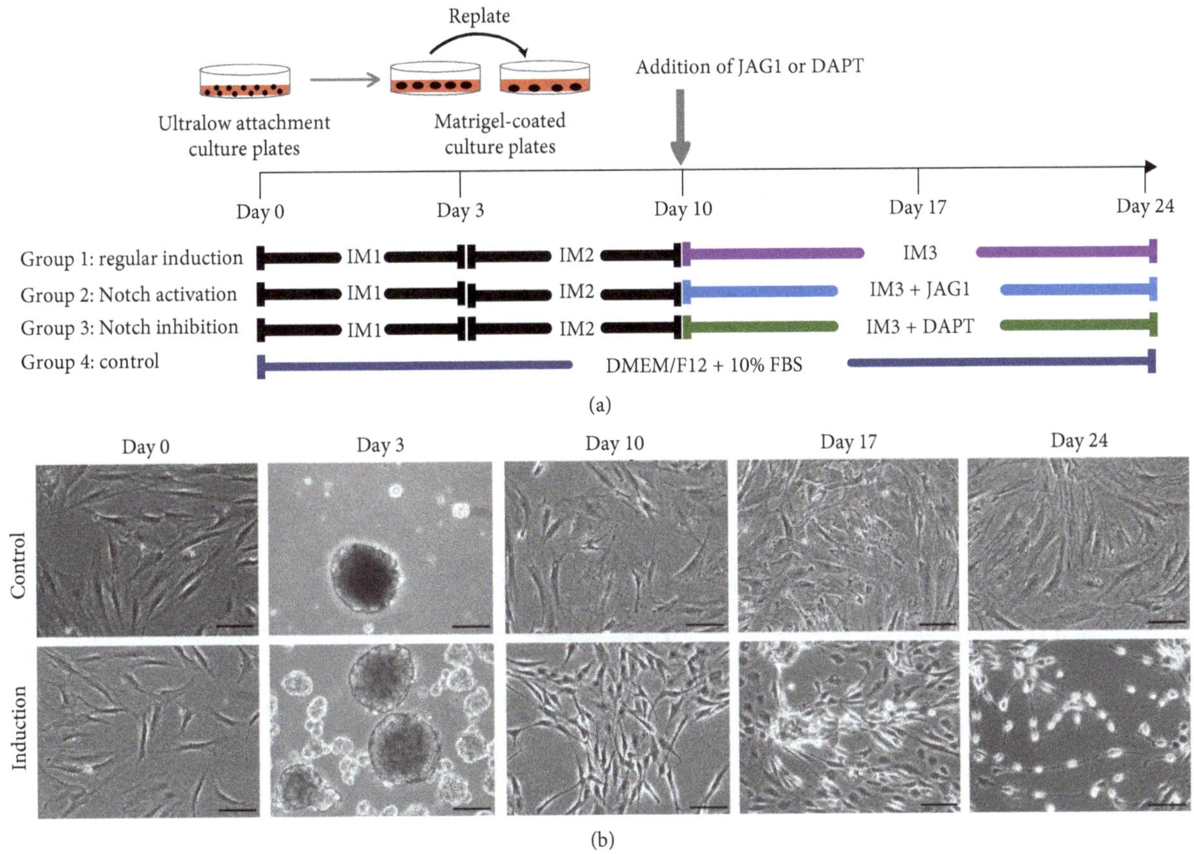

FIGURE 2: Induction treatment of human adipose-derived stem cells into the retinal lineage. (a) A schematic diagram of the induction treatment of human ASCs into the retinal lineage. Human ASCs were first aggregated in IM1 for 3 days and cultured on Matrigel-coated plates for 7 days in IM2 and 14 days in IM3. Notch signaling activation and inhibition were mediated by JAG1 and DAPT, respectively. The control cells were cultured with DMEM/F12 + 10% FBS for 24 days. (b) The morphology of human ASCs after retinal induction treatment at different time points. Upper: noninduction group (control). Lower: regular induction group. The cells in the regular induction group at Day 24 exhibited a neural-network-like morphology with condensed cell bodies, while the cells in the control group remained in a fibroblast-like shape. Scale bar: 100 μm.

neural-network-like morphology with condensed cell bodies (Figure 2(b)). In contrast, human ASCs in the negative control group remained in the fibroblast-like shape and proliferated continuously.

To verify the retinal differentiation capacity of human ASCs, the expression of retinal lineage markers was examined at Days 0, 10, 17, and 24 after induction. Gene expression analysis showed that the expression of RPC (*PAX6* and *NES*), photoreceptor (*CRX*, *NRL*, *RHO*, and *RCVRN*), and RGC (*ATOH7* and *TUBB3*) marker genes time-dependently increased along the retinal induction treatment period (Figure 3(a)). Sybr green PCR analysis demonstrated that, at Day 24, *PAX6* and *NES* genes were increased in the treated human ASCs by 38.03 ± 8.41-fold ($p < 0.05$) and 38.41 ± 4.12-fold ($p < 0.01$), respectively, compared to the expression at Day 0. Similarly, *CRX*, *NRL*, *RHO*, and *RCVRN* genes were increased by 15.46 ± 1.75-fold ($p < 0.05$), 3.94 ± 0.81-fold ($p < 0.05$), 14.25 ± 1.96-fold ($p < 0.05$), and 245.90 ± 15.46-fold ($p < 0.05$), respectively. Meanwhile, the expression of *ATOH7* and *TUBB3* genes in the retinal-induced ASCs at Day 24 were increased by 16.65 ± 3.35-fold ($p < 0.05$) and 1.75 ± 0.19-fold ($p < 0.05$), respectively. In contrast, all retinal marker genes showed no significant change in the negative control group throughout the treatment period.

Coherent to the gene expression results, the expressions of PAX6 and RHO protein were time-dependently upregulated in retinal-induced ASCs, with 3.06 ± 1.31-fold ($p < 0.01$) and 3.00 ± 0.53-fold increase ($p < 0.001$, Figure 3(b)) at Day 24, respectively, compared to the expressions at Day 0. Moreover, immunofluorescence analysis showed that the retinal-induced ASCs expressed PAX6 ($74.74 \pm 2.42\%$, $p < 0.001$), CRX ($40.72 \pm 7.01\%$, $p < 0.001$), POU4F2 ($35.10 \pm 7.86\%$, $p < 0.001$), and TUBB3 ($21.25 \pm 6.18\%$, $p < 0.001$; Figure 3(c)). In contrast, retinal marker expression was not observed in the ASCs of the negative control group.

The function of the retinal-induced ASCs was evaluated by the glutamate-evoked calcium response. A robust increase in fluorescence intensities was observed in the retinal-induced ASCs after glutamate stimulation, but only a very weak signal was observed in the negative control group (Figure 4, Supplemental Video 1 and Supplemental Video 2).

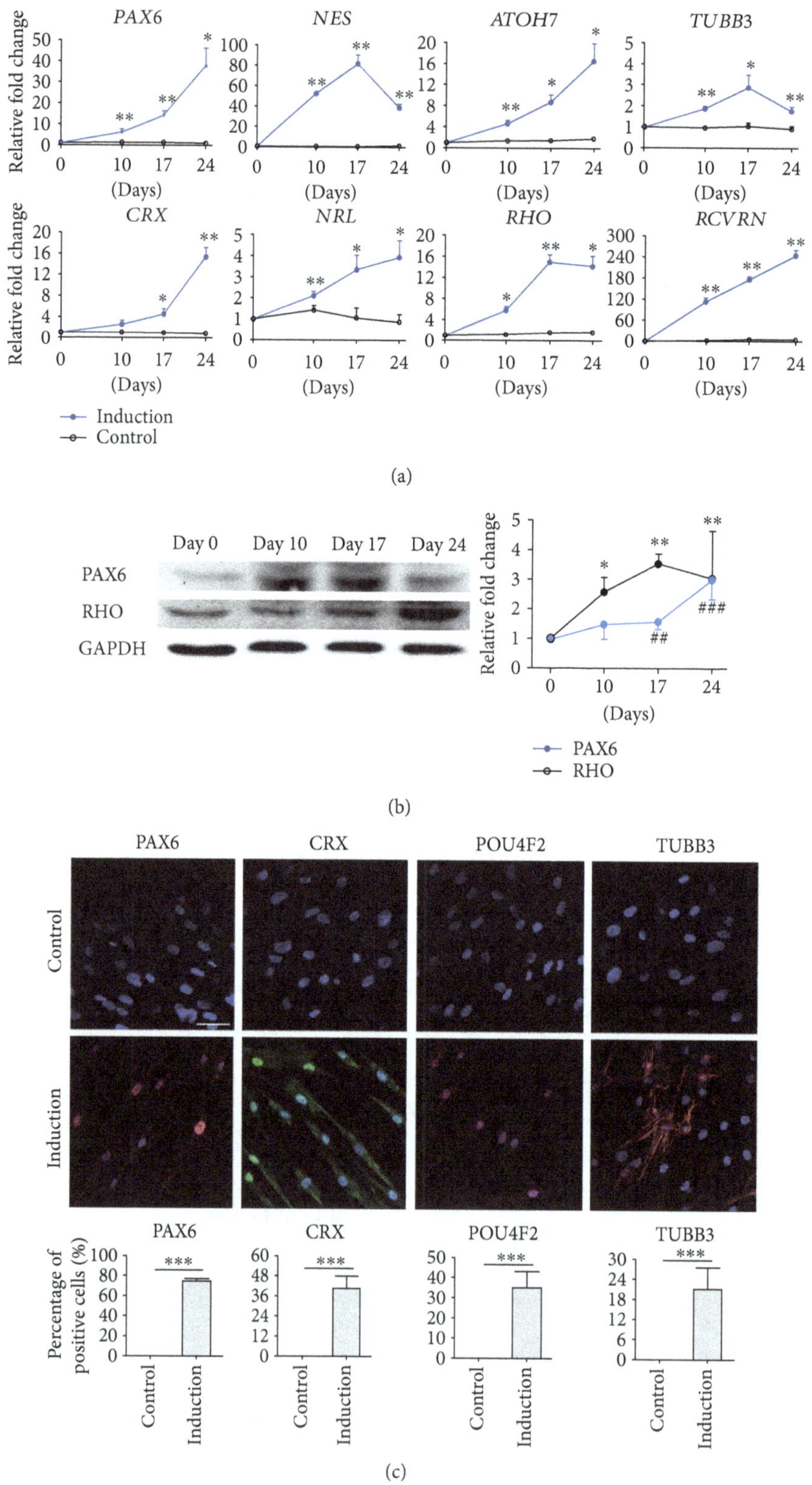

Figure 3: Retinal lineage marker expression in human adipose-derived stem cells after retinal induction treatment. (a) Gene expression analysis of retinal lineage markers: retinal progenitor cells (*PAX6* and *NES*), photoreceptor cells (*CRX*, *NRL*, *RHO*, and *RCVRN*), and retinal ganglion cells (*ATOH7* and *TUBB3*) ($^{*}p < 0.05$ and $^{**}p < 0.01$ compared to the control group). (b) Protein expression analysis of the retinal progenitor cell (PAX6) and photoreceptor marker (RHO) by immunoblotting analysis. GAPDH was used as the housekeeping protein for normalization ($^{*}p < 0.05$ and $^{**}p < 0.01$, compared to Day 0 in PAX6; $^{\#\#}p < 0.01$ and $^{\#\#\#}p < 0.001$, compared to Day 0 in RHO). (c) Immunofluorescence analysis of retinal lineage markers: retinal progenitor cell (PAX6; nucleus), photoreceptor precursor (CRX; nucleus), and retinal ganglion cell (POU4F2; nucleus and TUBB3). DAPI was used as the nucleus counterstain. Scale bar: 50 μm. The bar chats represent the percentage of expression of markers in the control and induction groups ($^{***}p < 0.001$).

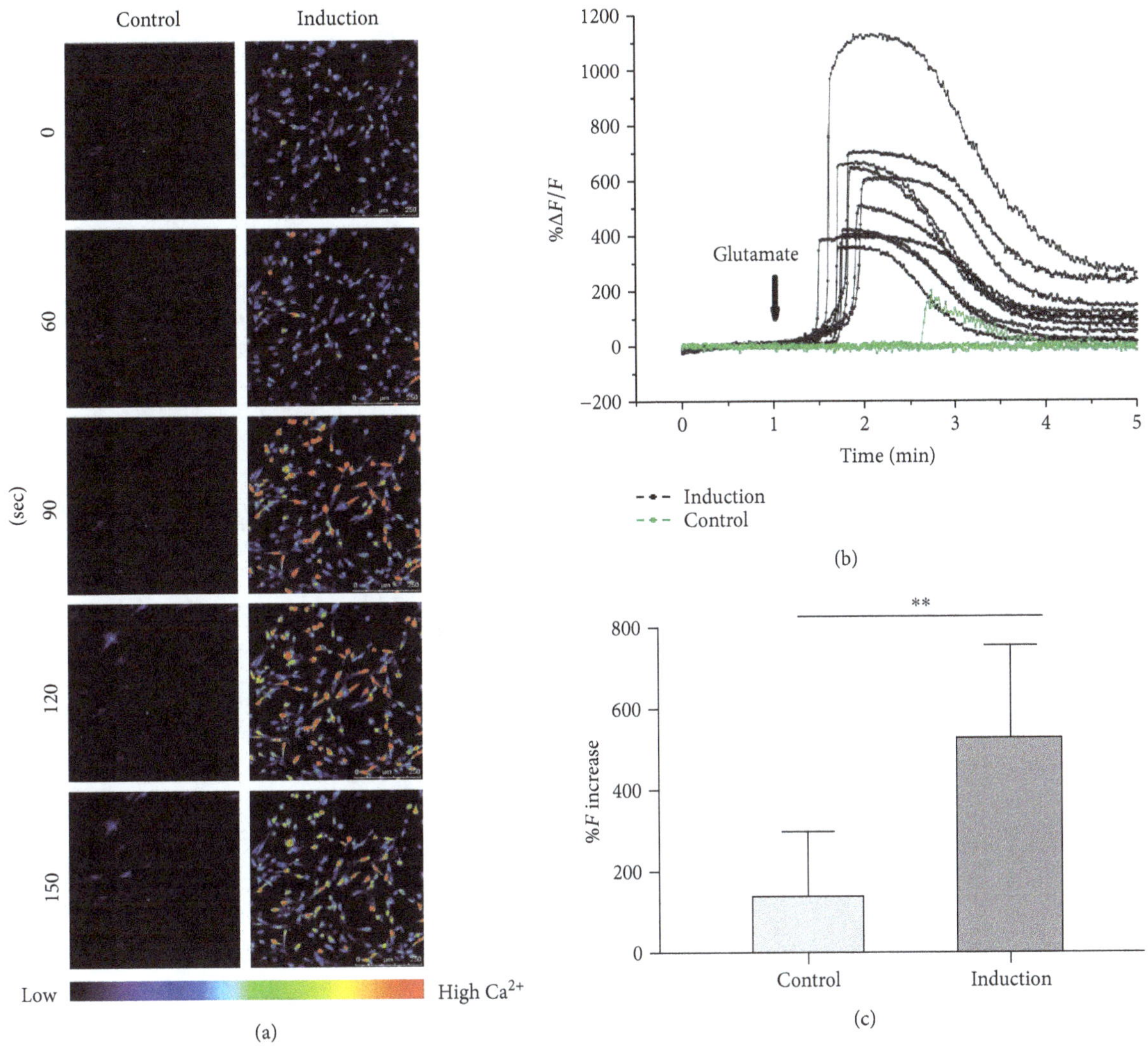

FIGURE 4: Glutamate-evoked calcium response in retinal-induced human adipose-derived stem cells. Human ASCs were treated under retinal induction treatment for 24 days. (a) Heat map images show the Fluo-4 AM fluorescence in the control and induction groups after 1 mM glutamate treatment for 0, 60, 90, 120, and 150 seconds. Scale bar: 250 μm. (b) Representative traces for spontaneous calcium transient profiles of retinal-induced ASCs (black) and control ASCs (green) are shown. (c) Peak calcium response (mean ± standard deviation) in the induction and control ASCs was compared to baseline levels ($^{**}p < 0.01$).

The fluorescence intensity changes ($\%\Delta F/F_0$) observed in the retinal-induced ASCs were 525.18 ± 228.80%, compared to 133.79 ± 159.82% in the negative control group ($p < 0.01$).

To confirm the specificity of retinal transdifferentiation, the retinal-induced ASCs were evaluated with the staining for adipogenesis and osteogenesis, and negative staining of lipid deposition, alkaline phosphatase, and calcium deposition was observed in the retinal-induced ASCs (Supplementary Figure 1). Collectively, our results indicated that human ASCs, upon noggin/Dkk-1/IGF-1 treatment, successfully and specifically transdifferentiated into functional retinal cells.

3.3. Notch Signaling Regulation in Retinal Differentiation of Human Adipose Tissue-Derived Stem Cells. To delineate the regulation of Notch signaling in the retinal differentiation of human ASCs, JAG1 (Notch signaling activator) and DAPT (Notch signaling inhibitor) were applied to the retinal induction medium (Figure 2(a)). The efficacy of Notch signaling modulators on human ASCs was confirmed by the expression of the Notch signaling downstream effector (*HES1* gene). In the JAG1 treatment group, the *HES1* gene was significantly upregulated by 1.50-fold at Day 24 ($p < 0.01$; Figure 5(a)), compared to the regular induction group, while, in the DAPT treatment group, the *HES1* gene was significantly downregulated by 1.43-fold at Day 24 ($p < 0.01$). Notably, the expression of the Notch signaling receptor (*NOTCH1* gene) was also upregulated in the JAG1 treatment group by 1.76-fold ($p < 0.01$), but not changed in the DAPT treatment group.

For the gene expression analysis on RPC markers, the expression of the *PAX6* gene was upregulated in the JAG1 treatment group by 1.93 ± 0.31-fold at Day 24 ($p < 0.001$), compared to the regular induction group. Similarly, the expression of the *NES* gene was also increased in the JAG1 treatment group by 1.37 ± 0.21-fold at Day 24 ($p < 0.05$). In

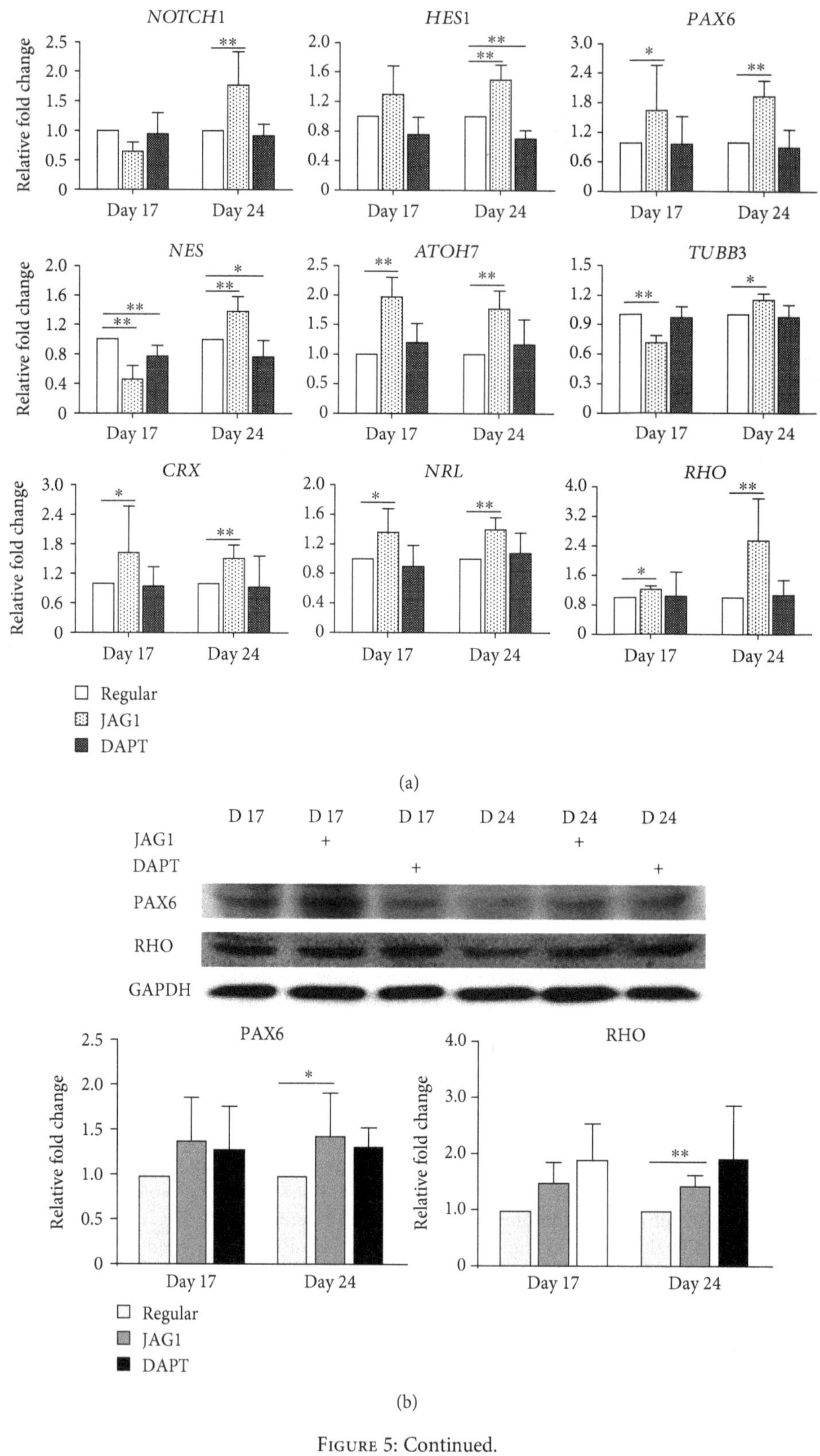

FIGURE 5: Continued.

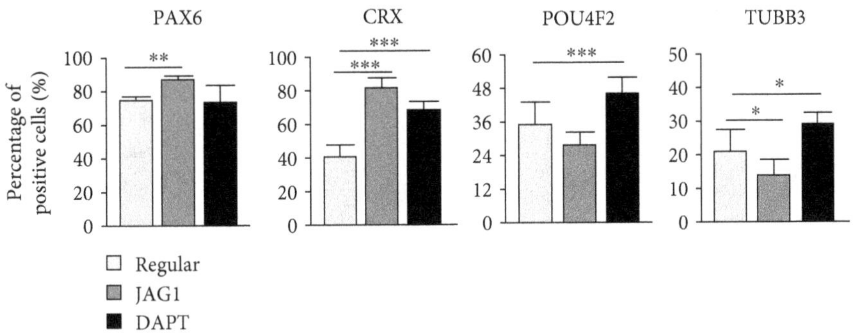

(c)

Figure 5: Retinal lineage marker expression in retinal-induced human adipose-derived stem cells upon Notch signaling modulation. (a) Gene expression analysis for markers upon Notch signaling modulation: Notch signaling effector *HES1* and Notch receptor *NOTCH1*; retinal progenitor cell markers *PAX6* and *NES*; photoreceptor cell markers *CRX*, *NRL*, and *RHO*; retinal ganglion cell markers *ATOH7* and *TUBB3*. Relative fold change was compared to the regular induction group at Days 17 and 24 ($^{*}p < 0.05$ and $^{**}p < 0.01$). (b) Immunoblotting analysis for the retinal progenitor marker (PAX6) and photoreceptor marker (RHO). GAPDH was used as the housekeeping gene for normalization ($^{*}p < 0.05$ and $^{**}p < 0.01$). (c) Immunofluorescence analysis of *PAX6*, CRX, POU4F2, and TUBB3 expressions in retinal-induced ASCs upon Notch signaling modulation treatments ($^{*}p < 0.05$, $^{**}p < 0.01$, and $^{***}p < 0.001$).

contrast, the expression of the *NES* gene was downregulated in the DAPT treatment group by 1.32 ± 0.22-fold ($p < 0.05$). For the photoreceptor markers, the expressions of *CRX*, *NRL*, and *RHO* genes were upregulated by 1.51 ± 0.28-fold ($p < 0.01$), 1.40 ± 0.17-fold ($p < 0.01$), and 2.55 ± 1.15-fold ($p < 0.001$), respectively, in the JAG1 treatment group at Day 24, compared to those in the regular induction group. For the RGC markers, the expressions of the *ATOH7* and *TUBB3* genes were increased in the JAG1 treatment group by 1.78 ± 0.31-fold ($p < 0.01$) and 1.15 ± 0.06-fold ($p < 0.05$), respectively, at Day 24, compared to the regular induction group. Human ASCs in the DAPT treatment group showed a similar retinal marker gene expression to that in the regular induction treatment group.

Coherent to the gene expression results, the immunoblotting analysis showed that the expression of the PAX6 protein was significantly upregulated in the JAG1 treatment group by 1.45 ± 0.33-fold at Day 24 ($p < 0.05$), compared to the regular induction group (Figure 5(b)). Similarly, the expression of the RHO protein was also upregulated in the JAG1 treatment group by 1.47 ± 0.17-fold ($p < 0.01$) at Day 24, compared to the regular induction group. Furthermore, the percentage of PAX6 nucleus-positive cells in the JAG1 treatment group (87.06 ± 2.69%, $p < 0.01$) was higher than that in the regular induction group (74.74 ± 2.42%; Figure 5(c)). The percentage of CRX nuclear-positive cells in the JAG1 treatment group (81.42 ± 6.49%, $p < 0.001$) was significantly higher than that in the regular induction group (40.72 ± 7.01%), and the percentage of CRX nuclear-positive cells was also significantly higher in DAPT treatment group (68.94 ± 4.77%, $p < 0.001$). The percentages of TUBB3-positive cells were lower in the JAG1 treatment group (14.23 ± 4.68%, $p < 0.05$), but higher in the DAPT treatment group (28.93 ± 3.40%, $p < 0.05$), compared to that in the regular induction group (21.25 ± 6.18%). In addition, the percentage of POU4F2 nuclear-positive cells was higher in the DAPT treatment group (46.12 ± 5.84%, $p < 0.01$) than that in the regular induction group (35.10 ± 7.86%).

Upon glutamate stimulation, the fluorescent intensity changes in the JAG1 treatment group (532.10 ± 191.77%; Figure 6(b)) were similar to those in the regular induction group (525.18 ± 228.80%; Figure 6(a)). On the contrary, the fluorescent intensity changes in the DAPT treatment group (369.36 ± 90.43%; Figures 6(c), 6(d)) were significantly smaller than those in the regular induction group ($p < 0.05$). Besides, the time response to the glutamate stimulation in the DAPT-treated cells was also significantly delayed (141.60 ± 16.24 sec, $p < 0.001$; Figure 6(e)), compared to the regular induction group (59.40 ± 10.29 sec). The JAG1 treatment did not affect the response of the induced ASCs to glutamate stimulation (60.30 ± 9.94 sec).

Collectively, our results suggested that Notch signaling activation further enhanced the expression of retinal markers and produced more RPCs and photoreceptor precursors without affecting the response to glutamate stimulation during the human ASCs' retinal differentiation process. In contrast, Notch signaling inhibition produced more RGCs but suppressed the response to glutamate stimulation.

4. Discussion

Stem cells isolated from adipose tissues are predominantly MSCs, and they can differentiate into adipocytes, osteoblasts, and chondrocytes *in vitro* upon induction (Figure 1). In addition to the mesodermal lineage, ASCs have also been reported to differentiate into the ectodermal lineage, including neuronal and retinal lineages, under specific induction conditions [18, 19]. Compared to the teeth, adipose tissues are more conveniently accessible and easily obtained by liposuction with minimal invasiveness. Furthermore, human ASCs can abundantly be isolated with a high proliferative capacity [20]. They also have a low risk of inducing teratoma after transplantation [7]. Human ASCs should be a promising cell source for retinal cell synthesis, *in vitro* disease modeling, and cell replacement therapy.

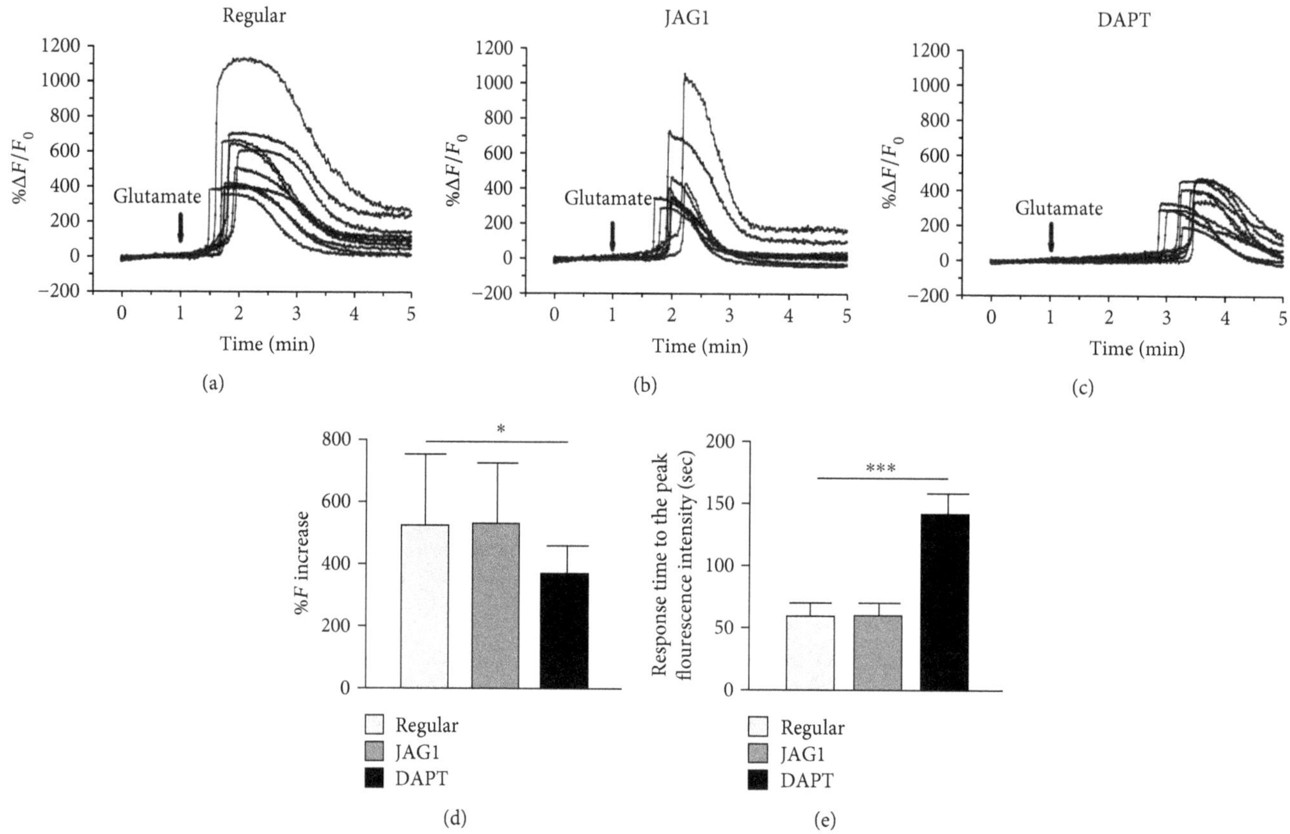

Figure 6: Glutamate-evoked calcium response in retinal-induced human adipose-derived stem cells upon Notch signaling modulation. Calcium transient profiles of retinal-induced ASCs in (a) the regular induction group, (b) JAG1 group, and (c) DAPT group. (d) Histogram showing the fluorescence intensity changes ($\%\Delta F/F_0$). (e) Histogram showing the response time to the peak fluorescence intensity after the addition of glutamate ($^*p < 0.05$ and $^{**}p < 0.01$).

The noggin/Dkk-1/IGF-1 protocol was originally developed for the retinal differentiation of human ESCs [3]. We have applied this protocol to induce human PDLSCs to the retinal lineage [5, 6]. Noggin and Dkk-1 are the respective inhibitors of the BMP and Wnt signaling pathways. Antagonizing the BMP and Wnt signaling pathways promote neural plate development and retinogenesis [21, 22], whereas the addition of IGF-1 specifies the retinal progenitor identity [3]. In this study, the noggin/Dkk-1/IGF-1 treatment reprogrammed human ASCs with distinct neuron-like morphology (Figure 2(b)). Cell aggregation promotes the induction into the neuronal lineage [23], whereas the Matrigel assists the maturation of neuronal cells [24]. In contrast, human ASCs, without the noggin/Dkk-1/IGF-1 treatment, retained the fibroblast-like morphology and are highly proliferative.

The noggin/Dkk-1/IGF-1 treatment on adult stem cells is specific. Our previous studies showed that, under noggin/Dkk-1/IGF-1 induction, human PDLSCs could express eye field transcription factors (*Pax6*, *Rx*, *Lhx*, and *Otx2*), photoreceptor markers (*Nrl*, *Rhodopsin*, and its kinase), and neuronal and retinal ganglion cell markers (*ATOH7*, *POU4F2*, *β-III tubulin*, *MAP 2*, *TAU*, *NEUROD1*, and *SIX3*). Moreover, the induced PDLSCs showed a significant response to excitatory glutamate [5, 6]. In this study, RPC (*PAX6* and *NES*), photoreceptor (*CRX*, *NRL*, *RHO*, and *RCVRN*), and RGC (*ATOH7* and *TUBB3*) markers were significantly upregulated during the induction treatment period in a time-dependent manner (Figure 3). In addition, as the inner retinal neurons possess the glutamate receptors [25, 26], the neurotransmission function of the retinal-induced ASCs was evaluated by the glutamate-induced calcium response (Figure 4). Similar to our previous study on human PDLSCs, a robust increase in fluorescence intensities was observed in the retinal-induced ASCs after glutamate stimulation, confirming that the retinal-induced ASCs possess an excitable membrane property, like the developing retinal neurons [26, 27]. Collectively, our results suggested that human ASCs can transdifferentiate into functional retinal cells under the noggin/Dkk-1/IGF-1 induction treatment. The noggin/Dkk-1/IGF-1 induction treatment is a chemical-based strategy with a precisely defined formula and condition for retinal differentiation, which can be adopted to synthesize the retinal cells for clinical applications.

Notch signaling is an evolutionarily conserved mechanism that is used by metazoans to control cell fates through local cell interactions [11]. In vertebrates, there are four Notch receptors (Notch-1, -2, -3, and -4) and two ligands (delta and jagged). The activation of Notch signaling induces the expression of transcriptional repressor genes, such as *HES1*, which represses the proneural gene expression and thereby inhibits neuronal differentiation. Thus, the activation of Notch signaling leads to the maintenance of the neural stem cell population, whereas the inactivation of Notch signaling induces neuronal differentiation and depletes the neural stem cell population [28, 29]. Downregulation of Notch-1 promotes neuronal differentiation of bone marrow-derived MSCs [30]. However, inactivation of Notch signaling leads to the complete loss of neural stem cells in both the developing and adult telencephalon, indicating an absolute requirement of Notch signaling for the maintenance of neural stem cells and a proper control of neurogenesis [29, 31].

In this study, we confirmed the efficacy of Notch signaling modulation with the upregulation of *HES1* in JAG1 treatment (as the Notch signaling activator) and its downregulation in DAPT treatment (as the Notch signaling inhibitor; Figure 5(a)). Notably, *NOTCH1* expression is also upregulated in the JAG1 treatment group, indicating that a positive feedback loop was established in human ASCs upon Notch signaling activation during the retinal differentiation process. Notch signaling activation by JAG1, on top of the regular noggin/Dkk-1/IGF-1 induction treatment, further enhances the expression of retinal progenitor and precursor markers (*PAX6*, *NES*, *CRX*, *NRL*, and *ATOH7*) as well as mature photoreceptor (*RHO*) and RGC (*TUBB3*) markers (Figures 5(a) and 5(b)). JAG1 treatment also produced more PAX6- and CRX-positive cells, but less POU4F2- and TUBB3-positive cells (Figure 5(c)), indicating that Notch signaling activation can enhance the maintenance or production of retinal progenitor and precursor markers during human adult stem cell retinal differentiation. Similar to previous reports on the retinal development of zebrafish, xenopus, chick, and mice, the role of Notch signaling is to preserve a pool of undifferentiated progenitor cells, acquire stem cell properties, and prevent differentiation [14–16, 32, 33]. In contrast, Notch signaling inhibition by DAPT downregulated the expression of the *NES* gene, but showed more POU4F2- and TUBB3-positive cells, suggesting that Notch signaling inhibition would reduce the RPC population but increase the production towards the retinal ganglion lineage. Yet, DAPT treatment also delayed the response of glutamate stimulation in the retinal-induced ASCs (Figure 6), suggesting that Notch signaling could be involved in the glutamate signaling transmission in retinal-induced ASCs. Apart from its direct regulation in the differentiation processes, Notch signaling could also interact with other signaling pathways, including the BMP and Wnt signaling pathways [34, 35], and the cell fate determination would be multifactorial [11]. Notch signaling promotes cyclic expression of both repressors and activators of proneural fate specification in progenitor cells [36, 37], indicating that the role of Notch signaling in progenitor cells is not static, but dynamic or oscillatory. Besides, the prolonged activation of Notch signaling would not interfere in the normal progression of progenitor temporal states [38], and a continuous supply of RPCs is required for the production of differentiated neurons and completes retinal development [39]. The molecular mechanisms of Notch signaling modulation in adult stem cell retinal differentiation and the optimal conditions of ASCs for retinal differentiation, as well as the neuroprotective effects of ASCs, require further investigations.

5. Conclusion

In summary, human ASCs possess the retinal differentiation potential upon noggin/Dkk-1/IGF-1 induction treatment, and the synthesis of retinal progenitor and precursor cells can further be enhanced by Notch signaling activation. Human ASCs should be a promising autologous source of adult stem cells for retinal cell synthesis, *in vitro* disease modeling, and stem cell replacement therapy in the future.

Authors' Contributions

Yuqiang Huang and Chong-Bo Chen mainly performed the experiments. Bing Huang and Jiajian Liang helped with the experiments. Yuqiang Huang recruited study subjects. Tsz Kin Ng, Chi Pui Pang, and Mingzhi Zhang supervised the project. Yuqiang Huang, Tsz Kin Ng, Chong-Bo Chen, and Chi Pui Pang interpreted the results and wrote the manuscript.

Acknowledgments

We express our deepest gratitude to all the participants in the study. This study was supported by the Natural Science Foundation of Guangdong Province of China (2016A030313063) and the Medical Scientific Research Foundation of Guangdong Province of China (A2015452).

References

[1] T. K. Ng, D. S. C. Lam, and H. S. Cheung, "Prospects of stem cells for retinal diseases," *Asia-Pacific Journal of Ophthalmology*, vol. 2, no. 1, pp. 57–63, 2013.

[2] Z. Tang, Y. Zhang, Y. Wang et al., "Progress of stem/progenitor cell-based therapy for retinal degeneration," *Journal of Translational Medicine*, vol. 15, no. 1, p. 99, 2017.

[3] D. A. Lamba, M. O. Karl, C. B. Ware, and T. A. Reh, "Efficient generation of retinal progenitor cells from human embryonic stem cells," *Proceedings of the National Academy of Sciences of the United States of America*, vol. 103, no. 34, pp. 12769–12774, 2006.

[4] C. B. Mellough, E. Sernagor, I. Moreno-Gimeno, D. H. W. Steel, and M. Lako, "Efficient stage-specific differentiation of human pluripotent stem cells toward retinal photoreceptor cells," *Stem Cells*, vol. 30, no. 4, pp. 673–686, 2012.

[5] L. Huang, J. Liang, Y. Geng et al., "Directing adult human periodontal ligament-derived stem cells to retinal fate," *Investigative Ophthalmology & Visual Science*, vol. 54, no. 6, pp. 3965–3974, 2013.

[6] T. K. Ng, J. S. Y. Yung, K. W. Choy et al., "Transdifferentiation of periodontal ligament-derived stem cells into retinal ganglion-like cells and Its microRNA signature," *Scientific Reports*, vol. 5, no. 1, article 16429, 2015.

[7] F. Ogura, S. Wakao, Y. Kuroda et al., "Human adipose tissue possesses a unique population of pluripotent stem cells with nontumorigenic and low telomerase activities: potential implications in regenerative medicine," *Stem Cells and Development*, vol. 23, no. 7, pp. 717–728, 2014.

[8] U. Vossmerbaeumer, S. Ohnesorge, S. Kuehl et al., "Retinal pigment epithelial phenotype induced in human adipose tissue-derived mesenchymal stromal cells," *Cytotherapy*, vol. 11, no. 2, pp. 177–188, 2009.

[9] Y. Zhang, D. Zhang, W. Wei et al., "Effects of RPE-conditioned medium on the differentiation of hADSCS into RPE cells, and their proliferation and migration," *Experimental and Therapeutic Medicine*, vol. 14, no. 4, pp. 3699–3707, 2017.

[10] H. Rezanejad, Z. S. Soheili, F. Haddad et al., "In vitro differentiation of adipose-tissue-derived mesenchymal stem cells into neural retinal cells through expression of human *Pax6* (5a) gene," *Cell and Tissue Research*, vol. 356, no. 1, pp. 65–75, 2014.

[11] S. Artavanis-Tsakonas, M. D. Rand, and R. J. Lake, "Notch signaling: cell fate control and signal integration in development," *Science*, vol. 284, no. 5415, pp. 770–776, 1999.

[12] E. A. Mills and D. Goldman, "The regulation of Notch signaling in retinal development and regeneration," *Current Pathobiology Reports*, vol. 5, no. 4, pp. 323–331, 2017.

[13] A. P. Jadhav, H. A. Mason, and C. L. Cepko, "Notch 1 inhibits photoreceptor production in the developing mammalian retina," *Development*, vol. 133, no. 5, pp. 913–923, 2006.

[14] K. Mizeracka, C. R. DeMaso, and C. L. Cepko, "Notch 1 is required in newly postmitotic cells to inhibit the rod photoreceptor fate," *Development*, vol. 140, no. 15, pp. 3188–3197, 2013.

[15] S. Reichman, A. Terray, A. Slembrouck et al., "From confluent human iPS cells to self-forming neural retina and retinal pigmented epithelium," *Proceedings of the National Academy of Sciences of the United States of America*, vol. 111, no. 23, pp. 8518–8523, 2014.

[16] A. O. Silva, C. E. Ercole, and S. C. McLoon, "Regulation of ganglion cell production by Notch signaling during retinal development," *Journal of Neurobiology*, vol. 54, no. 3, pp. 511–524, 2003.

[17] G. Dvoriantchikova, I. Perea-Martinez, S. Pappas et al., "Molecular characterization of Notch 1 positive progenitor cells in the developing retina," *PLoS One*, vol. 10, no. 6, article e0131054, 2015.

[18] P. A. Zuk, M. Zhu, P. Ashjian et al., "Human adipose tissue is a source of multipotent stem cells," *Molecular Biology of the Cell*, vol. 13, no. 12, pp. 4279–4295, 2002.

[19] J. L. Boulland, M. Mastrangelopoulou, A. C. Boquest et al., "Epigenetic regulation of Nestin expression during neurogenic differentiation of adipose tissue stem cells," *Stem Cells and Development*, vol. 22, no. 7, pp. 1042–1052, 2013.

[20] J. M. Gimble, A. J. Katz, and B. A. Bunnell, "Adipose-derived stem cells for regenerative medicine," *Circulation Research*, vol. 100, no. 9, pp. 1249–1260, 2007.

[21] P. Ybot-Gonzalez, C. Gaston-Massuet, G. Girdler et al., "Neural plate morphogenesis during mouse neurulation is regulated by antagonism of Bmp signalling," *Development*, vol. 134, no. 17, pp. 3203–3211, 2007.

[22] C. Houart, L. Caneparo, C. P. Heisenberg, K. A. Barth, M. Take-Uchi, and S. W. Wilson, "Establishment of the telencephalon during gastrulation by local antagonism of Wnt signaling," *Neuron*, vol. 35, no. 2, pp. 255–265, 2002.

[23] M. Yanagisawa, K. Nakashima, W. Ochiai et al., "Fate redirection of hippocampal astrocytes toward neuronal lineage by aggregate culture," *Neuroscience Research*, vol. 53, no. 2, pp. 176–182, 2005.

[24] Y. Li, M. Liu, Y. Yan, and S. T. Yang, "Neural differentiation from pluripotent stem cells: the role of natural and synthetic extracellular matrix," *World Journal of Stem Cells*, vol. 6, no. 1, pp. 11–23, 2014.

[25] S. Chen and J. S. Diamond, "Synaptically released glutamate activates extrasynaptic NMDA receptors on cells in the ganglion cell layer of rat retina," *The Journal of Neuroscience: The Official Journal of the Society for Neuroscience*, vol. 22, no. 6, pp. 2165–2173, 2002.

[26] M. Hoon, H. Okawa, L. Della Santina, and R. O. L. Wong, "Functional architecture of the retina: development and disease," *Progress in Retinal and Eye Research*, vol. 42, pp. 44–84, 2014.

[27] W. Sun, G. M. Seigel, and R. J. Salvi, "Retinal precursor cells express functional ionotropic glutamate and GABA receptors," *Neuroreport*, vol. 13, no. 18, pp. 2421–2424, 2002.

[28] E. R. Andersson, R. Sandberg, and U. Lendahl, "Notch signaling: simplicity in design, versatility in function," *Development*, vol. 138, no. 17, pp. 3593–3612, 2011.

[29] R. Kopan and M. X. G. Ilagan, "The canonical Notch signaling pathway: unfolding the activation mechanism," *Cell*, vol. 137, no. 2, pp. 216–233, 2009.

[30] L. Jing, Y. Jia, J. Lu et al., "Microrna-9 promotes differentiation of mouse bone mesenchymal stem cells into neurons by Notch signaling," *Neuroreport*, vol. 22, no. 5, pp. 206–211, 2011.

[31] I. Imayoshi, M. Sakamoto, M. Yamaguchi, K. Mori, and R. Kageyama, "Essential roles of Notch signaling in maintenance of neural stem cells in developing and adult brains," *The Journal of Neuroscience: The Official Journal of the Society for Neuroscience*, vol. 30, no. 9, pp. 3489–3498, 2010.

[32] R. A. Uribe, T. Kwon, E. M. Marcotte, and J. M. Gross, "Id2a functions to limit Notch pathway activity and thereby influence the transition from proliferation to differentiation of retinoblasts during zebrafish retinogenesis," *Developmental Biology*, vol. 371, no. 2, pp. 280–292, 2012.

[33] D. Henrique, E. Hirsinger, J. Adam et al., "Maintenance of neuroepithelial progenitor cells by Delta-Notch signalling in the embryonic chick retina," *Current Biology*, vol. 7, no. 9, pp. 661–670, 1997.

[34] T. Takizawa, W. Ochiai, K. Nakashima, and T. Taga, "Enhanced gene activation by Notch and BMP signaling cross-talk," *Nucleic Acids Research*, vol. 31, no. 19, pp. 5723–5731, 2003.

[35] M. Corada, D. Nyqvist, F. Orsenigo et al., "The Wnt/β-catenin pathway modulates vascular remodeling and specification by upregulating Dll4/Notch signaling," *Developmental Cell*, vol. 18, no. 6, pp. 938–949, 2010.

[36] R. Kageyama, Y. Niwa, H. Shimojo, T. Kobayashi, and T. Ohtsuka, "Ultradian oscillations in Notch signaling regulate dynamic biological events," *Current Topics in Developmental Biology*, vol. 92, pp. 311–331, 2010.

Permissions

All chapters in this book were first published in SCI, by Hindawi Publishing Corporation; hereby published with permission under the Creative Commons Attribution License or equivalent. Every chapter published in this book has been scrutinized by our experts. Their significance has been extensively debated. The topics covered herein carry significant findings which will fuel the growth of the discipline. They may even be implemented as practical applications or may be referred to as a beginning point for another development.

The contributors of this book come from diverse backgrounds, making this book a truly international effort. This book will bring forth new frontiers with its revolutionizing research information and detailed analysis of the nascent developments around the world.

We would like to thank all the contributing authors for lending their expertise to make the book truly unique. They have played a crucial role in the development of this book. Without their invaluable contributions this book wouldn't have been possible. They have made vital efforts to compile up to date information on the varied aspects of this subject to make this book a valuable addition to the collection of many professionals and students.

This book was conceptualized with the vision of imparting up-to-date information and advanced data in this field. To ensure the same, a matchless editorial board was set up. Every individual on the board went through rigorous rounds of assessment to prove their worth. After which they invested a large part of their time researching and compiling the most relevant data for our readers.

The editorial board has been involved in producing this book since its inception. They have spent rigorous hours researching and exploring the diverse topics which have resulted in the successful publishing of this book. They have passed on their knowledge of decades through this book. To expedite this challenging task, the publisher supported the team at every step. A small team of assistant editors was also appointed to further simplify the editing procedure and attain best results for the readers.

Apart from the editorial board, the designing team has also invested a significant amount of their time in understanding the subject and creating the most relevant covers. They scrutinized every image to scout for the most suitable representation of the subject and create an appropriate cover for the book.

The publishing team has been an ardent support to the editorial, designing and production team. Their endless efforts to recruit the best for this project, has resulted in the accomplishment of this book. They are a veteran in the field of academics and their pool of knowledge is as vast as their experience in printing. Their expertise and guidance has proved useful at every step. Their uncompromising quality standards have made this book an exceptional effort. Their encouragement from time to time has been an inspiration for everyone.

The publisher and the editorial board hope that this book will prove to be a valuable piece of knowledge for researchers, students, practitioners and scholars across the globe.

List of Contributors

Agnieszka Owczarczyk-Saczonek, Anna Kruszewska and Waldemar Placek
Department of Dermatology, Sexually Transmitted Diseases and Clinical Immunology, University of Warmia and Mazury in Olsztyn, Olsztyn, Poland

Magdalena Krajewska-Włodarczyk
Department of Rheumatology, University of Warmia and Mazury in Olsztyn, Olsztyn, Poland

Łukasz Banasiak
Department of Plastic, Reconstructive and Aesthetic Surgery, L. Rydygier Collegium Medicum in Bydgoszcz, Nicolaus Copernicus University in Torun, Toruń, Poland

Wojciech Maksymowicz
Department of Neurology and Neurosurgery, Faculty of Medical Sciences, University of Warmia and Mazury in Olsztyn, Olsztyn, Poland

Joanna Wojtkiewicz
Foundation for Nerve Cell Regeneration, University of Warmia and Mazury in Olsztyn, Olsztyn, Poland
Department of Pathophysiology, Faculty of Medical Sciences, University of Warmia and Mazury in Olsztyn, Olsztyn, Poland
Laboratory for Regenerative Medicine, Faculty of Medical Sciences, University of Warmia and Mazury, Olsztyn, Poland

Masahiro Nishikawa, Akihiro Inoue, Shohei Kohno, Shirabe Matsumoto, Satoshi Suehiro, Daisuke Yamashita, Saya Ozaki, Hideaki Watanabe and Takeharu Kunieda
Department of Neurosurgery, Ehime University Graduate School of Medicine, Toon, Ehime 791-0295, Japan

Takanori Ohnishi
Department of Neurosurgery, Washoukai Sadamoto Hospital, Matsuyama, Ehime 790-0052, Japan

Shiro Ohue
Department of Neurosurgery, Ehime Prefectural Central Hospital, Matsuyama, Ehime 790-0024, Japan

Hajime Yano and Junya Tanaka
Department of Molecular and Cellular Physiology, Ehime University Graduate School of Medicine, Toon, Ehime 791-0295, Japan

Hisaaki Takahashi
Division of Pathophysiology, Faculty of Pharmaceutical Sciences, Hokuriku University, Kanazawa, Ishikawa 920-1180, Japan

Riko Kitazawa
Division of Diagnostic Pathology, Ehime University Hospital, Toon, Ehime 791-0295, Japan

Ayu Suraya Ansari, Nur Qisya Afifah Veronica Sainik, Rabiatul Adawiyah Razali and Ruszymah Bt Hj Idrus
Department of Physiology, Faculty of Medicine, Universiti Kebangsaan Malaysia Medical Centre, Jalan Yaacob Latif, 56000 Cheras,Kuala Lumpur, Malaysia

Muhammad Dain Yazid
Tissue Engineering Centre, Universiti Kebangsaan Malaysia Medical Centre, Jalan Yaacob Latif, 56000 Cheras,Kuala Lumpur, Malaysia

Aminuddin Bin Saim
Ear, Nose & Throat Consultant Clinic, Ampang Puteri Specialist Hospital, 68000 Ampang, Selangor, Malaysia

Justin Elfman
Department of Biochemistry and Molecular Genetics, University of Virginia, 22903, USA

Hui Li
Department of Biochemistry and Molecular Genetics, University of Virginia, 22903, USA
Department of Pathology, University of Virginia, 22903, USA

Ayman Hyder
Faculty of Science, Damietta University, Damietta 34517, Egypt

Sabrina Ehnert
Siegfried Weller Institute for Trauma Research, Eberhard Karls University, Tübingen, Germany

Fred Fändrich
Institute for Applied Cell Therapy, University Hospital Schleswig-Holstein, Campus Kiel, Kiel, Germany

Hendrik Ungefroren
First Department of Medicine, University Clinic Schleswig Holstein, Lübeck, Germany

Guan Qun Zhu, Seung Hwan Jeon, Sae Woong Choi, Hyun Cheol Jeong, Kang Sup Kim, Hyuk Jin Cho, U. Syn Ha, Sung Hoo Hong and Ji Youl Lee
Department of Urology, College of Medicine, The Catholic University of Korea, Seoul, Republic of Korea

Woong Jin Bae and Sae Woong Kim
Department of Urology, College of Medicine, The Catholic University of Korea, Seoul, Republic of Korea
Catholic Integrative Medicine Research Institute, College of Medicine, The Catholic University of Korea, Seoul, Republic of Korea

Su Jin Kim
Department of Urology, Wonju College of Medicine, Yonsei University, Wonju, Republic of Korea

Eun Bi Kwon
KEMIMEDI, Seoul, Republic of Korea

Chandra Prakash Chaturvedi, Naresh Kumar Tripathy, Ekta Minocha, Akhilesh Sharma, Khaliqur Rahman and Soniya Nityanand
Stem Cell Research Facility, Department of Hematology, Sanjay Gandhi Postgraduate Institute of Medical Sciences (SGPGIMS), Raebareli Road, Lucknow 226014, India

A. G. E. Day, W. R. Francis, I. L. Pieper and Z. Xia
Institute of Life Science, Swansea University Medical School, Swansea SA2 8PP, UK

K. Fu
Department of Orthopaedic Surgery, The First Affiliated Hospital of Hainan Medical College, Hainan, China

O. Guy
College of Engineering, Swansea University, Swansea SA2 8PP, UK

Jie Cai, Ming Yue, Longfeng Jiang, Ruirui Xu, Lili Zhang, Jun Li and Chuanlong Zhu
Department of Infectious Disease, The First Affiliated Hospital of Nanjing Medical University, Nanjing 210029, China

Yongting Zhang
Department of Infectious Disease, The First Affiliated Hospital of Nanjing Medical University, Nanjing 210029, China
Department of Pediatrics, The Affiliated Hospital of Yangzhou University, Yangzhou 225000, China

Yuwen Li
Department of Pediatrics, The First Affiliated Hospital of Nanjing Medical University, Nanjing 210029, China

Wenting Li
Third Liver Unit, Department of Infectious Disease, The First Affiliated Hospital of Science and Technology of China, Hefei 230001, China

Jing-wan Luo, Ke-ke Zhang, Long-xiang Lin and Yu-long Sun
Center for Translational Medicine Research and Development, Shenzhen Institute of Advanced Technology, Chinese Academy of Sciences, Shenzhen 518000, China

Chang Liu
Center for Translational Medicine Research and Development, Shenzhen Institute of Advanced Technology, Chinese Academy of Sciences, Shenzhen 518000, China
Central Laboratory, Dalian Municipal Central Hospital, Dalian 116033, China

Ting Liang and Zong-ping Luo
Institute of Orthopaedics, Soochow University, Suzhou 215007, China

Yong-qing Zhuang
Shenzhen People's Hospital, Shenzhen, Guangdong, China

Yongjun Zheng, Xiaoming Fan, Yongqiang Xiao, Pengfei Luo, Yingying Liu, Li Wang, Zhenci Cui, Fei He, Shichu Xiao and Zhaofan Xia
Burns Center, Changhai Hospital, Second Military Medical University, Shanghai, China

Shiqing Zheng
Burns Center, Changhai Hospital, Second Military Medical University, Shanghai, China
No. 73051 Troop of the Chinese People's Liberation Army, Xiamen, China

Li Li and Yuhuan Liu
Department of Obstetrics and Gynecology, Changhai Hospital, Second Military Medical University, Shanghai, China

Ping Wang
Precision Health Program, Department of Radiology, College of Human Medicine, Michigan State University, East Lansing,MI 48823, USA

Aitor Aguirre
Division of Developmental and Stem Cell Biology, Institute for Quantitative Health Science and Engineering,Michigan State University, East Lansing, MI 48823, USA

Department of Biomedical Engineering, College of Engineering, Michigan State University, East Lansing, MI 48823, USA

X. Ambriz and J. R. Ambrosio
Departamento de Microbiologia y Parasitologia, Facultad de Medicina, UNAM, 04510 Ciudad de México, Mexico

P. de Lanerolle
Department of Physiology and Biophysics, College of Medicine, University of Illinois at Chicago, 60612 Chicago, Illinois, USA

Saifun Nahar and Jiro Fujita
Department of Infectious, Respiratory, and Digestive Medicine, Graduate School of Medicine, University of the Ryukyus, Okinawa 903-0215, Japan

Yoshiki Nakashima, Chika Miyagi-Shiohira and Hirofumi Noguchi
Department of Regenerative Medicine, Graduate School of Medicine, University of the Ryukyus, Okinawa 903-0215, Japan

Takao Kinjo
Department of Basic Laboratory Sciences, School of Health Sciences in the Faculty of Medicine, University of the Ryukyus,Okinawa 903-0215, Japan

Naoya Kobayashi
Okayama Saidaiji Hospital, Okayama 704-8192, Japan

Issei Saitoh
Division of Pediatric Dentistry, Graduate School of Medical and Dental Science, Niigata University, Niigata 951-8514, Japan

Masami Watanabe
Department of Urology, Okayama University Graduate School of Medicine, Dentistry and Pharmaceutical Sciences, Okayama 700-8558, Japan

Qingjie Fu, Shunsuke Ohnishi and Naoya Sakamoto
Department of Gastroenterology and Hepatology, Hokkaido University Graduate School of Medicine, Sapporo, Japan

Lingjia Yu, Zhenfei Huang, Yu He, Hai Wang and Guixing Qiu
Department of Orthopaedic Surgery, Peking Union Medical College Hospital, Peking Union Medical College and Chinese Academy of Medical Sciences, Beijing 100730, China

Bo Li
Department of Orthopaedic Surgery, Peking Union Medical College Hospital, Peking Union Medical College and Chinese Academy of Medical Sciences, Beijing 100730, China
Department of Orthopaedic Surgery, Fourth Clinical Medical College of Peking University, Beijing Jishuitan Hospital, Beijing 100035, China

Yuanhao Wu, Jieying Liu, Bupeng Ma and Yaqian Li
Central Laboratory, Peking Union Medical College Hospital, Peking Union Medical College and Chinese Academy of Medical Sciences, Beijing 100730, China

Zhihong Wu
Central Laboratory, Peking Union Medical College Hospital, Peking Union Medical College and Chinese Academy of Medical Sciences, Beijing 100730, China
Beijing Key Laboratory for Genetic Research of Bone and Joint Disease, Beijing, China

Martin Maldonado, Tianhua Huang, Jianying Chen and Ying Zhong
Reproductive Medicine & Genetics, Chengdu Jinjiang Hospital for Maternal & Child Health Care, Chengdu 610066, China

Yuqiang Huang, Chong-Bo Chen, Bing Huang, Jiajian Liang and Mingzhi Zhang
Joint Shantou International Eye Center of Shantou University and the Chinese University of Hong Kong, Shantou, Guangdong, China

Tsz Kin Ng
Joint Shantou International Eye Center of Shantou University and the Chinese University of Hong Kong, Shantou, Guangdong, China
Shantou University Medical College, Shantou, Guandong, China
Department of Ophthalmology and Visual Sciences, The Chinese University of Hong Kong, Hong Kong

Chi Pui Pang
Joint Shantou International Eye Center of Shantou University and the Chinese University of Hong Kong, Shantou, Guangdong, China
Department of Ophthalmology and Visual Sciences, The Chinese University of Hong Kong, Hong Kong

Index

www.ingramcontent.com/pod-product-compliance
Lightning Source LLC
LaVergne TN
LVHW060607210926
848485LV00005B/1385